Essentials of Clinical Psychiatry

Edited by

John I. Walker, M.D.

Clinical Associate Professor of Psychiatry
Duke University Medical Center
Durham, North Carolina

24 Contributors

Essentials of Clinical Psychiatry

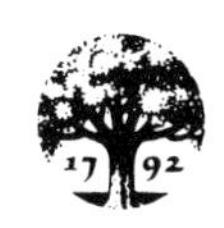

J. B. Lippincott Company Philadelphia

London Mexico City New York St. Louis São Paulo Sydney

Acquisitions Editor: William Burgower
Sponsoring Editor: Delois Patterson
Manuscript Editor: Lauren McKinney
Indexer: Sandra King
Art Director: Tracy Baldwin
Production Supervisor: Kathleen Dunn
Production Coordinator: George V. Gordon
Compositor: Bi-Comp, Inc.
Printer/Binder: R. R. Donnelley & Sons Company

Printed in the United States of America. For information write J. B. Lippincott Company, East Washington Square, Philadelphia, Pennsylvania 19105.

6 5 4 3 2 1

Library of Congress Cataloging in Publication Data
Main entry under title:

Essentials of clinical psychiatry.

Includes bibliographies and index.
1. Psychiatry. I. Walker, J. Ingram (John Ingram), 1944– . [DNLM: 1. Mental Disorders. 2. Psychiatry. WM 100 E777]
RC454.E82 1985 616.89 85-5167
ISBN 0-397-50642-2

The authors and publisher have exerted every effort to ensure that drug selection and dosage set forth in this text are in accord with current recommendations and practice at the time of publication. However, in view of ongoing research, changes in government regulations, and the constant flow of information relating to drug therapy and drug reactions, the reader is urged to check the package insert for each drug for any change in indications and dosage and for added warnings and precautions. This is particularly important when the recommended agent is a new or infrequently employed drug.

Contributors

Jack W. Barber, M.D.
Chief Resident in Psychiatry
Duke University Medical Center
Durham, North Carolina

Tracey Potts Carson, PH.D.
Clinical Psychologist
Veterans Administration Hospital
Clinical Assistant Professor
Duke University Medical Center
Durham, North Carolina

Douglas H. Finestone, M.D.
Associate in Psychiatry
Duke University Medical Center
Durham, North Carolina

E. Michael Kahn, M.D.
Assistant Professor in Psychiatry
Western Psychiatric Institute and Clinic
Duke University Medical Center
Durham, North Carolina

James E. Lee, M.D.
Associate, Child Psychiatry
Duke University Medical Center
Durham, North Carolina

Susan R. Levy, M.D.
Clinical Assistant Professor of Psychiatry
Duke University Medical Center
Durham, North Carolina

Steven Lipper, M.D., PH.D.
Associate Professor of Psychiatry
Duke University Medical Center
Durham, North Carolina

Stephen Mahorney, M.D.
Assistant Professor of Psychiatry
Duke University Medical Center
Durham, North Carolina

Richard D. Marciniak, M.D.
Fellow in Psychiatry and Law
Rush Presbyterian–St. Luke's Medical Center
Chicago, Illinois

Jacqueline J. Maus, M.D.
Resident in Psychiatry
Duke University Medical Center
Durham, North Carolina

James T. McCracken, M.D.
Fellow in Child Psychiatry
UCLA Neuropsychiatric Institute
Los Angeles, California

Gail McLeod
Psychiatric Social Worker
Veterans Administrations Hospital
Durham, North Carolina

Mark D. Miller, M.D.
Chief Resident in Psychiatry
Duke University Medical Center and Durham County General Hospital
Durham, North Carolina

Charles Nemeroff, M.D.
Associate Professor of Psychiatry and Professor of Pharmacology
Duke University Medical Center
Durham, North Carolina

John F. Steege, M.D.
Assistant Professor of Obstetrics and Gynecology
Duke University Medical Center
Durham, North Carolina

Roy M. Stein, M.D.
Chief Resident in Psychiatry
Veterans Administration Hospital and Duke University Medical Center
Durham, North Carolina

Michael G. Storck, M.D.
Psychiatrist
Fort Defiance Indian Hospital
Fort Defiance, Arizona

Anna L. Stout, PH.D.
Assistant Professor of Obstetrics and Gynecology
Duke University Medical Center
Durham, North Carolina

Marvin S. Swartz, M.D.
Associate in Psychiatry
Duke University Medical Center
Durham, North Carolina

Samuel B. Thielman, M.D.
Fellow in Geriatric Psychiatry
Center for the Study of Aging and Human Development
Duke University Medical Center
Durham, North Carolina

Michael R. Volow, M.D.
Assistant Professor of Psychiatry
Duke University Medical Center
Durham, North Carolina

Richard D. Weiner, M.D., PH.D.
Associate Professor of Psychiatry
Duke University Medical Center
Durham, North Carolina

David S. Werman, M.D.
Professor of Psychiatry
Duke University Medical Center
Durham, North Carolina

Floyd C. Wiseman, M.D.
Chief Resident
Durham County General Hospital and
Resident in Psychiatry
Duke University Medical Center
Durham, North Carolina

Preface

Essentials of Clinical Psychiatry grew from our efforts to teach the fundamentals of psychiatry to medical students. Residents and fellows who work with medical students on a day-to-day basis, and therefore who know the exact material these students need to become competent psysicians, have written the majority of the chapters in this book. Great effort has been made to condense a voluminous amount of material into a brief and concise yet comprehensive volume. The book is divided into three parts—"The Science of Human Behavior," "The Clinical Syndromes," and "The Therapies"—and contains numerous case examples and illustrations to clarify diagnostic and therapeutic issues. It is hoped that medical students will find this book informative and enjoyable reading.

John I. Walker, MD

Acknowledgments

We would like to thank the numerous medical students who gave suggestions and constructive comments during preparation of this volume. Special thanks goes to Frederick R. Hine for his help on the chapter "Theories of Personality and Psychopathology." Portions of the chapter "Child Psychiatry" and "Marital and Family Therapy" are available in altered form through the Dial Access Program of the Southern Medical Association; we thank Barbara Bedford for coordinating these efforts. We deeply appreciate the editorial assistance of Cecilia E. Burns, without whose help this volume would never have come to fruition.

Contents

Part I
The Science of Human Behavior

Samuel B. Thielman

1 Madness and Medicine: A Historical Perspective on the Medical Approach to Mental Disorders

If thou examinest a man having a gaping wound in his head, penetrating to the bone, smashing his skull, [and] rending open the brain of his skull, thou shouldst palpate the wound. . . . When it has happened . . . he discharges blood from both nostrils, [and] he suffers with stiffness in his neck. Thou shouldst say: "An ailment not to be treated." (The Edwin Smith Surgical Papyrus)

In about 2700 BC, some 200 years after the construction of Stonehenge, 700 years before the time of Abraham, and more than two millenia before the birth of Hippocrates, an Egyptian physician interested in surgical disease made the above observations about brain injury. His interest, exhibited so many years ago and in circumstances so vastly different from our own, demonstrates the amazing capacity of humans to think in rational terms not only about the role of physiologic processes in disease, but also about the role of the brain in governing the actions of the body. One of the oldest problems in medical thinking about mental disorders has been deciding to what extent madness is biologically based and to what extent nonbiological factors (*e.g.*, the soul or mind, life circumstances, society, culture) account for mental disorders.

A major concern in modern psychiatry is how to separate biochemically distinct behavioral syndromes from those that are primarily a result of intrapsychic, interpersonal, social, or cultural factors. This brief background chapter presents some historically important ways in which groups or individuals have tried to conceptualize mental disorders. The primary focus will be on how physicians have conceptualized biological and nonbiological influences on madness. A variety of approaches from the past are included, which will give the reader an idea of the diverse paths that physicians have taken in different eras in an effort to understand aberrant mental and behavioral phenomena.

Madness Defined

Although the notion of madness is a very old one, what different writers have meant when they have spoken of madness is often difficult to determine. As a general rule, madness has been viewed by physicians as any disorder that deprives a person of reason. Of the mental disorders spoken of by physicians of the past, mania, melancholia, and hysteria were mentioned most often, and even these terms were often used in a vague way. The idea that there are personality disorders is a relatively recent one, having its origins in the mid 19th century and becoming fully developed only in the 20th century. Nonetheless, for almost 3000 years humans have recognized that some individuals exhibit aberrant behavior for which they are not morally responsible and which can be attributed, at least in part, to physical abnormality.

Early Civilization

Though there are, in every age, people who attribute mental disorders to the direct influence of supernatural forces, the naturalistic view of mental disease emerges from records of a very early date. The oldest written medical sources dealing with madness are the tablets and papyri of the ancient Middle East that indicate the practice of Egyptian and Mesopotamian physicians. The Ebers Papyrus (ca 1500 BC), an Egyptian medical writing, contains some passages attributing aberrant mental phenomena to possession by gods or demons. One passage, for example, attributes "perishing of the mind" and confusion to the "breath" (spirit) of the activity of a priest, a "breath" that causes confusion as it enters the lungs. Nonetheless, the earliest Egyptian medical writing, the Edwin Smith Surgical Papyrus (ca 2500–3000 BC), quoted above, is conspicuously free of supernatural ideas about disease origins. Though this document does not mention mental disorders specifically, it nevertheless reveals a knowledge of the importance of the brain in relation to the rest of the body and suggests that the author had a rudimentary knowledge of cerebral localization.

Evidence that there were naturalistic conceptions of madness exists as early as the first millenium before Christ. In the Old Testament, which is noted for its lack of concern with demon possession, there are several recorded instances of apparent mental disorder. One of the most interesting of these is an incident recorded in I Samuel 21 (ca 1000 BC), where David, prior to his ascendancy to the throne of Israel, fled his predecessor, Saul, and ended up in Gath, a city whose king was unfriendly to Israelites. In an effort to escape harm, David pretended to be mad while in the presence of Achish, the king of Gath. The Bible records the event graphically:

> And David . . . greatly feared Achish king of Gath. So he disguised his sanity before them, and acted insanely in their hands, and scribbled on the doors of the gate, and let his saliva run down into his beard. Then Achish said to his servants, "Behold, you see the man behaving as a madman. Why do you bring

> him to me? Do I lack madmen, that you have brought this one . . . into my house. (I Samuel 21:12—15)*

Far from viewing David as a man possessed by the gods or by demons, the king of Gath regarded David with disdain and indicated to those around him that he viewed David as just one among many madmen in his kingdom. Thus, while notions of demonic possession and supernatural influence were present in many ancient medical writings of the Middle East, there is evidence, both from Egyptian medical papyri and the Old Testament, of naturalistic thinking about madness at a very early date, even among certain laymen.

The Greco-Roman World

One of the most extensive known discussions of insanity in the ancient world is that of Caelius Aurelianus (ca 500 AD), who wrote a treatise called *Acute and Chronic Diseases,* a book based on a similar writing by the prominent first century Roman physician, Soranus of Ephesus (ca 100 AD). Caelius, a member of the Methodist medical sect, rejected the humoralism of earlier physicians, which was espoused by many of the Hippocratic writings, and taught instead that disease was due to a different sort of alteration of bodily status. Some diseases were the result of excessive tension and dryness of the body, some to excessive relaxation and fluidity of the body, and some to a condition involving a combination of these two states. Caelius discussed both "mania" and "melancholia" in his work, teaching that mania was a state of stricture principally involving the head, while melancholia was a state of stricture and sometimes of looseness, involving primarily the esophagus. Mania, as understood by Caelius, probably included patients with a broad range of psychotic disorders with the symptom of physical excitement. "When mania lays hold of the mind," wrote Caelius, "it manifests itself now in anger, now in merriment, now in sadness or futility, and now . . . in overpowering fear of things which are quite harmless. Thus the patient will be afraid of caves or will be obsessed by falling into a ditch or will dread other things which may for some reason inspire fear."[1] Caelius was aware of arguments that madness arises from psychological aberrations, but he rejected that idea. "Those who imagine that the disease is chiefly an affection of the soul and only secondarily of the body are mistaken. For no philosopher has ever set forth a successful treatment for this disease; moreover, before the mind is affected, the body itself shows visible symptoms." Thus, physicians in the Greco-Roman era generally viewed mental disorders as being rooted in organic dysfunction. Philosophers, on the other hand, though often versed in medicine, gave primary consideration to phenomena of the "soul."

The Middle Ages

Though Galen of Pergamum (ca 130–201 AD), arguably the most influential physician of all time, wrote comparatively little that dealt specifically with madness,

* From the New American Standard Bible, the Lockman Foundation, 1960, 1962, 1963, 1968, 1971, 1972, 1973, 1975, 1977

Galenic medicine, with its emphasis on bodily humors and its system of therapeutics based on the "qualities" of particular remedies, had a profound impact on the practice of medicine throughout the Middle Ages, particularly after the 12th century. Not surprisingly, the Galenic system of medicine also exerted an important conceptual influence on the thinking of medieval physicians about madness.

Certain historians of psychiatry, most notably Gregory Zilboorg, have written that supernaturalism dominated medical thinking about mental disorders during this period; however, more recent scholarship has demonstrated that most physicians probably thought most mental disorders result from an imbalance of the humors, and that mental diseases were no more supernatural in origin than any other bodily disorders. This is not to say that medieval physicians thought that supernatural forces played no role in illness, for God and the devil were thought to be intimately involved in all the affairs of men; but mental disorders do not seem to have been singled out as being of particular supernatural importance.

One writer particularly illustrative of the medieval approach to understanding the interaction of biological and mental factors in behavioral disorders was Bartholomeus Anglicus, an English friar who lived in the 13th century. Bartholomeus's book dealing with medical subjects, *De Proprietatibus Rerum,* was widely circulated during the Middle Ages and during the early modern period. After the invention of the printing press, his work went through more than twenty editions.

Bartholomeus showed considerable concern with psychological concomitants of mental disorders, but seemed to view insanity primarily as a disorder of bodily function. Insanity, as he understood it, was of two types, mania and melancholia. Mania was a disorder of the imaginative faculty, melancholia a disorder of the ability to reason. There were many causes of these diseases. Meat with too much black bile could cause melancholia, and so could the use of strong wine. Sometimes mania was a result of overactivity or of preoccupation with deep thoughts. The bite of a mad dog or excessive inhalation of bad air could also produce mental disease. Insanity was seen as a disease of the brain, and treatment consisted of binding the patient so he could not hurt himself and seeing that the patient was able to be "refreshed and conforted" and isolated from anything that might be causing him to have overly serious thoughts. He should be kept occupied with pleasant activities, and music in particular might prove a useful treatment. In this medieval compiler of medical knowledge we find a conception of madness that is based primarily on a biological theory. Supernaturalism is absent from his account.

Paracelsus and Renaissance Thinking About Madness

The greatest preoccupation with supernatural influences on insanity came not during the Middle Ages, but during the Renaissance and Enlightenment. During the 15th and 16th centuries there evolved a new interest in the occult and the esoteric as keys to understanding the mysteries of disease. Sources that were particularly interesting to people who were thinking about medicine and natural philosophy were the writings of the alchemists from the Middle East. With the infusion of

Arabic knowledge in the 12th and 13th centuries came a number of important alchemical writings, and these writings assumed a place of particular importance as people began to challenge the Greek view of the natural world and to search for alternative solutions to understanding health and disease.

The complexity of the Renaissance approach to causes of insanity is illustrated by the views of Theophrastus Bombastus Phillipus von Hohenheim, or Paracelsus (1493–1541), an eccentric, influential physician of the 16th century. The son of a physician, Paracelsus traveled widely during his youth and spent time at many of the major universities of Europe, though whether he actually received a university degree in medicine is uncertain. Paracelsus violently opposed the teachings of Galen, and, like a number of other naturalists in his day, was a devotee of alchemy.

Paracelsus was deeply concerned with social, religious, and philosophical issues. Radically modifying the Aristotelian notion of elements, Paracelsus taught that natural objects were composed of three essential principles: sulfur, salt, and mercury. Man was a microcosm of the universe, the union of the visible and invisible worlds. The body existed in the world of matter; the mind and spirit existed in the celestial world. Both the material and celestial influences were important in understanding disease.

Paracelsus was particularly impressed by the influence of heavenly bodies on disease. Walter Pagel, the noted medical historian, observed that in Paracelsus's system, animal passions in man could be elicited by the stars. Viewing man as both a spiritual and material creature, Paracelsus not only recognized material causes of insanity such as poisoning, but also believed that emotions could cause insanity and that demon possession could account for loss of reason. In addition to prescribing chemical remedies for certain types of insanity, Paracelsus sometimes urged confession to the Church as a remedy.

Paracelsus's complex mixture of magical and natural understandings of insanity reflects the puzzling matrix of ideas that were abroad in medicine during the Renaissance. Indeed, this notion of an interaction of magical and natural elements in madness persisted well into the 17th century.

The Enlightenment

If the magical tradition in medical thinking about insanity continued into the 17th century, that century also saw the rise of mechanistic views of the human organism, a view inspired not only by the writings of men like René Descartes (1596–1650), but also by a general fascination with the idea of analogies between the natural world and the increasingly important machine. In the 17th century, most thinking on natural science was pervaded by a religious world view. At the same time, philosophers concerned with the nature of the mind often headed in intellectual directions that were different from religious thinkers of the past, opting for a more naturalistic understanding of mental processes.

John Locke (1632–1704), a physician by training as well as a philosopher, wrote that ideas were derived from the effect of sensations on the mind, and from the mind's reflection upon these sensations. An 18th-century physician, David

Hartley (1705–1757), built on the ideas of Locke and other philosophers and emphasized not only the importance of the association of sensations and ideas in mental processes, but also proposed a physiological theory of mental action based on the notion that the vibration of nerves is involved in the production of ideas.

By the late 18th century, the impact of philosophical ideas on physicians' thinking about insanity was increasingly noticeable. The American physician Benjamin Rush (1745–1813) exemplifies one facet of this influence. Rush was a general physician who made mental disorders an area of special study. Born near Philadelphia, Rush was educated at the College of New Jersey (now Princeton), served as an apprentice in Philadelphia, and then studied medicine at the University of Edinburgh in the late 1760s, where he came into contact with some of the greatest medical thinkers of the 18th century. Returning to Philadelphia in 1769, Rush established himself as a physician and eventually sought numerous reforms in the care of the insane at the Pennsylvania Hospital.

Rush's major work on mental disorders was *Medical Inquiries and Observations upon Diseases of the Mind* (1812). In this work, Rush distinguished clearly between mental and bodily influences in madness. Though Rush believed that insanity was fundamentally a disease involving inflammation of the blood vessels of the brain, he was nonetheless influenced by a number of contemporary philosophers as well as by philosophically oriented physicians like David Hartley. Rush's treatment for insanity, based on his notion that madness is fundamentally a physical disorder, involved purging, bleeding, and sedating. In addition, however, Rush advocated that the physician use mental techniques such as persuasion and diversion to address a patient's mental symptoms. Though based on now-obsolete physiology, Rush's essential approach, one viewing insanity as fundamentally a physical disorder with mental concomitants, has characterized American psychiatry throughout most of its history.

The Nineteenth Century

By the mid 19th century, medicine was coming to rely primarily on the clinicopathologic method of studying disease. This approach is the foundation of modern medicine, and it came about when a number of physicians, particularly of the "Paris Clinical School," began to seek to understand a patient's symptoms primarily through correlating symptoms with pathological anatomy. Whereas early 19th century thought about madness had generally reflected a concern with fusing a philosophical understanding of the mind with a concept of mental disease based on one of a number of systems for understanding disease, in the mid and later parts of the century physicians saw the development of an almost purely physiological understanding of disease.

Among the most important proponents of a fundamentally physiological understanding of mental disease was Wilhelm Griesinger (1817–1868), a German physician who made neurological and behavioral disorders an area of particular study. Very early in his medical career, Griesinger became convinced of the value of the new physiological understanding of mental disease for the practice of medicine. Griesinger became interested in the study of nervous and mental disease and at the age of twenty-eight published his textbook *Pathologie und Therapie der psychischen Krankheiten* (1845). He led a distinguished academic career until he died at the age of fifty-one.

Today Griesinger is remembered primarily for his dictum, "mental diseases are brain diseases." "What organ," asked Griesinger, "must necessarily and invariably be diseased where there is madness? . . . Physiological and pathological facts show us that this organ can only be the brain; we therefore primarily, and in every case of mental disease, recognize a morbid action of that organ."[2] Griesinger insisted that the study and treatment of mental disease were the domain of physicians alone and that philosophical approaches to psychiatric disorders were wholly inadequate.

> Insanity being a disease, and that disease being an affection of the brain, it can therefore only be studied in a proper manner from the medical point of view. The anatomy, physiology, and pathology of the nervous system, and the whole range of special pathology and therapeutics, constitute a preliminary knowledge most essential to the medical psychologist. All nonmedical, more particularly, all practical and ideal conceptions of insanity are as regards its study of the smallest value.[2]

Griesinger's references to "practical and ideal" conceptions are his response to German Romanticism of the early 19th century. Certain physicians in the German Romantic movement had deempasized the role of physical factors in mental disorders, and had instead explored the "spiritual" nature of madness. Griesinger clearly found such an approach to be useless.

Griesinger's approach was, however, quite complex, and this complexity reflects the multifaceted nature of German psychiatric thought during the later half of the 19th century. Griesinger believed that, though the soul, as he understood it, and the body were inseparable, the relationship between soul and body was unclear.

> From an empirical point of view the unity of the soul and body is indeed a fact primarily to be maintained, and the *a priori* investigation of the possibility of soul apart from body, of a bodiless soul, must be entirely dismissed, [for we must confine] ourselves to abstract considerations of its unity and oneness as distinguished from the endless modifications of matter. . . . How a material physical act in the nerve fibers or cells can be concerted into an idea, an act of consciousness, is absolutely incomprehensible. . . . The materialistic [hypothesis] offers fewer difficulties, obscurities and contradictions than any other. . . . Therefore, . . . it is scientifically admissible to connect the faculties of the soul with the body in the same intimate relation as exists between function and organ—to consider the understanding and the will as the function, the special energy of the brain, just as transmission and reflex action are considered the special function of the nerves and spinal cord, and to consider the soul primarily and preeminently as the sum of all cerebral states.[2]

This materialistic perspective on mental disorders has persisted in European and American psychiatry to the present day.

Griesinger's influence on the development of psychiatry in the 19th century was profound. Among the many individuals in Germany who came under Griesinger's influence, Sigmund Freud was the most significant. A detailed examination of Freud's understanding of the interaction of biological and psychological factors with the development of mental disorders is beyond the purpose of this chapter; however, a brief recounting of the influence of this perennial problem on the development of Freud's thought is in order.

Freud and After

Sigmund Freud (1856–1939), the second oldest child of a prosperous wool merchant, was born in Freiberg, Moravia (now Czechoslovakia). Freud's family moved to Vienna in 1860 after the wool market failed in Freiberg. Freud attended Sperl Gymnasium in Vienna, graduating with distinction in 1873. In that same year, Freud entered the University of Vienna, where he began a course of medical studies, eventually coming under the tutelage of Ernst Brücke (1819–1892), a renowned professor of physiology who headed the Physiological Institute. Freud became quite successful in his neuroanatomical work at the Institute, publishing significant studies on the crayfish. Because of the limited opportunity for advancement in the German university system, however, Freud left the Institute in 1882 to practice clinical medicine. He continued, nevertheless, to publish important research papers in the field of neurology, including papers on the structure of the medulla oblongata, childhood paralysis, and cocaine addiction.

In 1885 and 1886, with the help of Brücke, Freud obtained a government-sponsored fellowship to study with Jean-Martin Charcot (1825–1893), perhaps the greatest neurologist of the day, at the Salpetrière in Paris. With his investigations into the nature of hysteria through the use of hypnosis, Charcot stirred Freud's longtime interest in psychological phenomena. Thus, with a strong neurological background and a newly inspired interest in psychological phenomena, Freud became most interested in exploring psychological phenomena, particularly hysteria.

Freud's first great contribution to psychology came during the years 1885 to 1895, when he collaborated on investigations into hysteria with Josef Breuer (1842–1925). Particularly important to the development of Freud's thought was Breuer's work with a patient named Anna O. During the years 1881 and 1882, Breuer had treated Anna O, who had a number of severe psychological symptoms, using hypnosis to achieve emotional catharsis. Anna O experienced dramatic relief of her symptoms under Breuer's treatment, and Freud became so impressed with his colleague's results that in the late 1880s he began using Breuer's method with a number of patients. Freud eventually collaborated with Breuer on a work entitled *Studies on Hysteria* (1895), which described several of these cases. Freud disagreed with Breuer over the importance of sexuality in the "neuroses" shortly after the publication of their collaborative work.

Freud's investigations of "neurosis" during this early period reflected a desire not only to understand psychological processes in a more complete way, but to uncover a link between mental and neurophysiological processes. This desire is particularly evident in Freud's letters to his friend Wilhelm Fliess (1858–1928), a physician in Berlin with whom Freud corresponded from 1887 to 1902. Although Fliess had been trained as a nose and throat specialist, he had also developed certain biological theories about human behavior. Among these ideas was his "nasal reflex" theory of neurosis, in which Fliess proposed the existence of a neurosis caused by a disorder of the nose. Fliess also had an elaborate theory of the behavioral influence of biological rhythms. Freud was intrigued by these theories at the time, and he believed that Fliess's ideas on biological causes of mental disorders were of immense importance. For his part, Freud, in his letters to Fliess, evidenced an enthusiasm for exploring the relationship between psychological and physiological processes. For example, in a draft sent to Fliess in January, 1895, Freud made the following comments about melancholia:

> And now, how can the effects of melancholia be explained? They can best be thus described: *psychical inhibition* [is] *accompanied by* [an] *instinctual impoverishment, and* [there is psychic] *pain that this should be so.* We can imagine that, if the psychical sexual group [of ideas] suffers very great loss in the amount of its excitation, this may lead to a kind of *indrawing in the psyche,* which produces an effect of suction upon the adjoining amounts of excitation. The neurones associated [with the group] are obliged to give up their excitation, and this *produces pain.* The uncoupling of associations is always painful. There sets in an impoverishment of excitation—of reserve stock—in a way that resembles *internal bleeding,* and this shows itself in the other instincts and functions. This indrawing process has an inhibiting effect and operates like a wound, in a manner analogous to pain. . . .[3]

Thus, during this period Freud wrestled with the problem of how the brain produces pathological mental processes. Later in his scientific career, Freud became almost exclusively concerned with psychological mechanisms.

Freud made monumental contributions to 20th century psychiatry through his theories of the role of the unconscious in human behavior. As Freud's ideas developed, however, a number of people who acknowledged the importance of a number of Freud's views were nonetheless dissatisfied with various aspects of his approach.

Among the many individuals who took exception to Freud's ideas in the early part of the 20th century, two Americans deserve special consideration. Harry Stack Sullivan (1892–1949) rejected many of Freud's formulations of the psyche and emphasized interpersonal factors in forming the individual's personality. Adolph Meyer (1866–1950), a Swiss-born American immigrant, believed that emphasis should be placed on the individual as a complex biological organism interacting with his environment. Sullivan, Meyer, and many other significant contributors to 20th-century psychiatry departed from earlier thinking that had struggled with the relation of the mind to the body, and sought instead to weave increasingly sophisticated notions of brain function, individual psychology, sociology, and anthropology into a more comprehensive understanding of how people become behaviorally aberrant, and when and how intervention of the physician is appropriate.

The study of mental disorders is a very complicated endeavour, as is demonstrated by the variety of approaches physicians have taken toward them in the past. Indeed, mental disorders exhibit a degree of complexity that is unique among the problems addressed by physicians. Nonetheless, the conviction of a large number of physicians during many different periods of history has been that an adequate understanding of aberrant thoughts and behaviors must include consideration of both mental and biological processes.

References

1. Drabkin IE (ed): Caelius Aurelianus on Acute and Chronic Diseases, p 539. Chicago, University of Chicago Press, 1950
2. Griesinger W: Mental Pathology and Therapeutics, p 7. New York, William Wood, 1882
3. Freud S: The Origins of Psycho Analysis, Letters to Wilhelm Fliess, Drafts and Notes: 1887–1902, pp 107–108. New York, Basic Books, 1954

Bibliography

Ackerknecht EA: A Short History of Psychiatry. Wolff S (trans): New York, Hafner, 1968

Breasted J: The Edwin Smith Surgical Papyrus. Chicago, University of Chicago, 1930

Ellenberger HF: The Discovery of the Unconscious: The History and Evolution of Dynamic Psychology. New York, Basic Books, 1970

Ghalioungui P: The House of Life Per Ankh: Magic and Medical Science in Ancient Egypt. Amsterdam, B.M. Israel, 1973

Kroll J: A reappraisal of psychiatry in the Middle Ages. Arch Gen Psychiatry 29:276–283, 1973

Neugebauer R: Medieval and early modern theories of mental illness. Arch Gen Psychiatry 36:477–483, 1979

Pagel W: Paracelsus: An Introduction to Philosophical Medicine in the Era of the Renaissance. New York, S Karger, 1982

Sigerist HE: A History of Medicine, Vol 1. New York, Oxford University Press, 1951

Sulloway FJ: Freud, Biologist of the Mind: Beyond the Psychoanalytic Legend. New York, Basic Books, 1979

Walsh JJ: Bartolomeus Anglicus. Medical Life 40:449–602, 1933

Zilboorg G: A History of Medical Psychology. New York, WW Norton, 1941

Charles B. Nemeroff

2 Biological Psychiatry

We may now believe that in the interstitial tissues of the gonads special chemical substances are produced, which when taken up in the blood stream, charge definite parts of the central nervous system with sexual tension.[1]

The above statement by Freud reveals that the "father of psychoanalysis" was cognizant of the importance of biological factors in human behavior. During his lifetime the now burgeoning science of neurobiology was in its infancy and there was little in terms of a rationally developed, somatic treatment to alleviate the suffering of patients with major mental disorders. In the past 25 years, remarkable advances in neuroanatomy, neurochemistry, neurophysiology, neuropharmacology, and neuropsychology have occurred, and these have now been increasingly applied in an interdisciplinary manner in order to gain a better understanding of psychiatric and neurological disease. These advances, especially in neuroradiology (*e.g.*, computed tomography, nuclear magnetic resonance, and positron-emission tomography), genetics, neuroendocrinology, and neurochemistry, have provided compelling evidence that the major psychiatric disorders (*e.g.*, major depression with melancholia or psychosis, schizophrenia) are, in fact, disorders of the central nervous system (CNS). Stated another way, the brain is, truly, the organ of the mind, and not surprisingly diseases of the brain frequently present with disturbances of mood and cognition and changes in personality. The remainder of this chapter summarizes certain of the available evidence concordant with the hypothesis that the vulnerability to develop major affective illness (manic–depressive illness) and schizophrenia are, most certainly, biologically determined. In fact, it is now clear that the term *biological psychiatry* is redundant—all of psychiatry is, and must be, considered biological. Thus, as recently recounted by Bleuler, the various theories of the humors and their role in the etiology and pathogenesis of mental illness (*e.g.*, melancholia) postulated in the 17th and 18th centuries have reemerged in the 20th century with the demonstration that neurotransmitters, neuromodulators, and hormones play important roles in the brain and consequently influence both normal and abnormal behaviors.[2]

Genetics in Psychiatry

Genetic analysis of the prevalence and hereditability of the major psychiatric disorders has corroborated the view that the diatheses for these diseases are, undoubtedly, biologically determined.[3,4] The controversy surrounding the nature–nurture conundrum regarding vulnerability to manic–depressive illness and schizophrenia has been well publicized. There seems to be little doubt that these disorders occur in increased rates in those who have family members so affected—the controversy surrounds the interpretation of the data. Are the increased rates of major depression in offspring of parents who have been diagnosed to have this affective illness due to an inherited vulnerability, or are they due to the consequences of upbringing in a "depressive" (*i.e.*, depressogenic) environment? Similar data on schizophrenia are available. Several strategies have been employed, and much of the available data are discussed in detail in the chapters on schizophrenia and affective disorders (Chapters 6 and 7). However, because this chapter subserves a propaedeutic function, certain of the genetic data will be briefly described.

The rate of mood disorders among first degree relatives of manic–depressive patients (especially bipolar patients) is considerably higher than that observed in the general population. The twin studies are of particular interest. In essence they attempt to eliminate the confounding variable of environmental influence by comparing the concordance rates of the illness under study in monozygotic and dizygotic twins (both in twins reared in the same environment and in twins separated at birth). Table 2-1 illustrates the much higher concordance rate of major affective disorders in monozygotic (when compared to dizygotic) twins both for unipolar and bipolar affective disorder. These data strongly support the view that inherited

Table 2-1
Concordance Rates in Twins With Major Affective Disorders

Category	Concordance Rates by Index Diagnosis	
	Bipolar	*Unipolar*
Dizygotic	14	11
Monozygotic	72	40
Monozygotic : dizygotic ratio	5.0	3.6

Note: Data are pooled from reviews of nine published reports. Overall concordance rates for manic or depressive illness, regardless of polarity, are 68% and 19% for monozygotic and dizygotic twins, respectively (monozygotic : dizygotic ratio = 3.6). The groups above include more than 100 twin pairs. Among the rate instances (12 pairs) of monozygotic twins reared separately, the concordance rate for manic–depressive illness is 75%. (From Baldessarini RJ: Biomedical Aspects of Depression and Its Treatment. Washington, DC, American Psychiatric Press, 1983. With permission.)

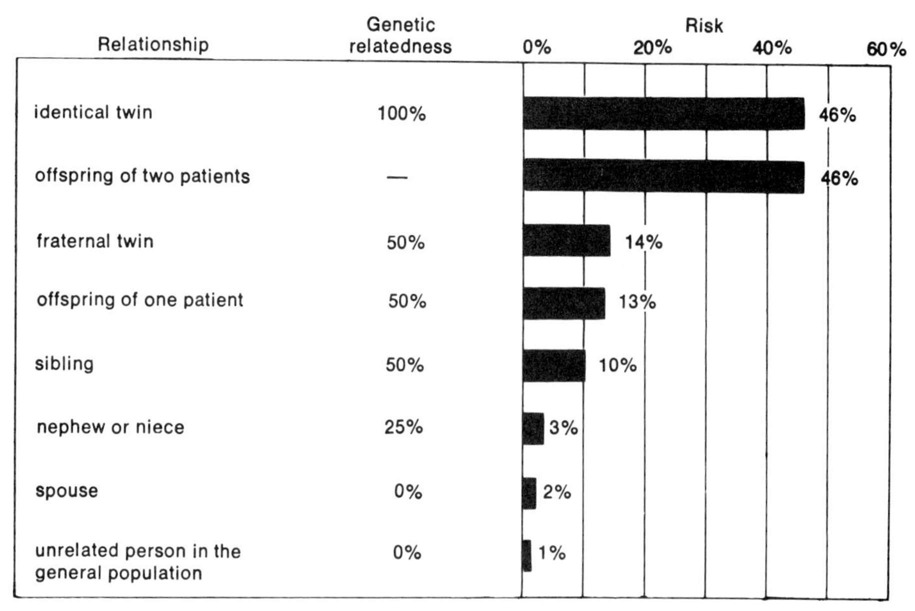

Figure 2-1. Lifetime risks of developing schizophrenia are largely a function of how closely an individual is genetically related to a schizophrenic, and not a function of how much their environment is shared. The observed risks, however, are much more compatible with a multifactorial polygenic theory of transmission than with a mendelian model or one involving a single major locus, especially after allowance is made for some unsystematic environmental transmission. In the case of an individual with two schizophrenic parents, genetic relatedness cannot be expressed in terms of percentage, but the regression of the individual's "genetic value" on that of the parents 1, is the same as it is for identical twins. (From Nicol, Gottesman: Clues to the genetics and neurobiology of schizophrenia. Am Scientist 71:398, 1983. With permission.)

(*i.e.*, biological) factors play an important role in risk of affective illness. Similar findings for schizophrenia have been reported.[4,5]

There seems to be little doubt that the risk of schizophrenia to relatives of schizophrenics is substantially increased with the degree of genetic relatedness (Fig. 2-1). The importance of environmental factors is highlighted by the fact that somewhat less than half the identical twins of schizophrenics develop the disease, though they share an identical genetic makeup with them. Whether the mode of transmission of risk for these psychiatric illnesses is inherited in a simple single dominant or recessive gene or in a polygenic fashion is unknown. Whether the risk to develop any of the less well-studied psychiatric diseases (*e.g.*, anxiety disorders, personality disorders) is genetically determined is presently not known.

Psychopharmacology

One of the final chapters in this book describes antipsychotic and antidepressant drugs, lithium, anxiolytics, and sedative–hypnotics. In the limited space available, only a superficial outline of the neurobiological basis of modern psychopharmacology can be described. As noted previously, considerable advances in the past three decades have dramatically increased our understanding of CNS function. A variety of putative neurotransmitters, neuromodulators, and neuroregulators have been identified:[6]

Acetylcholine
Adenosine
Adrenocorticotropic hormone (ACTH)
Angiotensin
Aspartate
ATP
β-Endorphin
Bombesin
Calcitonin
Carnosine
Cholecystokinin (CCK)
Corticosteroids
Corticotropin-releasing factor (CRF)
Delta sleep-inducing peptides (DSIP)
Dimethoxyphenylethylamine (DMPEA)
Dimethyltryptamine (DMT)
Dopamine
Dynorphin
Epinephrine
Estrogens
5-Hydroxydimethyltryptamine (bufotenin)
5-Methoxydimethyltryptamine
5-Methoxytryptamine
FRMF amide
γ-Aminobutyric acid (GABA)
γ-Hydroxybutyrate (GHB)
Gastrin
Gastrin-releasing peptide
Glucagon
Glutamate
Glycine
Growth hormone
Growth hormone-releasing hormone (GHRH)
Histamine
Insulin
Kytorphin
Leu-enkephalin
Luteinizing hormone
Luteinizing hormone-releasing hormone (LHRH)
Melanocyte-stimulating hormone
Melatonin

Met-enkephalin
Motilin
Neuropeptide Y
Neurotensin
Norepinephrine
Octopamine
Oxytocin
Pancreatic Polypeptide
Phenylethanolamine
Phenylethylamine
Proctolin
Prolactin
Prostaglandins
Quinolinic acid
Secretin
Serotonin (5-hydroxytryptamine)
Somatomedin
Somatostatin
Substance P
Taurine
Testosterone
Tetrahydroisoquinolines
Thyroid hormone
Thyrotropin
Thyrotropin-releasing hormone (TRH)
Tryptamine
Tryptolines
Tyramine
Vasoactive-intestinal polypeptide (VIP)
Vasopressin

These include the monoamine and amino acid neurotransmitters as well as the more recently discovered neuropeptides. As more information on the distribution, synthesis, release, inactivation, and effects of all these endogenous substances became available, it became evident that the activity of certain of these chemically defined neural circuits is altered by many of the psychotropically active drugs. A complete review of the neurochemical pharmacology of these well-defined circuits is beyond the scope of this chapter, but is described in detail elsewhere (see Cooper). A brief discussion of brain dopamine (DA) systems is provided to subserve a generic function. Figure 2-2 illustrates the major DA-containing neural systems in the mammalian brain. Three arise in the midbrain: (1) the nigroneostriatal system with cell bodies in the substantia nigra that project to the striatum (caudate nucleus, putamen, and globus pallidus); (2) the mesolimbic system with cell bodies in the ventral tegmental area (VTA) that project to the nucleus accumbens, olfactory tubercles, amygdala, and septum; and (3) the mesocortical system with cell bodies in the VTA that project to the frontal and temporal cortex. Additional DA-containing systems have been described: the tuberoinfundibular system

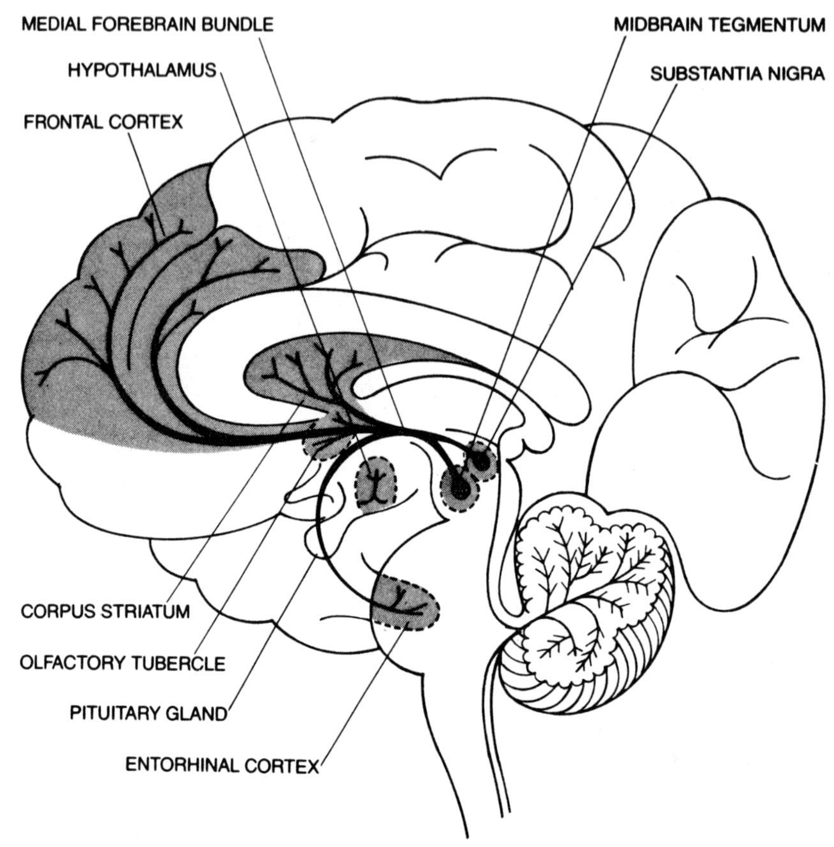

Figure 2-2. Dopamine pathways in the human brain are shown here schematically. The neurons that contain dopamine have their cell bodies clustered in two small regions of the midbrain, the substantia nigra and the tegmentum. These neurons send out widely branching fibers that terminate in the corpus striatum, which regulates motor activity; and in the limbic forebrain, which is involved in emotion. A small set of dopamine neurons in the hypothalamus also regulates secretion of hormones from the pituitary. Dopamine has been associated with two brain disorders: A deficiency of the transmitter in the corpus striatum causes the rigidity and tremor of Parkinson's disease; and an excess of dopamine in limbic forebrain may be involved in schizophrenia. (From Iversen LL: The chemistry of the brain. In: The Brain. San Francisco, WH Freeman, 1979. With permission.)

with cell bodies in the arcuate and periventricular nuclei of the hypothalamus that project to the median eminence and posterior pituitary, and a newly discovered incerto-hypothalamic system, which projects from the zone incerta to the hypothalamus. Finally, a retinal DA system has also been discovered. The synthesis and metabolism of DA and norepinephrine (NE) are illustrated in Figure 2-3. These

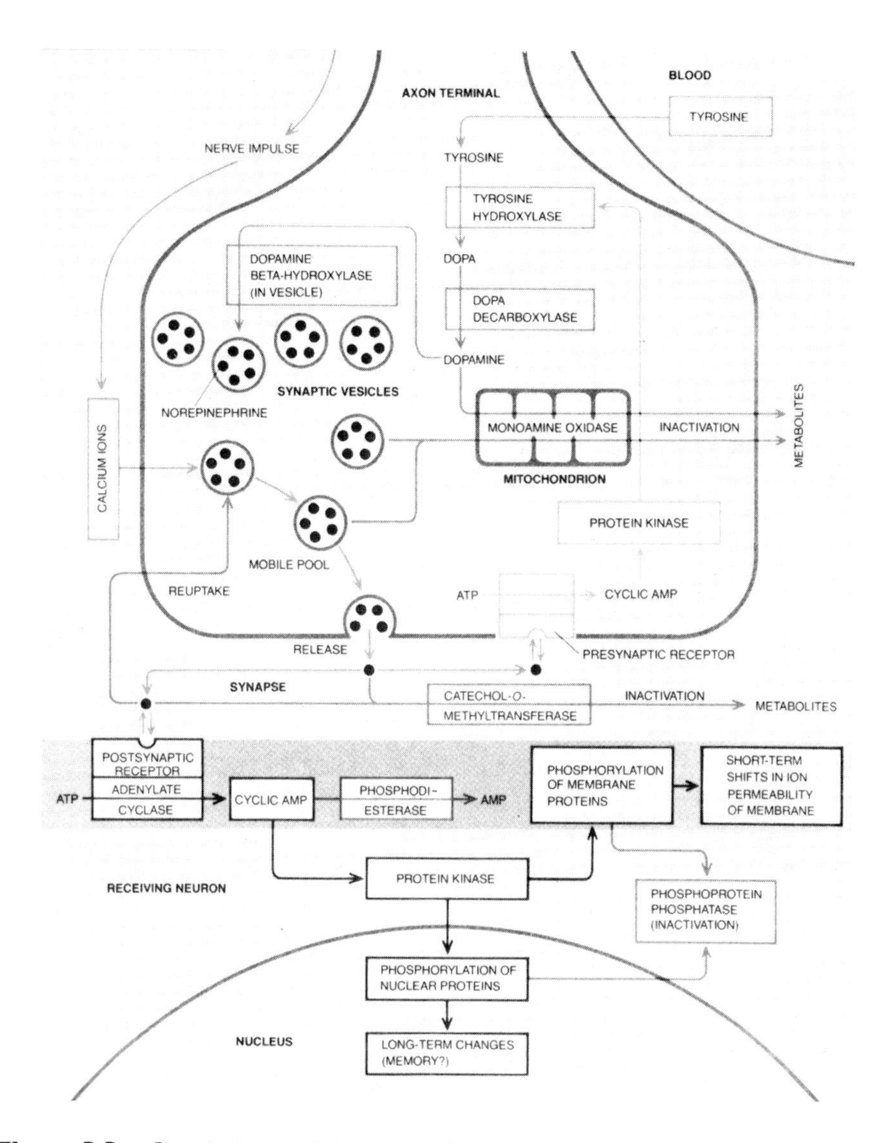

Figure 2-3. Chemical transmission across the synapse, the narrow gap between two neurons in the brain, involves an elaborate sequence of molecular events. Here the process of transmission at a norepinephrine synapse is diagrammed. First, norepinephrine is manufactured from the amino acid tyrosine in three steps, each of which is catalyzed by an enzyme. The transmitter is then stored with membrane-bound vesicles in association with storage proteins. The arrival in the axon terminal of a nerve impulse triggers an influx of calcium ions, which induces the release of norepinephrine from the vesicles into the synaptic space. The liberated transmitter molecules bind to specific receptor proteins that are embedded in the postsynaptic membrane, triggering a series of reactions that culminate in short-term (electrical and long-term effects on the receiving neuron. The action of norepinephrine is then terminated by a variety of means, including rapid reuptake of the transmitter into the axon terminal, and degradation by enzymes. The release of some norepinephrine into the synaptic space activates presynaptic receptors on the axon terminal, initiating production of cyclic AMP, which activates protein kinase, thus stimulating more norepinephrine production. (From Iversen LL: The chemisry of the brain. In: The Brain. San Francisco, WH Freeman, 1979. With permission.)

catecholamines are synthesized from tyrosine, an amino acid taken up by the brain from the blood by a carrier-mediated process. The rate-limiting step in the biosynthesis of DA and NE is the conversion of tyrosine to L-dopa, catalyzed by tyrosine hydroxylase, an enzyme present in catecholamine-containing cell bodies and nerve terminals. L-Dopa is converted to DA by the action of a relatively nonspecific aromatic amino acid decarboxylase. In NE-containing neurons, DA is converted to NE by the action of dopamine β-hydroxylase. DA is released from presynaptic DA nerve terminals in a calcium-dependent manner by the action of a depolarizing nerve stimulus, and the neurotransmitter, once released into the synaptic cleft, acts on postsynaptic DA receptors (of which four subtypes have been described). At least one of these postsynaptic DA receptors is linked to activation of adenylate cyclase, with the consequent enhanced production of the second messenger, cyclic AMP. Although enzymes that degrade DA are present both intraneuronally (monoamine oxidase) and extraneuronally (catechol-O-methyltransferase), the primary mode of inactivation of released DA is reuptake into the presynaptic terminal.

Each of the DA circuits is believed to modulate different physiological and behavioral functions. The tubero-infundibular DA system is known to modulate the secretion of prolactin from the anterior pituitary gland; enhanced release of DA from the median eminence inhibits prolactin release. The nigroneostriatal system is believed to modulate aspects of movement; when this system degenerates, as it is known to do in Parkinson's disease, resting tremor, rigidity, and bradykinesia result. The functions of the mesolimbic and mesocortical DA systems are less well understood but, based on preclinical data, have been hypothesized to modulate emotion, reward, motivation, and responses to stress.

The psychopharmacology of the DA systems has been studied in detail. Considerable evidence has accumulated that is consistent with the view that antipsychotic drugs (*e.g.*, chlorpromazine, haloperidol, thiothixene) act by blocking DA receptors. Although these drugs exert a variety of effects on other neural circuits, there is strong evidence that their antipsychotic properties are due to blockade of forebrain DA receptors (probably in mesolimbic or mesocortical DA terminal areas). The neurologic side effects of these major tranquilizers (*i.e.*, acute extrapyramidal effects and tardive dyskinesia) are believed to be mediated at nigroneostriatal DA receptor sites whereas the hyperprolactinemia induced by these drugs is due to blockade of the action of DA at tubero-infundibular DA receptor sites. These findings and others (*e.g.*, psychomotor stimulants such as d-amphetamine that increase DA release also exacerbate the symptomatology of many schizophrenics) led to the formulation of the DA hypothesis of schizophrenia,[7] which states that hyperactivity of certain DA systems, especially the mesolimbic DA circuits, may in fact represent the primary pathophysiological "lesion" in schizophrenia. More data support the DA theory of antipsychotic drug action than the DA theory of schizophrenia.[7,8] It is evident that although much can be learned about the action of clinically effective drugs by studying their neural substrates, it is quite another matter to draw conclusions about the primary etiology of a psychiatric disorder from such psychopharmacological data.

Sleep

It may seem less than obvious to the student reader why a section on sleep is included in a chapter entitled *Biological Psychiatry*. The reasons are multifactorial, but suffice it to say that (1) sleep disturbances rank high on a list of frequently cited symptoms for which patients complain both to psychiatrists and primary-care physicians; (2) insomnia with early morning awakening is a cardinal feature of major depression; (3) disordered sleep, as assessed by electroencephalographic (EEG) recordings (*i.e.*, shortened rapid eye movement [REM] latency), is a characteristic of major depression but not of other psychiatric illnesses; and (4) the existence of several distinct sleep disorders (*e.g.*, narcolepsy, sleep apnea, and night terrors) and specific treatments for them make it imperative for physicians to properly diagnose these entities and not, as often occurs, treat them as symptomatic of another psychiatric disorder, such as depression, anxiety, or personality disorders. Several excellent descriptions of sleep physiology and pathology are available (see Hartman for review). This concatenation of findings, as well as the longstanding interest that psychoanalytically oriented psychotherapists have in dream interpretation, and the often-made observation that schizophrenia is like the breaking through of dreams into conscious life, has rendered sleep physiology, pathology, and pharmacology an important area of psychiatric research.

EEG recordings have revealed the presence of different sleep stages. These are illustrated in Figure 2-4. The waking state is often termed *stage 0,* and brief awakenings occur several times during the course of a night's sleep. In stage one the subject experiences light sleep and is easily awakened, and the EEG pattern is one of low voltage and fast activity. In stage 2 the subject is still sleeping lightly, and frequent spindle-shaped tracing and high-voltage spikes (K complexes) are seen. Stage 3 is characterized by the presence of high voltage δ waves that become the predominant part of the tracing in stage 4. Stages 1 to 4 are called *non-REM* or *synchronized sleep,* and stages 3 and 4 are *slow-wave* or *deep sleep*. After stage 4, *REM* or *paradoxical sleep* is observed. The EEG pattern is similar to that observed in stage 1 and the sleeper is easily awakened, but this stage is characterized by heightened autonomic activity (*e.g.*, increased heart rate and blood pressure) and dreaming. Figure 2-5 shows the sleep pattern of an average, healthy, young adult over an 8-hour period. Note that REM sleep occurs three to five times per night at 90- to 110-minute intervals. An interesting and unexpected observation is the finding that in human infants (and neonatal mammals), not only do the young spend more time sleeping than do adults, but that they spend much of their time in REM sleep (Fig. 2-6).

The great unanswered question is, of course, what function does sleep serve? The effects of sleep deprivation and selective REM sleep deprivation have been studied to provide some clues to the importance of sleep, but the results have been difficult to interpret.[9] The relation of sleep to mental illness remains obscure but is of interest. The reduced sleep latency seen in major depression is one of the most reliable biological markers in psychiatry. A potentially related and interesting ob-

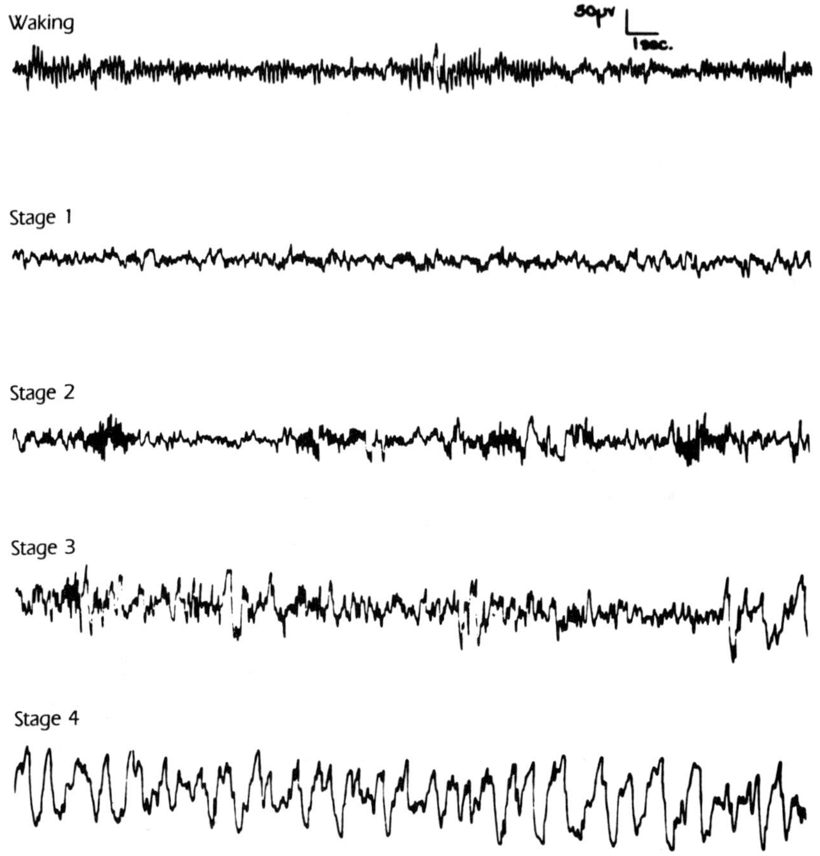

Figure 2-4. The electroencephalogram of sleep in a human adult. A single channel of recordings—a monopolar recording from the left parietal area, referred to as the ears for a neutral reference point—is shown for each stage. (From Hartman EL: Sleep. In: Kaplan HI, Freedman AJ, Sadock BJ (eds): Comprehensive Textbook of Psychiatry III, 1, 3rd ed. Baltimore, Williams & Wilkins, 1980. With permission.)

servation recently made by investigators in both Europe and the United States is that sleep deprivation produces a short-lived but reproducible antidepressant effect. As noted above, some of those in the field have postulated that schizophrenia is, in fact, the intrusion of dreams into conscious life; however, schizophrenics invariably show normal sleep patterns.

Much of the uncertainty about sleep resonates with our ignorance of its neuroanatomical and neurochemical substrates. There is considerable evidence that both serotonergic and noradrenergic circuits modulate sleep. In the past several years, extracts of brain, blood, and cerebrospinal fluid (CSF) from animals (both sleep-deprived and non-sleep-deprived) have been evaluated for sleep-promoting properties. Several crude, chemically impure preparations were originally discov-

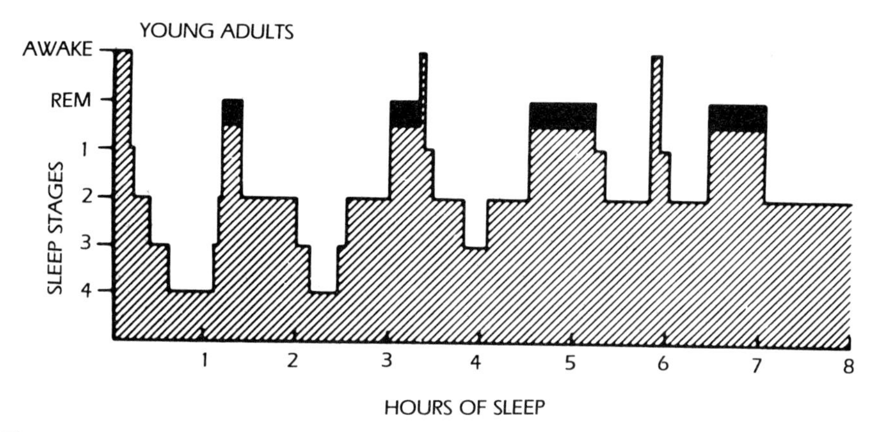

Figure 2-5. Stages of sleep. (From Berger R: The sleep and dream cycle. In: Kales A (ed): Sleep: Physiology and Pathology. Philadelphia, Lippincott, 1969. With permission.)

ered, and one such substance, delta sleep-inducing peptide (DSIP), a nonapeptide, has been sequenced and synthesized. The pharmaceutical utility of such an agent would be great, especially if the drug had no abuse liability.

The major sleep disorders are narcolepsy, sleep apnea, night terrors, somnambulism, and enuresis. Narcolepsy is characterized by excessive daytime sleepiness, sleep attacks, cataplexy (decreased muscle tone resulting in weakness, usually induced by strong emotion or physical exertion), and hypnagogic hallucinations (hallucinations experienced upon falling asleep). Narcolepsy has been mistaken for alcohol intoxication. The primary pathophysiologic defect appears to be the abrupt onset of REM sleep during the day. Sleep apnea is characterized by apnic periods of 10 to 60 seconds followed by snoring, gasping, and rapid breathing. Sleepwalking is common in children and is dangerous because of risk of injury. Night terrors, a familial disorder, is the occurrence of extreme fear and terror, and the patient (often a child) is difficult to awaken. Unlike nightmares, these occur in stage 4 sleep. Enuresis (involuntary discharge of urine), a common condition in children, usually occurs during stage 4 sleep, and it is treated quite successfully with imipramine.

Neurochemistry of Behavior

The elucidation of many chemically defined neurotransmitter systems in the brain has led to the study of their role in behavior. The use of a variety of newly discovered, specific lesioning techniques (6-hydroxydopamine to destroy catecholamine circuits, 5,7-dihydroxytryptamine to destroy serotonergic circuits, kainic acid and other excitotoxic amino acids to destroy neuronal perikarya, but not axons in passage) has allowed investigators to evaluate the contribution of these circuits in a variety of physiological and behavioral functions including eating, sexual behavior, sleep, thermoregulation, learning and memory, reward, and so forth.

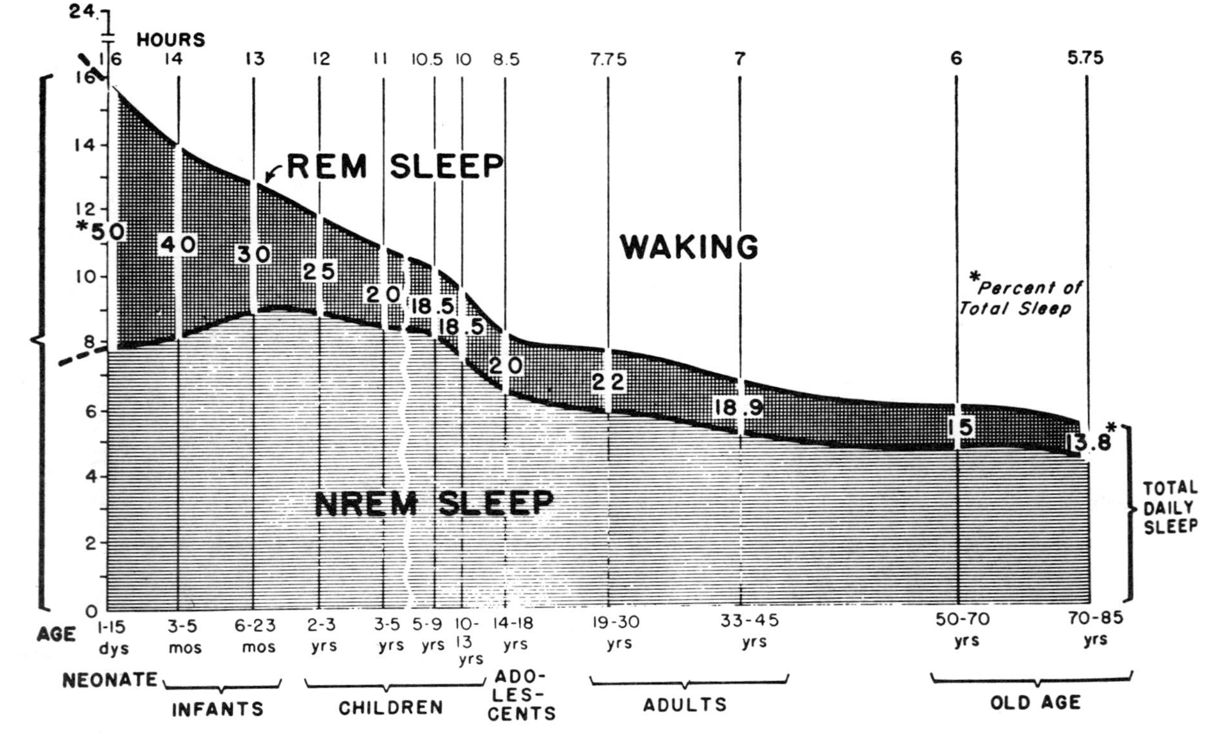

Figure 2-6. Changes, with age, in total amounts of daily sleep, daily REM sleep, and in the percentage of REM sleep. Note the sharp diminution of REM sleep in the early years. REM sleep falls from eight hours at birth to less than one hour in old age. The amount of NREM sleep throughout life remains more constant, falling from 8 hours to 5 hours. In contrast to the steep decline of REM sleep, the quantity of NREM sleep is undiminished for many years. Although total daily REM sleep falls steadily during life, the percentage rises slightly in adolescence and early adulthood. This rise does not reflect an increase in amount; it is because REM sleep does not diminish as quickly as total sleep. (Data for the 33–45-year group and the 50–90–year group are taken from Strauch, Kales et al (1967), Feinberg et al (1967), and Kahn and Fisher (1969), respectively.) (From Roffwarg HP, Muzio JN, Dement WC: Ontogenetic development of the human sleep–dream cycle. Science 152:604, 1966. With permission.)

Another experimental approach has been the measurement of changes in neurochemical constituents associated with behavioral changes (*e.g.*, monoamine turnover, changes in nucleic acid, and protein metabolism). These studies are difficult to conduct because of problems in choosing appropriate controls and the interpretation of the data obtained. See Dunn for discussion of the problems associated with the study of the neurochemistry of learning and memory.

An often-used experimental technique is to microinject endogenous substances into particular brain areas using stereotaxic surgery in an attempt to mimic the endogenous concentration of the substance after its synaptic release. The behavioral changes observed might reflect the normal physiological function(s) of the injected compound. This technique is also fraught with potential problems—spread of the compound after injection, use of supraphysiological concentrations, action of the substance at sites where it normally does not act, and so forth. When used judiciously, valuable information has been obtained with this method.

A comprehensive review of neurochemistry and behavior is beyond the scope of this chapter, but an illustrative example might be instructive. Angiotensin II (Asp-Arg-Val-Tyr-Ile-His-Pro-Phe-OH) is an octapeptide that is almost certainly involved in drinking behavior. Fifteen years ago, Epstein and colleagues reported that microinjection of small quantities of angiotensin II (0.05 μg to 2.0 μg) into the hypothalamus of conscious, unrestrained, non-water-deprived rats induced drinking. The description of the behavior of these animals is informative:

> The animal is clearly motivated to drink. After an injection it stops whatever it is doing, proceeds to the water spout and starts drinking. If the water bottle is removed from its usual place in the cage, the rat searches for it and licks up any spillage that may have occurred. The rat continues looking for water at least 10 min. after the injection, and if water is restored at the end of this time, it starts to drink avidly. A starving animal which has just been allowed to start eating, but which has only taken a few mouthfuls of food, stops eating when injected with angiotensin and then starts to drink after the usual latency. On one occasion a sleeping animal was awakened by the injection and started to drink. Intracranial angiotensin is a sufficiently powerful stimulus of drinking to make a rat, which is manually restrained, struggle and overcome its natural fear of men in order to reach the water spout.[10]

Much work since then has sought to determine the specificity and neuroanatomical loci of actions of antiotensin. Other neuropeptides such as vasopressin, bradykinin, neurotensin, and cholecystokinin do not produce this effect. The subfornical organ, a circumventricular organ, is one site where extraordinarily small quantities of angiotensin are dipsogenic; several researchers have reported that the drinking observed after intraventricular application of angiotensin is blocked by subfornical organ lesions. The anterior part of the third ventricle adjacent to the organum vasculosum laminae terminalis is another angiotensin-sensitive site. From an evolutionary perspective, it is of interest that angiotensin is a potent dipsogen in many vertebrate species including the rat, dog, cat, sheep, opossum, chicken, pigeon, and iguana. What has not yet been resolved is whether angiotensin normally plays a physiological role in drinking behavior. This example should serve to

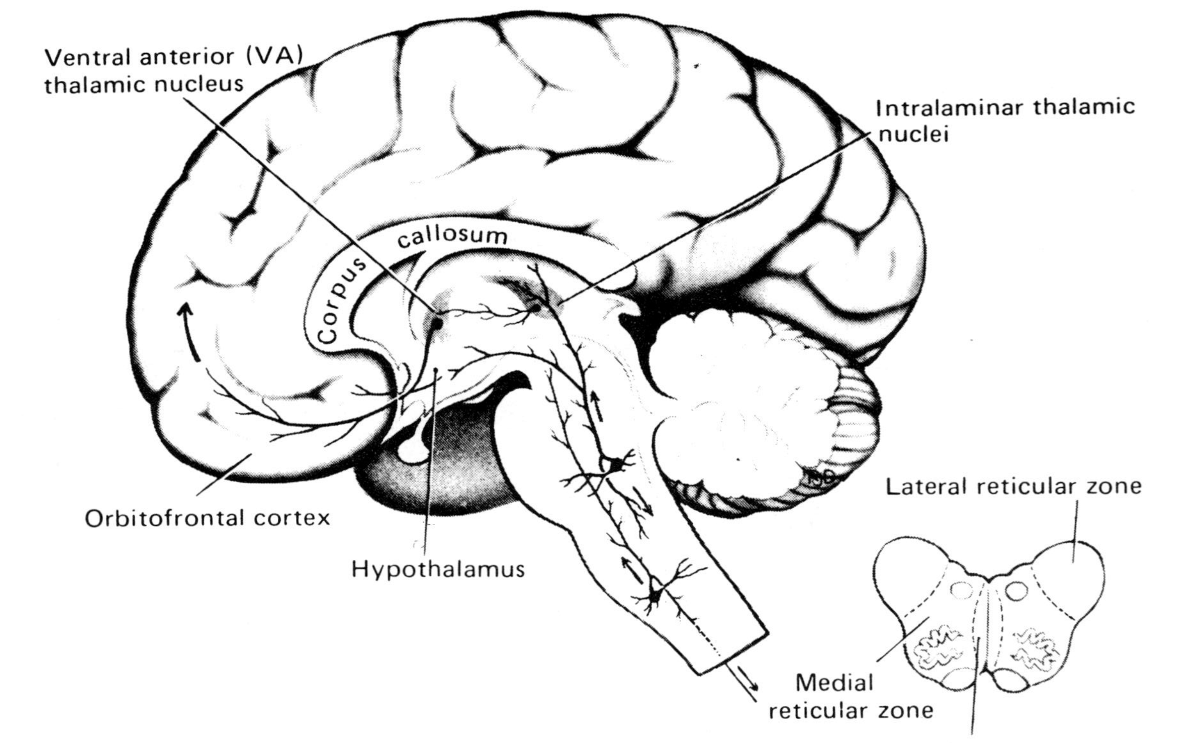

Figure 2-7. Schematic representation of the ascending projections of the ascending reticular pathway system. In general, the multineuronal, multisynaptic relays of the brain stem reticular formation (located in the tegmentum) extend rostrally into two telencephalic regions: (1) posteriorly into the intralaminar, ventral anterior, and dorsomedial thalamic nuclear complexes, and (2) anteriorly into the subthalamic and hypothalamic complexes. The thalamic component projects, by way of the VA thalamic nucleus, to the orbitofrontal cortex.

The cross section through the brain stem (medulla) illustrates the division of the brain stem reticular formation into a midline raphe or paramedian zone, a medial reticular or "motor" zone, and a lateral reticular or "sensory" zone. (From The Nervous System: Introduction and Review, by CR Noback, RJ Demarest. Copyright © 1972. Used with permission of McGraw-Hill Book Company.)

demonstrate that even evaluation of what at first seems to be a relatively simple, well-defined problem (Does angiotensin play a physiological role in drinking behavior?) is, in fact, quite a complex and difficult question to answer.

Similar approaches have been taken to study the role of dopamine, norepinephrine, serotonin, acetylcholine, γ-aminobutyric acid (GABA), and other neurotransmitters in a myriad of behaviors. In conducting such studies it is important to remember that not only are neurochemical changes able to produce behavioral alterations, but that behavioral changes (*e.g.*, stress, hyperactivity) can also result in neurochemical changes.

Neurophysiology of Behavior

The neurophysiology of behavior covers a wide scope of research areas ranging from studies of invertebrate behavior and its electrophysiological basis (pioneered by Kandel) to assessment of the behavioral effects of electrical stimulation of specific brain loci in animals and humans.

One area of intense study has been the reticular activating system (RAS), an ill-defined anatomical collection of heterogenous cell types enmeshed in a complex fiber network in the central portion of the brain stem (Fig. 2-7). The reticular formation includes part of the medulla, pons, and midbrain, and comprises the caudal segment of the RAS while the diencephalon comprises the rostral portion. Electrical stimulation of parts of the RAS produce, in animals, EEG patterns that are similar to those observed during arousal. The behavioral signs of increased alertness were observed to occur concomitant with these electrophysiologic changes. The neuroanatomical connections of the RAS are extremely complex—it appears to receive afferents from all the sensory pathways and projects to a diverse number of areas, including the cerebral cortex. The RAS is said to modulate a bewildering number of behavioral and physiologic processes, including attention, memory, sensory habituation, and sleep. Most of these conclusions have been drawn using the relatively crude electrolytic lesion and electrical stimulation techniques available in the 1950s and 1960s. Use of newly developed research tools with greater specificity and resolution will almost certainly provide more detailed mechanistic information on the role of specific anatomically defined homogenous subpopulations of neurons in the RAS in specific behaviors. Similar studies, which grew out of the work of Papez (Fig. 2-8), have been conducted to elucidate the function of the limbic system, a group of structures that are anatomically and functionally interrelated (*e.g.*, amygdala, hippocampus, cingulate gyrus, and septum). These ill-defined heuristic concepts of structure–function relations were helpful in organizing the available data concerning the brain circuits that modulate fear, rage, and aggression.

Research advances have now allowed for what was once considered impossible—single-unit, intracellular recordings of CNS neurons in the conscious unrestrained cat. The increased resolution of modern electrophysiological, neuroanatomical, and neurochemical techniques, when applied to studies correlating brain structure and behavior, will undoubtedly result in a better understanding of brain–behavior relations.

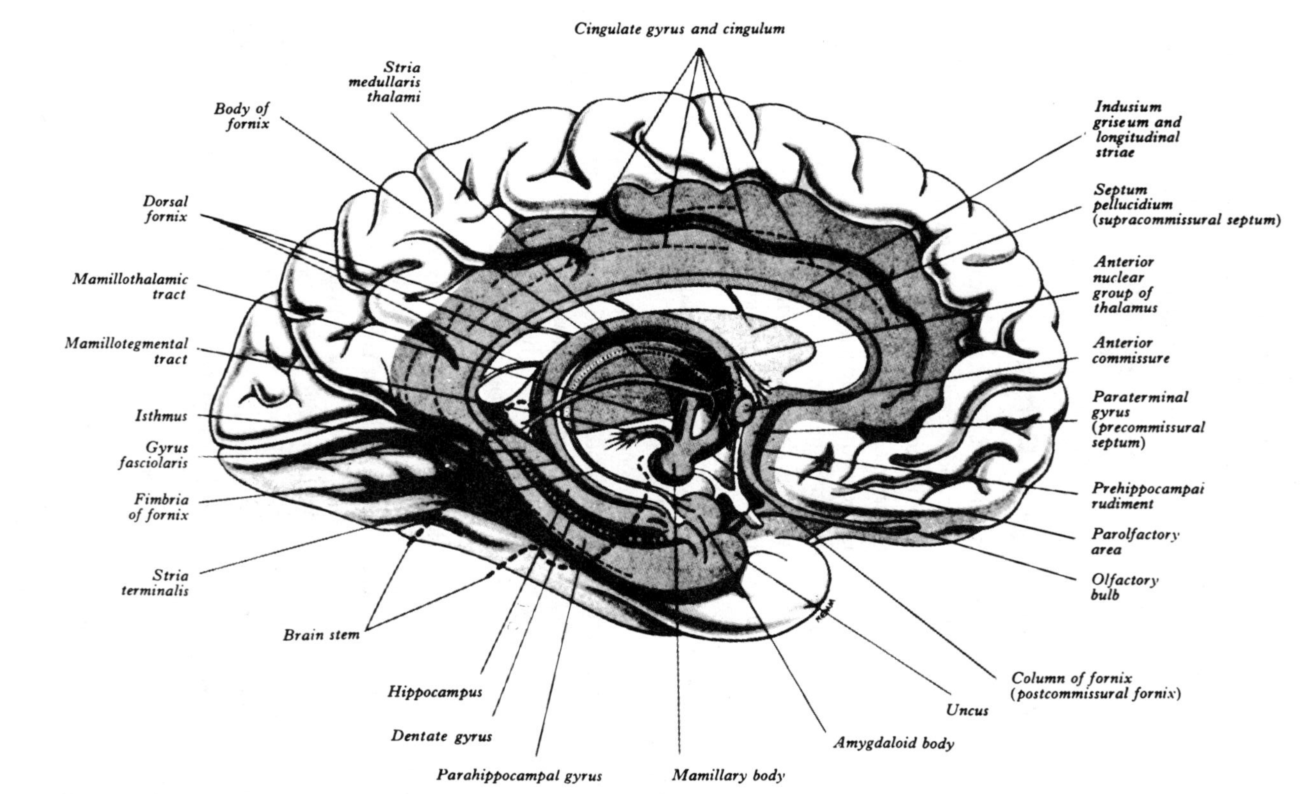

Figure 2-8. The limbic system. A diagram of a dissection of the medial aspects of a cerebral hemisphere to demonstrate the majority of the structures included under the term *limbic system.* The anterior nuclear group of the dorsal thalamus is included with the limbic system. The approximate position of the brain stem that was removed in the course of dissection is outlined in a heavy dashed line. (From Warwick R, Williams PL (eds): Gray's Anatomy, 35th ed. New York, Longman Group, 1973. With permission.)

Biological Markers

If the major psychiatric disorders are, in fact, biologically based, and evidence from several disciplines (genetics, neurophysiology, psychopharmacology) is concordant with this hypothesis, there should be alterations in biological systems that can be measured in these patients. Such biological abnormalities may either be associated with the fundamental pathophysiologic alteration of the disease or epiphenomenonologically associated with it. In the latter case, the physiologic abnormality might, for example, be due to altered expression of a sequence of DNA in close proximity to the sequence associated with the primary defect. In major depression, several biological markers have been identified, including (1) hyperactivity of the hypothalamic–pituitary–adrenal axis as, for example, evidenced by lack of suppression of serum cortisol after administration of the synthetic glucocorticoid, dexamethasone (See Carroll for a comprehensive review of the dexamethasone suppression test [DST]); (2) a blunted thyrotropin (TSH) response to exogenous administration of thyrotropin-releasing hormone (TRH) (See Loosen and Prange for a thorough review of this area); (3) reduced binding of radiolabeled imipramine to platelets; (4) decreased onset of REM sleep (*i.e.*, REM latency); and (5) reduced content of somatostatin (SRIF) in cerebrospinal fluid. Many of these findings are discussed by Baldessarini (1983). Others have reported reduced secretion of growth hormone in response to provocative stimuli and altered concentrations of urinary or CSF monoamine metabolites (*e.g.*, 3-methoxy-4-hydroxyphenolglycol [MHPG]) in depression.

The reproducibility of these findings and their usefulness as adjuncts in the diagnosis of affective disorders depend on their sensitivity and specificity, and these issues are still being debated. Similarly, it is unclear whether these represent *state* or *trait* markers, that is, markers of the state of being depressed vs the trait of being genetically predisposed to the disease. The DST has been the most closely scrutinized and appears to be a state marker.

Biological markers in schizophrenia, unlike in the affective disorders, have not been as easily identified. A few studies have reported reduced platelet monamine oxidase (MAO) activity in schizophrenics, though this has not been confirmed by others. A variety of other putative biological markers have been reported in schizophrenics, but the majority were found to be artifactual, such as the "pink spot" in urine. The findings of abnormalities in smooth eye pursuit in schizophrenics have been repeatedly confirmed.[11] In a recent study, the cerebrospinal fluid concentration of a neuropeptide neurostransmitter candidate, neurotensin, was found to be reduced in drug-free schizophrenics.[12] There is no doubt that one of the major problems associated with the discovery of biological abnormalities in schizophrenia, as compared to affective disorders, is the heterogeneous mixture of patients who are diagnosed as schizophrenic. One of the most salient, but difficult to interpret, findings in schizophrenia is the large range and variance around the mean observed in this mental disorder when compared to normal controls or other psychiatric disorders. This was observed in early studies and more recent ones.[13] This may reflect the diagnostic heterogeneity of schizophrenia or a fundamental disturbance of homeostatic mechanisms in this disease.

Conclusion

In a letter to his friend and colleague Wilhelm Fliess, Freud wrote, In 1898, after all his attempts at integrating his descriptions of mental phenomena with CNS function,

> I have no desire at all to leave the psychology hanging in the air with no organic basis. But beyond the feeling of conviction (that there must be such a basis), I have nothing, either theoretical or therapeutic, to work on, and so I must behave as if confronted by just psychological factors only.[14]

This chapter was introduced with a quote from Freud and it concludes with another. Both quotes document his conviction that behavioral phenomena shall ultimately be described in neurophysiological and neurochemical terms. It is indeed ironic that this view is endorsed by the founder of the school of thought (psychoanalysis) that is often considered the antithesis of biological psychiatry. There is no doubt that the goal alluded to in Freud's letter to Fliess is now being realized.

References

1. Freud S: Three contributions to the theory of sex (1905). In Brill AA (ed): The Basic Writings of Sigmund Freud. New York, The Modern Library, 1938
2. Bleuler M: The development of psychoendocrinology. In Beaumont PJV, Burrows GD (eds): Handbook of Psychiatry and Endocrinology. Amsterdam, Elsevier Biomedical Press, 1982
3. Baldessarini RJ: Biomedical Aspects of Depression and Its Treatment. Washington, DC, American Psychiatric Press, 1983
4. Rosenthal D: Genetic Transmission in Schizophrenia. In Matthysse S (ed): Psychiatry and the Biology of the Human Brain. New York, Elsevier/North Holland Press, 1981
5. Nicol SE, Gottesman II: Clues to the genetics and neurobiology of schizophrenia. Am Scientist 7:398, 1983
6. Barchas JD, Akil H, Eliot GR, et al: Behavioral neurochemistry: Neuroregulators and behavioral states. Science 200:964, 1978
7. Baldessarini RJ: Does biological research lead to clinical progress or does clinical progress lead to biological research? A psychopharmacologist's perspective. In Matthysse S (ed): Psychiatry and the Biology of the Human Brain. New York, Elsevier/North Holland Press, 1981
8. Lipton MA, Nemeroff CB: An overview of the biogenic amine hypothesis of schizophrenia. In Fann WE, Karacan I, Pokorny AD, et al (eds): Phenomenology and Treatment of Schizophrenia. New York, Spectrum Publications, 1978
9. Hartman EL: Sleep. In Kaplan HI, Freedman AJ, Sadock BJ (eds): Comprehensive Textbook of Psychiatry II, 3rd ed. Baltimore, Williams & Wilkins, 1980
10. Epstein AN, Fitzsimons JT, Simons BJ: J Physiol (Lond) 196:98–104, 1968
11. Holtzman PS, Proctor LW, Hughes DW: Eye-tracking patterns in schizophrenia. Science 181:179, 1973
12. Widerlöv E, Lindström LB, Besev G, et al: Subnormal CSF levels of neurotensin in a subgroup of schizophrenic patients: Normalization after neuroleptic treatment. Am J Psychiatry 139:1122, 1982

13. Linnoila M, Ninan PT, Schainin M, et al: Reliability of norepinephrine and major monoamine metabolite measurements in CSF of schizophrenic patients. Arch Gen Psychiatry 40:1290, 1983
14. Meissner WS: Theories of personality and psychopathology: Classical psychoanalysis. In Kaplin HI, Freedman AM, Saddock BJ (eds): Comprehensive Textbook of Psychiatry II, p 632. Baltimore, Williams & Wilkins, 1980

Bibliography

Carroll BJ: Neuroendocrine diagnosis of depression: Dexamethasone suppression test. In Clayton PJ, Barrett JE (eds): Treatment of Depression: Old Controversies and New Approaches. New York, Raven Press, 1983

Copper JR, Bloom FE, Roth RH: The Biochemical Basis of Neuropharmacology, 4th ed. New York, Oxford University Press, 1983

Dunn AJ: Neurochemistry of learning and memory: An evaluation of recent data. Ann Rev Psychol 32:343, 1980

Hartman EL: Sleep. In Kaplan HI, Freedman AJ, Sadock BJ (eds): Comprehensive Textbook of Psychiatry III, 3rd ed. Baltimore, Williams & Wilkins, 1980

Loosen PT, Prange AJ Jr: Serum thyrotropin response to thyrotropin-releasing hormone in psychiatric patients: A review. Am J Psychiatry 139:405, 1982

Michael G. Storck

3 Theories of Personality and Psychopathology

The basic unit in psychiatry is the individual human. Psychologically, people are similar in some ways and different in others. How are the patterns, tendencies, styles, and reactions of humans derived? What determines and maintains these differences and similarities? The elucidation of personality has demanded career-long efforts on the part of many thinkers in this century. This chapter will focus on the modern notions of the psychological organization of the person.

Conceptual Models of Personality

Personality theory had its formal beginning with the classical Greeks, who described character types and proposed explanatory models for understanding their differences. Hippocrates theorized that there are four major personality types, based on humoral theory: sanguine, melancholic, phlegmatic, and choleric. The roots of the term *personality* may be in the Greek word *persona*, denoting a theatrical mask; or in such Latin constructs as *peri soma* (around the body) or *per se una* (self-containing). A medical dictionary adds requirements of internal organization and individuality in defining personality as being the unique self; the organized system of behavioral predispositions and attributes by which one impresses and forms relationships with others. Other features of personality listed in definitions include a self-concept, dynamic organization, reactiveness, capacity for development, and dependence on biological and cultural factors.

Theories of personality are formed by the use of two processes, observation and conceptualization. Observation of personality includes looking out and looking in (extraspection and introspection). The observation of others (extraspection) has been a human activity since the beginning of groups. Controlled experimental observation has been pursued only in the last hundred years. Introspection (observing oneself) is also a major tool in personality theory formation and verification.

Observations are woven together with hypotheses to form theories. Hypotheses are derived by using intuition (the tacit and inarticulate sensing of significant connections) and reasoning (the dialectic process of forming inferences). Some of the theories are more grounded in one activity (observation, intuition, or reasoning) than another.

Salvatore Maddi (1933–), a contemporary scholar of comparative theories of personality, proposes three major types of conceptual models in personality theory: the *conflict model,* in which the central force in personality formation is the struggle within the individual between two opposing systems of demand; the *fulfillment model,* in which the individual is steered by one unified system of directives; and the *consistency model,* in which the core features of a person are arrived at by consistent internal balancing of either physiologic, behavioral, cognitive, or learning patterns. These models will be referred to as we evaluate the specific theories of personality.

Freudian Theory

The lifetime of Sigmund Freud (1856–1939) spanned a period of tremendous progression of ideas in the field of psychiatry. Freud's influence was formative in this evolution. In 1886, only several years out of medical school, Freud journeyed from Vienna to Paris to study neuropathology under the great neurologist Charcot. Charcot and his pupil Janet were studying hysteria, a neurologic disorder for which no neuropathologic lesion could be found. Janet explained hysteria (a sudden impairment of function) as being caused by an hereditary deficiency of the nervous energy that is necessary for maintaining personality. Within several years of returning to Vienna, Freud proposed that mental forces acting within the individual are responsible for hysterical symptoms. He conceived hysteria to be a defense against unconscious sexual or aggressive conflicts, and thus the psyche was seen as a dynamic entity.

Freud's first full theory of the nature of the psyche was the topographic model formulated in the first years of this century. The psyche was conceived as having three zones: the *conscious,* which contains cognitions (thoughts, memories, and feelings) and is present in awareness; the *preconscious,* which contains cognitions that can readily be brought into awareness; and the *unconscious,* which contains cognitions kept from awareness by mental forces or defenses.

Freud conceived the individual as being governed by three principles; *psychic determinism,* which holds that no mental events are random and that causal connections exist between all mental events; the *consistency principle,* which argues that an organism tries to conserve psychic energy and maintain equilibrium; and the *instinct principle,* in which innate life-threatening (aggressive) and life-preserving forces (appetitive and sexual) drives motivate actions of the individual. In the topographic model, an unacceptable drive could be defended against in the individual by, for example, repression (banishing the content of the drive from consciousness to the unconscious or to dream states).

The structural model proposed several years later by Freud moved metaphorically from a psychical map to a psychical apparatus model. This is the model principally held to today by Freudians. The apparatus is composed of id, ego, and superego. The id is a completely unconscious and unorganized constellation of drives grounded in the basic biological requirements of self-gratification and preservation. It blindly seeks discharge on the basis of its ever satisfaction-seeking "pleasure principle." Freud also posited that the id can be driven by destructive or aggressive instincts. The energy of these drives Freud termed *libido.*

The ego is the part of the apparatus that is charged with perceiving reality and organizing the organism's adaptation to it. This task is accomplished through the use of such conscious and unconscious functions as motor control, language, perception, memory, thinking, and defense mechanisms. Defense mechanisms are the mental processes by which an individual protects itself from threatening impulses and cognitions. They will be discussed more completely in Chapter 4.

The superego is charged with directing the ego. It is viewed as an offshoot of the ego that arises from identification with, and incorporation of the attitudes of, parents and society. Serving as judge, the superego is the source of conscience. It includes both unconscious and conscious elements.

The psychic apparatus is conceived as evolving from birth when only id is present. Superego develops as the individual faces the constraints placed on selfish instinctual–biological drives. Herein lies a central feature of Freud's view of the human as caught between the demands of the instincts and society.

Ego development proceeds through five psychosexual stages: oral, anal, phallic, latent, and genital (see Chapter 14). Full adult psychosexual function (termed *genital maturity*) depends on resolution of the pregenital and genital conflicts, culminating in the ability to love and work.

Neuroses result when the ego cannot successfully resolve a conflict between libidinal drives and superego demands. Anxiety, a hallmark of neurosis, and maladaptive defense mechanisms persist. Character disorders result when primitive patterns remain fixed and produce relatively little anxiety. Character disorder types include oral, anal, and phallic fixations. For example, a man who is consistently and disruptively angry could be understood, using Freud's model, as having a mixture of oral and phallic traits, which are manifested by his projection of blame onto others, identification with aggressors, and reaction formation (anger in response to the threat of feeling trust or intimacy). These traits would serve to defend him from the more massive threat of feelings of inferiority and exclusion.

In the Freudian system, treatment of disorders necessitates the establishment of an environment whereby an individual can rework his developmental deviations. The primary model of therapy is psychoanalysis, a lengthy one-to-one process using free association of thoughts, dream interpretations, and understanding of the therapist–patient relationship. Psychoanalysis brings a clarified sense of meaning and an understanding of oneself.

Freudian psychoanalytic understandings of the human use all three methods of study referred to in the introduction: observation, intuition, and reasoning. Freud's elaborately detailed case studies demonstrate unsurpassed observational techniques, but he has been faulted for relying too heavily on patient contact for his theories. The psychoanalytic method, though, relies heavily on introspection by both the patient and therapist. In summary, Freud's pioneering study methods provided new access to the nuances of behavior and cognition, and brought the psyche more into the scope of science.

In Maddi's system of personality theory classification, Freud's psychology is a representative of the psychosocial conflict model. An individual, as protected by his ego, is caught in conflict between the appetites of the instinctual drives and the demands of society. While total mastery of the conflicts is not possible, the healthy personality is able to sustain a dynamic equilibrium.

Early Dissenters to Freudian Theory

The pioneering exploration of the human psyche by Freud and his followers in the Vienna Psychoanalytic Society has served as the point of reference for nearly every other theory of personality posed in this century. Significant dissention first arose within the Freudian school in the early 1900s. Jung, Adler, and Rank were three major theorists who broke off from Freud's inner circle before 1925. Their central shared objection was to Freud's overly mechanistic and biological view of the human and psychological conflict.

Jung

Perhaps the most notable dissident was Carl Jung (1875–1961), who at one point had been considered Freud's successor. Jung's theory held to some of the central concepts of Freud's, such as his acceptance of the unconscious, the importance of dreams, and the relationship between biological and mental events. On the specifics of libido, though, Jung parted ways, hypothesizing it to be a generalized life energy rather than primarily sexual or aggressive. He also considered the unconscious to have two parts, a personal and a collective aspect. The personal unconscious, similar to the Freudian concept, is the gathering place of forgotten or avoided cognitions. The collective unconscious is the deeper layer of the psyche that holds the universal experiences and wisdom of humanity that have been passed down through the ages. Jung labeled these inherited symbolic modes of unconscious thought *archetypes*. They are symbols through which we grasp and transmit our heritage. Dreams, myths, and artistic creations are examples of the processes whereby archetypes become manifest in consciousness.

A central goal for the individual in Jungian theory is the attainment of selfhood, which comes from exploring the depths in one's psyche. This process evolves by understanding one's shadow, anima–animus, and persona. The shadow acting in a person's life represents the basic (primitive) urges that humans have in the trials of life. Anima–animus represents the archetypes of bisexuality within each person. The persona is derived from the Greek term for *mask* and refers to the social face that a human presents to the world. Jungian psychotherapy brings to awareness the archetypes, forces, and relationships at work in the individual's life. The goal is self-awareness.

Despite the spiritualistic and almost archaeologic concepts in Jung's theory, he presents a clear formulation of personality typology based on polarities that exist within each person. He postulated six functions within the personality: introversion and extraversion (which are polar opposites), thinking, feeling, sensing, and intuiting. These six functions are in a flux in each person's life. Each individual will have dominant modes involving primarily two or three functions. Pathology exists when the patterns of functioning are rigid.

In Maddi's system, Jung presents an intrapsychic conflict model of personality, since in that system the directives for an individual come from within. With Jung's fascination and respect for the spiritual dimension and his call for a self-searching approach to life, he also embraces some of the attributes of the fulfillment theories of personality discussed later in this chapter.

Adler

Alfred Adler (1870–1937) turned against Freud's heavy emphasis on infantile sexuality and its derivative conflicts. Adler considered the individual to be purposive and striving for self-realization. He initially proposed that the major force in childhood development derived from the infant's initial state of helplessness and inferiority. The child, trying to master the "inferiority complex," strives for superiority through the use of determination and will. Adler later dropped the emphasis on inferiority and argued that the individual is born with an innate striving for powerfulness.

Striving is modulated in a healthy person by another trait, social interest. Social interest and social usefulness are developed through empathy and identification with significant others. Healthy self-esteem both ensues from and fosters an effective balance between striving for power and social interest. Adler argues that many forms of psychopathology are attempts to protect self-esteem that nonetheless result in impairment of the individual's social usefulness. Passivity, superiority complexes, and bizarre or grand thoughts are examples of socially ineffective ways of protecting self-esteem.

Every individual, according to Adler, develops a unique lifestyle or pattern of adaptation to his or her social matrix. A child's birth order and family constellation are major factors in the resultant lifestyle. Adler's concern with the quality of the home environment for children led to the development of the "child guidance center" concept that became a social institution in America in the middle of this century.

Psychotherapy involves helping a patient mobilize creative and self-analyzing resources so as to be able to study his childhood, family constellation, dreams, attitudes, and goals. The Adlerian therapist is more directly optimistic and encouraging than the others we have discussed.

Adler's theory, in summary, embraces dimensions of both conflict and fulfillment models. He conceives the individual as being placed in a struggle between self and society; however, ultimate guidance is derived from social needs.

Rank

Otto Rank (1884–1939), the third significant rebel from Freud's circle, produced his first book, *The Trauma of Birth,* in 1924. He proposed that childhood conflicts are due to the anxieties of becoming a separate individual rather than to libidinal frustrations. Birth, Rank argued, is the first source of anxiety. Rank believed that man exists between two poles—a striving for union and a striving for separation. In union with others one discovers likeness, self-worth, and assimilation. In separateness, one finds identity and clarity of self-view. The fear of too much union (death fear) is dialectically opposed to the fear of too much separation (life fear). Life is a series of alternations between union and separation, and one passes through four stages in the quest for individuality: family life, society life, artistic life, and spiritual life.

Maddi categorizes Rank as an intrapsychic conflict theorist. Rank argued that a self-directing, organizing force, which he called *will,* resolves intrapsychic conflict by spurring creativity. He maintained that there are three personality types: artistic, average, and neurotic. The ideal personality, the artist, is a person who can creatively forge the tensions between life fear and death fear into growth-oriented relationships with society. The average person can achieve adjustment but without the capacity for growth. The neurotic is unable to master separation or develop an effective will. Rankian psychotherapy emphasizes the uniqueness of the individual. Therapy, a re-creation of the union–separation challenge in life, centers on the patient–therapist relationship and the issues of independence fears and dependence fears. Rank designed his therapy to take a significantly shorter period of time than Freudian psychoanalysis.

Evolution of Freudian Theory

While Jung, Adler, and Rank were founding their own theories of personality, the classical psychoanalytical movement was not stagnating. There were steady amendments to the dogma. Melanie Klein (1882–1960) is noted for reworking the psychodynamic concepts of the first years of life. Psychic processes regarded by Freud as beginning in midchildhood, Klein perceived as occurring in infancy. The rudiments of conscience (superego) develop, Klein argued, as the infant experiences the effects of its aggression towards its mother. Klein theorized that the infant experiences the mother as either a positive, nurturing object (mother as "good breast"), or as a negative, withholding bad object (mother as "bad breast"). The infant's destructive drives projected onto mother bolster this split view of mother as good or bad. Integration of these two views should normally be completed by the age of two.

Wilhelm Reich (1889–1957), a later follower of Freud, contributed to the understanding of the function of character. In his view character is armor-like (defensive and protective) for the ego, protecting it from both internal (libidinal) and external (societal) threats. Character remains flexible in healthy persons, but becomes rigidly automatic in neurotic persons.

The work of Franz Alexander (1891–1964) also bears mentioning. Noted for developing and experimentally refining a set of lasting hypotheses relating specific personality mechanisms to specific somatic illnesses, Alexander argued that each of seven psychosomatic disorders (essential hypertension, rheumatoid arthritis, ulcerative colitis, neurodermatitis, bronchial asthma, peptic ulcer, and thyrotoxicosis) is due to the damming-up of a specific emotion. For example, poorly processed aggression could lead to hypertension, and unresolved dependency with guilt could lead to a peptic ulcer. Alexander's hypotheses are significant because they remind us of the grounding of Freudian theory in biological processes.

Cultural, Interpersonal, and Adaptational Theories

Several theorists noted for their elucidation of cultural, interpersonal, and adaptational determinants of personality will be discussed here.

Horney

Karen Horney (1885–1952), trained in the psychoanalytic tradition, came to view the human as growth-oriented. Her theory has been labeled as holistic because of her insistence that individuals and their environments be understood as being mutually influential. She is the first theorist who perceived personality as a balance between intrapsychic and interpersonal forces.

Horney theorized that, with the right balance of challenge and support, the child acquires a real self—a spontaneous, resilient, self-realizing core of strength and source of growth in life. If the early environment lacks warmth, acceptance, or flexibility, the real self cannot mature, and instead settles into a stance of basic anxiety.

Maladaptive solutions to the basic anxiety result in a pseudo-unity of the personality. Horney terms these maladaptive solutions *neurotic*. There are three neurotic subtypes commonly found in our society: the compliant, aggressive, and detached. The compliant subtype is generally self-effacing; the aggressive, expansive; the detached, resigned and withdrawn. The neurotic strives to have needs met but is prevented from this by the very tactics exerted. A vicious cycle often ensues whereby defensive postures provoke reactions in others that only serve to drive the individual further into the alienating stance.

Horney described two other processes used by neurotics, the pride system and the tyranny of the "should." The pride system is a defensive idealization of the self that protects and prevents the individual from realistic self-appraisal. The tyranny of the "should" refers to the power of restrictive unchallenged inner dictates, to which the real self is subservient. Isolation and self-hatred result from the self-defeating efforts of the neurotic as in the following example.

☐ Mrs. A, a 40-year-old housewife, grew up in a home with an alcoholic father and a bitter, overwhelmed mother. As the oldest of three children, Mrs. A feels as though she was never accepted but still heavily depended upon by all in her family. Compliance and self-effacement became her mode in early life, and it extended into her 15-year marriage. Her idealized self-view is "I'm always loving, hardworking, and available to my family." Some of the tyrannical shoulds governing her life are "You must always place others first," "Do not assert your own views or needs," and "Never be angry." Underneath the external shell is a despairing, insecure, indignant self, struggling to pull off a deceit—to present the facade of an effective person. Her efforts serve to alienate those around her or increase their demanding behavior, thus perpetuating the spiral of indignation and self-sacrifice. Mrs. A's complaint personality is caught between a demanding world, her trampled real self, the pride system, and "shoulds" that have developed.

Horney's personality theory presents a blending of conflict and fulfillment approaches. The above example demonstrates the role of conflict in personality formation. Horney's approach in therapy demonstrates the fulfillment orientation. In therapy, an individual is supported and guided to reacquire a more resilient, accepting, and growth-oriented self. The individual's early history is less emphasized than in Freudian therapy. The corrective process requires active engagement between the therapist and the patient's interacting personality matrix. This added dimension hints at the approach conceived by the next theorist we will consider.

Sullivan

Harry Stack Sullivan (1892–1949), noted for his interpersonal theory of personality, viewed the interpersonal situation, not the individual, as the unit of study in personality. In addition to emphasizing the interpersonal situation, Sullivan also proposed a relatively detailed, biologically grounded, model of the individual. Sullivan contended that the individual has two sets of needs, general and zonal. General needs include sleep, rest, breathing, and eating; zonal needs include oral, anal, and phallic desires (reflecting Freud's influence). Needs create tension in the infant, which in turn creates tension in the mother, causing the mother to satisfy the need and bring security to the infant. If the mother does not relieve the tension, she becomes anxious, and the anxiety is transmitted to the infant, resulting in infant anxiety and insecurity.

Sullivan imagined the infant beset with the task of integrating several parts of the self. The parts are: *good me*—the self that gathers around the experience of satisfaction of tensions; *bad me*—the self caused by anxieties; and *not me*—the self derived from extreme anxiety. As the child matures, these separate personifications must be integrated into one self system for the purpose of mastering anxiety.

Sullivan conceptualized the self system as a dynamism—a unique, consistent, and enduring pattern of behavior. Sullivan's notion of the self-dynamism (with patterns of tendencies, attitudes, and defenses) is fundamental to his definition of personality, which, simply stated, is "the relatively enduring pattern of recurrent situations which characterize a human life."[1] Sullivan's view of the structure of personality differs sharply from Freud's. Freud's model is based on the structural concept (id, ego, and superego), whereas Sullivan's is based on patterns and situations.

According to Sullivan, the maturation of personality takes 15 to 20 years. Needs, tasks, perceptions, and defenses evolve from birth to maturity. Individuals manage anxiety by using a wide range of patterns. A partial list of these patterns (or dynamisms) includes emotion (direct expression of feelings), dissociation (separating specific feelings or ideas from the rest of one's cognitions), hypochondriasis (exaggerated concern about one's health), obsession (persistent preoccupation), the paranoid condition (protective delusions), and sublimation (productive muting and rechanneling of impulses). Sullivan called these patterns or dynamisms *security operations,* that is, they secure the individual from anxiety. The healthy adult may use any one or many of these dynamisms when threatened. Dependence on primarily one dynamism, however, signifies rigidity, poor mastery of anxiety, and evidence of psychopathology.

In contrast to other personality theorists, Sullivan studied schizophrenic patients extensively. He maintained that schizophrenia results from early arrest in psychosocial development and that schizophrenics demonstrate a dissociative dynamism, or autistic withdrawal. This dynamism is a rigid transformation of personality that protects the individual from anxiety. Autistic withdrawal serves as an interpersonal strategy against the threat of becoming close to others and the threats that would ensue from more fully experiencing the early deficits and conflicts over needs, wants, and limitations.

In therapy, Sullivan viewed himself as a participant–observer, an active factor in his patient's therapy and in his patient's life. Sullivan argued for thorough history-taking and encouraged vigilence for signs, in the interpersonal process, of anxiety or security operations. The goal of Sullivanian therapy is a rediscovering and reworking of the self system to enable the patient to leave behind the rigidifying parts of the *not me* and the *bad me* that had persisted.

Sullivan introduces consistency (or homeostasis-seeking) dimensions to personality theory while emphasizing self-directiveness and basic conflict in life; thus his theory does not fit neatly into any one of our three general conceptual models. Like Sullivan, the next two theorists, Rado and Hine, emphasize adaptational dimensions of personality functioning; thus their theories do not fall neatly into one of Maddi's conceptual models.

Rado

Sandor Rado (1890–1972) labeled his personality formulation *adaptational psychodynamics*. Grounded in classical psychoanalytic training, Rado set out to posit a more medically useful, biological adaptational model of the psyche. He maintained that there are four levels of the psyche:

1. Hedonic, self regulation, geared around pain and pleasure
2. Preverbal brute emotion, which includes emergency emotions, such as fear and rage; and welfare emotions, such as affiliation, satisfaction, and joy

3. Emotional thought
4. Unemotional thought, or reason

Each of these levels corresponds to a separate dimension of human adaptation. The part of the psyche charged with integrating these levels into a self-aware, intentionally acting whole is called the *action self.* The action self has been compared to the ego in Freudian psychology.

Rado maintained that psychologically healthy people are those who effectively perform their biological and psychosocial functions. They have a relative predominance of welfare emotions—affiliation, satisfaction, and joy. The overuse of emergency emotion, especially fear, indicates maladaptation. The goal of therapy follows directly: Enhance the role of the welfare emotions and decrease the influence of emergency emotions. Rado emphasized the role of therapists as educators.

Hine

The work of Frederick Hine (1925–   ) expands Rado's view of unrealistic fear as central to psychopathology. Hine, adapting Leary's formulation of interpersonal theory, posits that there are four basic directions of personality function: dominance and independence; submission and dependence; trust and affiliation; and aggression and disaffiliation. This concept can be schematically represented on perpendicular axes, as in Figure 3-1. Each direction has a healthy and an unhealthy range. For example, healthy submission might include appropriately allowing oneself to be cared for, unhealthy submissiveness would include inflexible, inappropriate passivity and helplessness. Fighting for one's civil rights can be an example of

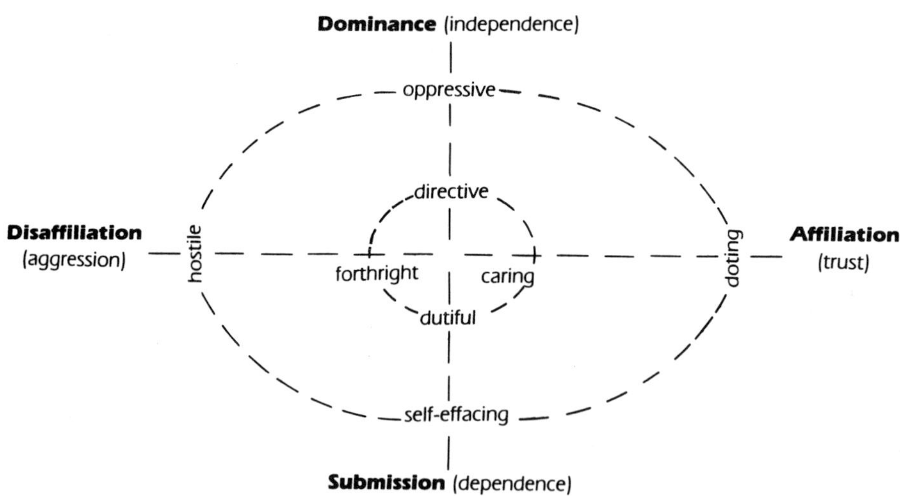

Figure 3-1. Basic directions of personality functioning. The terms in parentheses indicate functions to manage. The inner circle represents healthy functioning and the outer circle represents unhealthy, fear-based functioning. (Adapted from Hine FR: Introduction to Psychodynamics: A Conflict–Adaptational Approach, Durham, Duke University Press, 1971; and Leary T: Interpersonal Diagnosis of Personality, New York, Ronald Press, 1957)

healthy aggression, whereas violating another's trust would exemplify unhealthy disaffiliation.

Personality disturbances, according to Hine, consistently involve the inhibition of one or more of the four behavior functions by exaggerated, unrealistic fears. Personalities differ on the basis of variations in the prevailing fear patterns as observed in the person's assumptions about himself and others and in his resulting interpersonal behavior. Individuals may be influenced by any combination of conflicts: submission–fear, independence–fear, affiliation– or trust–fear, or aggression–fear. Because the fear behavior is inhibited, contrasting opposite behaviors are typically exaggerated; this defense called *reaction formation*. Mrs. A, presented earlier, may be understood as having deep fear of being appropriately aggressive or independent; thus she compensates by being doting and self-effacing. A submission–fear conflicted individual (perhaps someone who grew up in a violent, unloving home) might be repetitively angry and seek to dominate others for fear of being brutalized or abandoned again if he were to get close to someone. The trust–fear conflicted person will be compromised in the ability to form close, interpersonal relationships, and will tend to express disaffiliative behavior such as hostility and bitterness, or shy withdrawal. Hine agrees with Horney in emphasizing that these fear patterns tend to be cyclically maintained and often spirally worsened because of the impact they have on others. The more the above individual is defensively hostile, the more he drives people away, and, in turn, becomes more isolated and more convinced that his fears of getting close to others are justified.

Object-Relations and Ego Theories

Two related extensions of classical psychoanalytic theory are object-relations theory and ego psychology. Ego theories emphasize the central role of the ego (in contrast with id and superego) in personality functioning. The ego is conceptualized as more efficacious than in Freudian theory. Object-relations theory is the psychoanalytic formulation of the process of the development and internalization of interpersonal relations. It posits that the evolving psychological challenges of the infant and child are best understood as centering around the negotiation of interpersonality. Again, drives and instincts are deemphasized.

Three branches of personality theory include the varied ideas of many contributors over the last fifty years. Early theorists include Hartman, Fairbairn, and Winnicott.

Heinz Hartman (1884–1970) proposed that instead of the ego evolving from the id, as Freud hypothesized, the ego arises from a common matrix with the id. The ego is thus autonomous.

Ronald Fairbairn (1889–1964) further theorized that instead of just being a referee between id and superego demands, the ego directs the other components of the psyche. The healthy person is thus not just a constellation of defenses but is fundamentally self-seeking and other-seeking (or object-seeking).

Donald Winnicott (1897–1971), a pediatrician influenced by Melanie Klein, emphasized the importance of the early interactions between mother and child in ego development. The child's successful transition from total dependence to em-

Table 3-1
Erikson's Formulation of Epigenetic Ego Development*

Chronological Stage	Psychosexual Stage	Psychosocial Conflict	Mastered Ego Functions
1. Birth to 1 year	Oral–sensory	Basic trust vs. mistrust	Drive and hope
2. 1–3 years	Muscular–anal	Autonomy vs. shame and doubt	Self-control and willpower
3. 3–5 years	Locomotor–genital	Initiative vs. guilt	Direction and purpose
4. 5–11 years	Latency	Industry vs. inferiority	Method and competence
5. 12–21 years	Puberty and adolescence	Identity vs. role confusion	Devotion and fidelity
6. 21–40 years	Young adulthood	Intimacy vs. isolation	Affiliation and love
7. 40–60 years	Adulthood	Generativity vs. stagnation	Production and care
8. 60 years and older	Maturity	Ego integrity vs. despair	Renunciation and wisdom

* Erikson intends for his staging of ego development to serve as a general (not strict) guide.
(Adapted from Erikson EG: Childhood and Society, 2nd ed, p 273–274. New York, WW Norton, 1963.)

erging independence is contingent on what he called "good enough mothering," which consists of consistent and empathic involvement by the mother. He also developed the concept of *transitional object,* which ties together central facets of object-relations theory. The child negotiates separation and differentiation from the mother by transferring feelings of security from mother onto special belongings (transitional objects). The image of a forlorn child clutching a tattered blanket to its cheek provides an example. The blanket serves as a representation (and thus a transitional source) of safety, security, and warmth. Relying on this symbol when the real mother is not available is a step toward acquiring the object-relationships of an independent self.

Current ego and object-relations personality theories are provided by the works of Kernberg, Erikson, Kohut, and Berne.

Kernberg

Otto Kernberg (1928–) is noted for his theories on the defense processes and disordered object relationships that form in response to early psychosocial deprivation. He maintains that an infant growing up in a psychologically unsafe environment develops initially helpful but ultimately maladaptive defenses in an effort to stabilize its internal world. The child, for example, of ambivalent and hostile parents, according to Kernberg, may unconsciously strive to keep separate the good and bad inner images of the parents. This defense mechanism, known as *splitting,* fosters the child's illusion of inner security and interpersonal constancy. The needed "good parent" is thus preserved.

Splitting may be used by many children temporarily in early ego development, as Melanie Klein argued. If the psychosocial environment, though, does not support the acquisition of more realistic views of self and others, the individual will be unable to resolve the inevitable challenges in negotiating adult object-relationships. Stable self-esteem and full interpersonal relationships are contingent on being able to weave together positive and negative perspectives of oneself and others. Adults who continue to use defenses like splitting are often impulsive, frightened of intimacy and isolation, and have low self-esteem. Kernberg considers these individuals as having primitive or borderline personality organizations (see Chapter 11), and he uses intensive, long-term, psychoanalytically oriented psychotherapy in their treatment.

Erikson

Erik Erikson (1901–) considers the ego as forming throughout the whole life of the individual by eight psychosocial conflicts that must be mastered for optimal development. In his model, id and ego evolve contemporaneously. In each successive stage of development, the individual is faced with a conflict and the challenge to master another ego function (Table 3-1). Erikson's formulation that ego development continues throughout the lifespan is revolutionary.

Erikson is also credited with another addition to personality theory, his concept of identity. Identity is a multidimensional concept that involves a conscious sense of selfhood and uniqueness, an unconscious striving for continuity in life, and a grounding in the ideals of the group of which one is a part. Identity emerges with mastery of the psychosocial challenges of adolescence and early adulthood.

Kohut

Heinz Kohut (1913–1982) argued that drives are not as central as experiences in personality development. Kohut believed that the child uses two processes in developing a stable personality (or sense of self); mirroring and idealization. Mirroring is the process whereby the child, usually through the mother, experiences admiration and approval. The mother reflects back to the child the good feelings she has for him. This process is necessary for the child's later capacity to sustain healthy ambitions such as a career, family, and self-expression. Idealization is the process whereby the child, usually through the father, admires and identifies with the power of the parent. This is necessary for the later sustenance of goals and ideals.

Narcissistic personality disturbances are primary pathologies of the self that may stem from either inadequate or excessive parental involvement in the mirroring and idealizing processes. Behaviorally, individuals with narcissistic problems may appear as approval-hungry or as ideal-hungry. Their neediness may drive others away. The chief task in therapy is reworking of the mirror and idealization needs. It is a process that depends heavily on the therapist–patient relationship.

Berne

Transactional analysis is the theory rooted in ego psychology, and was developed by Eric Berne (1910–1970) in the 1950s and 1960s. Berne's popular psychology characterizing interpersonal dynamics is centered around the premise that within each person are three variably active ego states: the child, the adult, and the parent. The child ego state represents feelings, thoughts, and behaviors that are fixed early in childhood and remain active throughout life. The adult ego state is directed toward reason and objective problem-solving. The parent ego consists of feelings, thoughts, and behaviors internalized from the parents' value system. All three states are necessary for full functioning in relationships.

Other key concepts in transactional analysis are transactions, games, basic position, and scripts. When two people communicate, any of the three ego states can predominate. A transaction is a stimulus from one person to another. A complimentary transaction occurs when the initiator's ego state matches the recipient's. A crossed transaction occurs when the ego states do not match. The overt statements in a transaction may appear to be complimentary, but the latent or psychological levels may differ. For example, if a husband says to his wife, "I can't balance this checkbook," and the wife says, "You've never balanced the checkbook," on the social or overt level these may be rational, thus adult-level, communications. However, the husband's latent meaning might be, "Why do I always get this stupid job?" (demonstrating a child ego state), to which his wife is latently answering, parentally, "You should be more responsible in life."

Games occur between two people when the social level and psychological level of communication are consistently at odds. Generally in a game there is a shifting among the participants between one of three positions of what is called the *drama triangle*. The positions are victim, persecutor, and rescuer. If the husband above were to next tell his wife, "I've had it with your silly moralizing," he has moved from being victim to persecutor. If she responds, "Honey, you do work hard, I'm sorry I got on you," she has shifted from persecutor to rescuer.

Life scripts are generally unconscious, pervasive attitudes discerned about oneself early in life. They provide the basis for Berne's typology of personalities. A life script forms the foundation of an individual's basic position in life. The four basic positions in life are: "I'm OK and you're OK"; I'm OK and you're not OK"; I'm not OK but you're OK; and "Neither of us is OK." An individual raised to be able to experience trust and act altruistically demonstrates the basic position, "I'm OK, you're OK." Chronically depressed and suicidal individuals may have internalized from childhood the injunctive script, "Don't exist," with the resulting basic position, "I'm not OK, you're OK."

The process of therapy (often conducted in groups) uses high involvement by the therapist to foster transactions whereby the patient can understand his or her games and scripts. Berne believed strongly in intuition as a method for understanding life. To detect the subtle games and scripts at work in one's life requires heavy use of this faculty. Confrontation, permission to disobey parental injunctions, therapist's stroking, and guided fantasy are some methods used to help the patient unravel the troubled matrix, make new decisions, and redirect and rebuild a healthier self.

The object-relations and ego theories we have discussed are classified by Maddi as conflict models. However, especially in the theories of Berne and Erikson, we see elements that suggest that human life, though grounded in conflict, is a growth or fulfillment process.

Humanistic Theories

The humanistic theorists reject what they consider as biological and psychoanalytic reductionism. Instead, they view the human as autonomous, self-directing, and uniquely creative.

Allport

Gordon Allport (1897–1967), an esteemed American psychologist, maintained that humans direct their lives with functional autonomy. Subjective experiences and motivations are not reducible to biological or historical explanations. The individuality of each person was such a core concept for Allport that he felt that few generalizations about personality would be tenable.

There are several key personality concepts, for Allport, though, that do apply transpersonally. He viewed personality as an open system that tends toward progressive organization and creative involvements in the world. He described two sets of functions in the human, opportunistic and propriate. Opportunistic functions maintain biologic survival. The notion of *proprium,* or propriate functioning, is the central concept of his theory.

The maturing individual evolves proprium (or self-functioning) as he advances into adulthood. Propriate functions include self-identity, self-esteem, self-extension, rational coping, and striving. Allport believed that higher-level propriate functions, such as aspirations, are strong effectors in life. The self is thus pro-active and future oriented. The mature individual, in Allport's view, is emotionally secure and empathetic and has such traits as enthusiasm, insight, a personal conscience, and a unifying philosophy of life.

Maslow

Abraham Maslow (1908–1970), like Allport, is a fulfillment theorist using Maddi's classification. He regarded the human as striving for self-actualization. Man is basically good. While not totally opposed to mechanistic scientific approaches to the human, Maslow felt that such approaches obscured vital aspects of the human, such as morality, consciousness, purpose, and human potential. Maslow considered man as seeking fulfillment of a hierarchy of intrinsic needs as follows. The most basic need is survival, motivated and activated by deficiency. The higher-level needs are growth-motivated, and they are the pursuits that bring meaning to life. The highest need of all is found in the desire for self-transcendence.

Needs may be satisfied hierarchically. For Maslow, satisfaction of physiological needs is a prerequisite for being able to address the next higher level, safety needs. As safety needs are met, other less powerful, though more actualized, needs can be addressed, such as belonging and self-esteem. The human faces choices and conflicts between physiological and growth needs as he moves toward actualization. Other conflicts can arise, for example, between dependence and independence needs, regression and progression, and security and growth. The traits that strengthen an individual's growth process are spontaneity, creativity, humor, independence, problem-centeredness, and self-acceptance. The process is also aided by what Maslow called "peak experiences"—ineffable experiences of heightened understanding, euphoria, and transcendence. Historical examples of those whom Maslow considered to be fully actualized individuals include Lincoln, Beethoven, Thoreau, and Eleanor Roosevelt.

Maslow did not propose any substantial theories of psychopathology, except to acknowledge that there can be hindrances to self actualization. Therapy for those inhibited from the actualizing process involves provision of a supportive environment conducive to trust, reflectiveness, a building of higher functions, and peak experiences.

Phenomenological Theories

Phenomenological theorists believe that behavior is determined by the way the subject perceives reality, and not by objective reality as described in physical terms.

Gestalt Theory

Gestalt psychology originated in Germany and found its most popular expression in the therapy of Frederick Perls (1893–1970). According to Gestalt theory, the organism exists as a unified, interrelated whole, and a relationship between itself and the environment is maintained in a balance. The perceptual experience of the organism is of configurations, not of atomistic sets of parts. The Gestalten (holistic perceptions) are influenced not just by external reality but also by the inner phenomenal state.

Gestalt therapy emphasizes that a person's phenomenal world is organized around needs. The most heavy emphasis in therapy is on the immediate or "here and now" perceptions of the individual. The goal of therapy is to remove the blocks to full perception and awareness of oneself and one's relationships.

Field Theory

Kurt Lewin (1890–1947), influenced by Gestalt concepts, formulated field theory to define personality. He conceptualized that person and environment are parts of the same psychological field. The environment does not necessarily correspond with external reality, but to the psychological milieu as the person interprets it. Behavior is a function of the person and this environment. The emphasis in field theory (in contrast to Gestalt theory) is not on subjective perception but on the interplay of personal and environmental meanings and forces.

Rogers

Carl Rogers (1902–   ) has provided perhaps the most popular nonpsychoanalytic approach to understanding the human. His primary concern is with psychotherapy. He argues strongly for the fulfillment model and is grounded in a phenomenological view of the person. For Rogers, the phenomenal field for the individual is the totality of experience. The self, which develops during childhood, becomes a differentiated and conscious part of the individual's phenomenal field. This subjective experience of efficacy and being is preeminently meaningful according to Rogers, despite whatever reductionistic laws science may say govern the individual.

Rogers, to further the contrast between him and Freud, believes that the person does not necessarily exist in conflict with society. Rogers maintains a devoutly optimistic view of the human. He believes that the central tendency in life is to strive to actualize one's potentials. The basic needs that must be met for a person to be self-actualizing are the need for positive regard and positive self-regard.

If a person receives unconditional positive regard while growing up, he will evolve, without defensiveness, to self-actualization. This individual is said to be congruent with his potentialities and will be flexible, spontaneous, trusting, and freely choosing his course in life. If the regard received in childhood is conditional, the self-concept will be incongruent with the potentialities. Incongruence breeds defensiveness, distortion, anxiety, and interpersonal conflicts.

Rogers insists that therapy provide a safe environment based on genuineness, empathy, and unconditional positive regard by the therapist for the client. This environment slowly facilitates self-acceptance, trust, and feelings of safety for the client, which allows for the gradual attainment of congruence and a self-actualizing direction in life.

Existential Theory

The existential approach to the person is based on several philosophical tenets: (1) self-awareness is the most primary experience in life, (2) human existence is unchosen (birth is not chosen), (3) human nature is not predetermined, and (4) humans must, thus, choose and be responsible for their paths in life.

Human growth, in existential theory, is based on facing the ontological anxiety of being thrown into life as a limited being without a prescribed essence. This demands that which existentialists call authenticity and courage. Authenticity is achieved by fully recognizing that to fulfill one's responsibility to humanity, one must embrace one's freedom and responsibility. This process is demanding and difficult and calls for courage. Inauthenticity occurs when one avoids, through self-deception, one's responsibilities and the demands of freedom.

The goal of therapy is to help a person achieve clarity of self-view and authenticity. The existential therapy approach demands that the therapist strive to experience the view of the client. The therapist, as in the Rogerian framework, must accept the client unconditionally. Progress comes not from therapist interpretation or intervention but in providing an affirming and safe environment for the client to become aware of his existential situation. It is a mutual search for the client's authentic self-view. Karl Jaspers (1883–1969) is a representative existential theorist.

Consistency and Learning Theories

The last group of theories take a more operational look at the human. Not all the perspectives discussed here represent full theories of personality. Their views, though, may help to clarify the complex functioning of the human.

Consistency Models

The consistency theories as classified and described by Maddi consider human functioning as being best understood as a feedback process based on interaction with the environment. Information processing and emotional state modulation are core operations in consistency models. This is in contrast to the humanists' emphasis on inherent attributes and goals and the Freudian theorists' emphasis on an intrapsychic apparatus. In these models, cognitive processes are at the center of personality functioning.

Kelly

In the theory of George Kelly (1905–1967), cognitive processes are used in the never-ending attempt by the individual to predict and control experiences. The intellect actively construes rather than passively receives. Intrapsychic constructs (such as concepts, beliefs, and anticipations) are the elements in Kelly's accuracy-demanding, homeostasis-seeking psychological system. The goal of the system is tension reduction and avoidance of cognitive conflict.

Maddi

Maddi's own model posits that the primary function of personality is to maintain for the organism a consistent and customary level of physiologic and psychological activation. Humans have varying customary activity levels. Some humans are highly active and outwardly directed, whereas others are passive and introspective. Each individual, though, strives (through such operations as anticipation and self-correction) to maintain his own unique homeostasis.

Learning Paradigms

Perhaps the most parsimonious theory of personality is the stimulus-response model, behaviorism. Like Freud's psychoanalytic theory, it arose early in this century, and was influenced by the positivist shifts in the philosophy of science. Behaviorism, in its most radical position (as associated with BF Skinner [1904–]), considers such concepts as consciousness, needs, drives, habits, lifestyle, and even personality to be unnecessary in the understanding of the organism. The organism, instead, according to behaviorism, should be defined by its observable outputs in response to environmental stimuli. The environment, not the organism, is seen as the selective force in behavior, in contrast with the humanist's insistence on self-directedness. Behaviorism is a strictly extraspective approach, as opposed to the phenomenologists' introspective emphasis. It seeks to operationalize a functional understanding of an organisms' output.

Classical and Operant Conditioning

Classical and operant conditioning are two key behavioral constructs. Classical or respondent conditioning—as immortalized by Pavlov's dog, who salivated to the ringing of a bell after the bell had been paired with the presentation of a steak—demonstrates that learning occurs by association. Operant or consequence–governance conditioning—as exemplified by Skinner's rat learning to press the bar to receive food—demonstrates the impact of environment on the shaping of behavior.

Some maladaptations are examples of classical conditioning. For example, a boy who encounters a mean dog in the park on his way home from school may come to experience anxiety in parks even if no dogs are around. Here a previously neutral stimulus come to elicit a fear response on its own. Operant conditioning or solution learning, in EH Mowrer's formulation, is at work when the boy is rewarded (no fear) for finding an alternate route home from school. Mowrer observed that both conditioning modes often occur together in complex functioning.

Dollard and Miller

A moderate formulation of behaviorism that grew from the work of John Dollard (1900–) and Neil Miller (1909–) also seeks to delete subjective concepts from explanations of human behavior. They offer a translation of Freud's intrapsychic terminology into such concepts as drive, cue, response, reinforcement, and habit. They thus disagree with Skinner's complete exorcism of the concept of intrinsic psychological forces acting within the organism.

Humans respond to primary and secondary drives from within, according to Dollard and Miller. Primary drives include hunger, avoidance of pain, and sex. Secondary or learned drives (*e.g.*, fear) are derived from primary drives. Fear is considered a drive because in itself it can motivate and impel. It is considered a secondary (learned) drive because it derives from the primary drive, self-preservation, in association with a threat initially paired with a neutral cue. The new motivation (secondary drive) for the above-mentioned boy on his way home from school is to find a new way home avoiding the parks. More complex examples of the function of the secondary drive, fear, were seen in the elucidation of Hine's theory earlier.

Bandura

The most comprehensive modern statement of the role of behavior and learning in human personality function is provided by social learning theory. Albert Bandura (1925–), a major theorist in this school, posits that psychological functioning is best understood as a reciprocal interaction between behavioral, cognitive, and environmental influences.

Cognitive processes are used in observation, judging, and self-regulation. Bandura notes that much of human learning is accomplished through activities in which responses cannot be observed directly, but where learning can still be inferred from later observation of the individual. Humans learn through vicarious experiences (*e.g.*, television viewing) and modeling. Imitation is a form of learning, with implied cognitive components, not reducible to a stimulus–response model.

As the child develops it learns, with its evolving cognitive capacities, to negotiate a self-regulated status. Norms and values are acquired through parental and societal modeling.

The view of the human as self-evaluative, self-determining, and able to actively construe events and experiences with meaning is central to social learning theory. The social learning theorists strive to ground these previously discounted or vaguely described processes in a scientific and operationally useful explanatory model.

Behavioral, cognitive, and learning processes can obviously be parameters in psychopathology. Phobias (unrealistic and intense fears of an object of a situation), for example, involve maladaptive learning processes and can hold pervasive roles in the lives of individuals. Cognitions can define and sustain disturbed functioning. Behavior therapy for phobias, systematic desensitization, as used by Joseph Wolpe, employs behavioral, cognitive, and learning modalities. An individual is trained from a relaxed state to progressively imagine and then experience increasingly threatening exposures to the phobic situation until fearfulness can be held in check.

From social learning theory we might surmise that personality disturbances can be related to inadequate parental–societal modeling. This is consonant with Kohut's theory explaining narcissistic disorders as resulting from impairment of the mirroring and idealization processes in early childhood. Bandura, further, observed that perceived self-efficacy is a better predictor of an adaptive response to an

Table 3-2
Summary of Theories of Personality and Psychopathology

Theory	Theorist	Central Feature or Goal of Personality Function	Key Concepts
Psychoanalytic Theory	Freud	Resolving psychosocial conflict between instinctual drives and societal demands	Structural model of the psyche The unconscious Five psychosexual stages of development Neurosis as unresolved conflict Defense mechanisms
Analytic Psychology	Jung	Attainment of selfhood and transcendence	Libido as life force Unconscious includes a collective unconscious Archetypes and other connections with history Introversion–extroversion and four functions
Individual Psychology	Adler	Striving towards powerfulness and self-realization	Individual as purposive Motivation by social interest Lifestyle as characteristic mode of function
An intrapsychic conflict model	Rank	Resolution of tension between striving for union and striving for separation	Anxiety as due to conflicts over individuation and dependence Will as a self-directing force
Interpersonal Theory	Sullivan	Building a unified self system capable of interpersonal functioning	Personality is a function of interpersonal relationships Self-dynamism using security operations Good me/bad me/not me Mother–child anxiety cycle
A Psychodynamic–cultural theory	Horney	Management of psychosocial conflicts so as to achieve the enrichment of the "real self"	Real self is oriented toward growth Pride system is a pseudo-unity of self resulting from unresolved anxiety Personality is a balance of intrapsychic and interpersonal forces

(*Continued*)

Table 3-2
Summary of Theories of Personality and Psychopathology (Continued)

Theory	Theorist	Central Feature or Goal of Personality Function	Key Concepts
Adaptation theorists	Rado Hine	Management of biological and psychosocial needs, demands, and conflicts	Rado: action-self integrates a hierarchy of biopsychical levels Health is predominance of welfare emotions Hine: four directions of personality functioning, fear is central to maladaptation
Object-relations theory	Klein (forerunner) Fairbairn Winnicott Kernberg	The development of stable internalized and interpersonal object relationships	Ego as: 1) object- (relationship-) seeking, and 2) independent of id Role of transitional objects Role of persistence of primitive defenses
Ego theorists	Hartman Erikson Kohut	Full autonomous ego and self-development and resolution of psychosocial conflict	Ego as autonomous Erikson: maturation of the ego through the lifespan Kohut: mirroring and idealization as necessary for self-development
Transactional analysis	Berne	Mastery of psychosocial conflicts so as to enhance meaning and satisfaction	Three ego states Transactions and games involve hidden ego states Scripts as fixed internalized messages Drama triangle
Humanistic theorists	Allport Maslow	Self-actualization	Biological needs must be met first. Higher self functions are more important and growth-motivated The human is autonomous and basically good
A phenomenological approach	Rogers	Self-actualization	Optimistic view: man does not need to exist in conflict Congruence vs incongruence Importance of unconditional positive regard in development and therapy

Existential theorists	Jaspers	Achievement of authenticity	Responsibility and freedom must be embraced Avoidance is inauthenticity Therapy involves seeing the world through the experience of the client
Consistency theory	Kelly Maddi	Maintenance of homeostasis and tension reduction	Homeostasis is individualized Kelly: cognition is the most critical function of personality Cognitive constructs enable anticipation
Behaviorism	Skinner Pavlov	No central goal—the organism is viewed as a product of the environment	Rejects dynamic and internal constructs Seeks to operationalize output (behavior) Classical/operant conditioning and their role in more complex learning
Learning theory	Dollard and Miller Bandura Beck	Dollard and Miller: management of drives Bandura and Beck: self efficacy through effective cognitive capacities	Dollard and Miller: learned drives such as fear are major effectors of behavior Reciprocal interaction of behavior, cognition, and environment defines functioning Beck's cognitive therapy: changing distorted cognitions

unfamiliar threat than is past performance, implying that self-concepts (be they positive or negative) are strong effectors of psychological functioning.

Beck

AT Beck (1921–) has further highlighted the importance of cognitive processes in psychiatric disorders. He considers the uncovering and clarification of patients' private meanings, "automatic thoughts" (recurrent distorted cognitions), self-evaluations, and assumptions about danger as central vehicles in psychological assessment. Distorted cognitive representations of self or relationships (along with the accompanying unreasonable fears) can contribute to such stances as chronic depression or chronic isolation. Beck, for example, proposes that a cognitive triad of distortions accompanies chronic depression: (1) negative conceptions of oneself, (2) negative interpretations of experiences, and (3) hopeless view of the future.

Integration

There have been recent efforts to integrate principles of social learning, behavioral, cognitive, and psychoanalytic theory. Paul Wachtel (1940–), a theorist trained in psychoanalytic and learning theory, argues for conceptually weaving together these previously disparately perceived models of psychological functioning. He finds that psychoanalytic and learning paradigm techniques can be complementarily used in psychotherapy.

Conclusion

This chapter has presented a broad range of selective models and approaches to the study of the nature, functioning, and malfunctioning of human personality. Table 3-2 provides a condensed summary of these orientations. The diversity of emphases and perspectives included here affirms the complexity of the human and points to the benefits and necessity of individual theoretical synthesizing.

Reference

1. Sahakian WS (ed): Psychology of Personality: Readings in Theory, p 160. Chicago, Rand McNally, 1965

Bibliography

Allport GW: Personality, a Psychological Interpretation. New York, Hokd, 1937
Arieti SW (ed): American Handbook of Psychiatry, pp 1417–1455. New York, Basic Books, 1959
Bandura A: The self system in reciprocal determinism. Am Psychol 33:344–358, 1978
Beck AT: Cognitive Therapy and the Emotional Disorders. New York, International Universities Press, 1976
Brenner C: An Elementary Textbook of Psychoanalysis. New York, International Universities Press, 1955
Erikson EG: Childhood and Society, 2nd ed. New York, WW Norton & Company, 1963
Hall CS, Lindzey G (eds): Theories of Personality. New York, John Wiley & Sons, 1970

Hine FR: Introduction to Psychodynamics: A Conflict–Adaptational Approach. Durham, Duke University Press, 1971
Horney K: Neurosis and Human Growth: The Struggle Toward Self-Realization. New York, WW Norton & Company, 1950
Kaplan HI, Freedman AM, Saddock BJ (eds): Comprehensive Textbook of Psychiatry, 3rd ed, pp 378–393, 729, 847, 868–894. Baltimore, Williams & Wilkins, 1980
Leary T: Interpersonal Diagnosis of Personality. New York, Ronald Press, 1957
Maddi SR: Personality Theories: A Comparative Analysis, 4th ed. Homewood, Illinois, Dorsey Press, 1980
Nicholi AM (ed): Harvard Guide to Modern Psychiatry, pp 115–172. Cambridge, Massachusetts, Belknap Press, 1978
Wachtel PL: Psychoanalysis and Behavior Therapy: Toward an Integration. New York, Basic Books, 1977

Douglas H. Finestone

4 Psychodynamics: Defense Mechanisms and Symptom Formation

Psychodynamics, the study of the mental forces responsible for our thoughts, feelings, and actions, recognizes the roles of psychological, social, and biological factors in the development of the mind. According to psychodynamic theory, behavior results from a conflict between internal psychic forces and the limitations of external reality. An understanding of these mental forces will be approached through the discussion of defense mechanisms and symptom formations.

Defense Mechanisms

Defense mechanisms, the cornerstone of psychodynamics, are unconscious mental processes designed to protect an individual from anxiety resulting from sexual or aggressive impulses. We are born as helpless infants with needs that we are dependent on our world to fulfill. These needs, or drives, of sexuality and aggression exist throughout life. The fulfillment of these drives is influenced by others. Since we are social animals, our sexual and aggressive drives cannot be fulfilled without regard to our external reality. We are guided by our parents and other important figures in our world to develop within us prohibitions and oppositions to certain expressions of aggression or sexuality.

All animals have biologically based reflex mechanisms of fight or flight to deal with danger. As humans, we must deal not only with external dangers but also with internal sexual and aggressive conflicts that, at times, cause us to feel shame, guilt, disgust, or anxiety. Defense mechanisms allow us to indirectly satisfy sexual or aggressive needs without unpleasant effects. Although defense mechanisms are unseen, their expression is observable in our thoughts, feelings, actions, and dreams.

A developmental perspective is necessary to understand defense mechanisms. At different periods of our childhood, certain defense mechanisms are normal and adaptive. At these periods, these defense mechanisms are the best available means for us to express our sexual and aggressive needs. Normal adults use a wide variety of defense mechanisms in a flexible, adaptive manner that allows our basic needs to be expressed in an acceptable but fulfilling way. Psychopathology or abnormal behavior exists when previously adaptive defense mechanisms of an earlier period of life are extensively used in a later period when they are maladaptive, or when only a limited number of defense mechanisms are used in a restrictive and rigid way, resulting in primitive, unacceptable, or unfulfilling behavior.

This section will review the development of the concept of defense mechanisms. A number of established defense mechanisms will be defined and their function in mental life will be illustrated. The role of defense mechanisms in symptom formation will be reviewed.

History of Defense Mechanisms

Sigmund Freud first introduced the concept of defense mechanisms in his 1894 paper, "The Neuropsychoses of Defense (An Attempt at a Psychological Theory of Acquired Hysteria, of Many Phobias and Obsessions, and of Certain Hallucinatory Psychoses)." He hypothesized that certain defense mechanisms are associated with hysteria, phobias and obsessions, and psychoses. Freud viewed defense mechanisms as a means of keeping incompatible ideas out of consciousness. Throughout his career, he formulated various defense mechanisms from his work with patients.

In 1936, with the publication of "The Ego and the Mechanisms of Defense," Anna Freud made a major contribution to the theory of defense mechanisms. Miss Freud was the first theorist to catalog mechanisms of defense used by the ego in opposing sexual and aggressive drives. She listed ten methods of defense: regression, repression, reaction formation, isolation, undoing, projection, introjection, turning against the self, reversal, and sublimation. The first nine defense mechanisms are associated with the symptoms of neurosis in adults, but are normal in children. The tenth mechanism of defense, sublimation, allows the normal expression of drives by adults.

Otto Fenichel, in *The Psychoanalytic Theory of Neurosis* (1945), catagorized defenses as unsuccessful or successful. Unsuccessful defense mechanisms ward off drives from direct expression, but require constant effort by the ego to oppose drives, restricting the ego's functioning. Fenichel, like Anna Freud, recorded several unsuccessful defense mechanisms. In contrast, the successful defense mechanism of sublimation allows acceptable expression of drives.

In 1961, Arthur Valenstein and Edward Bibring published a *Glossary of Defenses*. They listed 24 basic defense mechanisms and an additional 15 complex defenses consisting of a mixture of defense mechanisms and behaviors. George

Vaillant, in "A Theoretical Hierarchy of Adaptive Ego Mechanisms" (1971), listed 18 defense lifestyles or behavior patterns. Valenstein, Bibring, and Vaillant acknowledged that their expanded listings of defense mechanisms included complex behaviors and defensive lifestyles, as well as specific unconscious mental processes.

Types of Defense Mechanisms

There is no set number of defense mechanisms. Each author's list varies not only in number but also in complexity of defense mechanisms. The following list of defense mechanisms closely resembles Anna Freud's own compilation. Each one has been recognized ever since defense mechanisms were first conceptualized. As previously defined, each of the following defense mechanisms is a simple and distinct mental process. More complex defense mechanisms, behaviors, or lifestyles are combinations of these basic defense mechanisms. Many mental processes are specific examples of defense mechanisms, and in the following list they are recorded under their individual mechanism.

Denial is the disavowal or refusal to acknowledge an unpleasant reality. The reality denied may be an idea, feeling, memory, or perception. If an unpleasant event that is witnessed is denied, it is as if it were never seen.

Projection is the attribution of one's thoughts or feelings to another. It is a negation or splitting of a part of oneself, an externalization of something within oneself onto the outside world. A delusion or hallucination may be a projection of one's thoughts or feelings.

Introjection is the taking into oneself part of the outside world. An example of introjection is incorporation, the psychological swallowing of something external. The complex processes of internalization and identification involve the use of introjection.

Regression is the return to an earlier pattern of behavior. Regression is viewed from a developmental perspective and is a retreat in functioning to an earlier period in life.

Turning against the self is the change in the object of a drive towards oneself. Instead of expressing the drive onto another person, it is reversed in direction onto oneself. Self-inflicted pain may be a turning against the self.

Reaction formation is the expression of a thought or feeling that is opposite to that actually felt. The expressed feeling, thought, or behavior is excessive and forced; it is the antithesis of the implicit drive.

Isolation is thought without feeling. It is the expression of a drive without associated feelings of significance. Examples of isolation are intellectualization, extremely logical thinking; rationalization, justifying the expression of a drive; and displacement, placing feelings about one object onto another object.

Undoing is the performance of an action that serves as a magical expiation of a distressing thought that has been previously experienced. A ritual may be an example of undoing by symbolically making amends for a disquieting thought.

Repression is the banishment of a thought or feeling from awareness. Repression is equivalent to forgetting; what is on the tip of one's tongue or in the back of one's mind is repressed.

Sublimation is the successful expression of a drive. Sublimation may involve the substitution of one object for another in the expression of a drive, it may allow a drive to be expressed through love, or it may allow the expression of a drive through socially acceptable means, such as work, art, study, or recreation.

Classification of Defense Mechanisms

Besides listing defense mechanisms, several authors have attempted to classify them. Anna Freud hypothesized that a chronological order exists for defense mechanisms. She reasoned that certain defense mechanisms develop in response to a person's sexual drive, while other defense mechanisms evolve in response to a person's aggressive drive. She also postulated that individual defense mechanisms come into existence at specific psychosexual developmental stages of a child's life. During each of these stages, particular forms of sexual or aggressive drives predominate, and specific defense mechanisms develop to deal with them. Miss Freud cautioned that a chronological classification of defense mechanisms is only generally applicable. Several defense mechanisms are present at different psychosexual developmental stages. She emphasized that the best way to study and understand defense mechanisms is to observe how and when they are used.

George Vaillant ranked defense mechanisms according to a hierarchy of adaptability, and delinated four categories of defense mechanisms, ordered in increasing adaptability. Narcissistic defense mechanisms are those used by children or psychotic individuals, immature defense mechanisms are used by adolescents, and neurotic defense mechanisms are used by adults under stress. Mature defense mechanisms are used by adults as the most adaptive means of dealing with drives. As a person develops, he does not completely replace early defense mechanisms with more adaptive ones, but increases the range and flexibility of his use of the same ones.

According to Vaillant's studies, those people who had lasting marriages, a satisfying career, the ability to enjoy recreational pursuits, and good physical health used mature defense mechanisms more often than immature defense mechanisms. In addition to sublimation, mature defense mechanisms include altruism, suppression, anticipation, and humor. Altruism, constructive service to society that satisfies instinctive needs, allows one to receive appreciation and affection from others. Suppression, the conscious decision to delay paying attention to an unpleasant conflict, prevents unconstructive rumination, allowing one to be more productive. Anticipation, goal-directed planning for the future, helps one to establish priorities while preventing anxious pondering. Humor releases tension and allows one to tolerate life's misfortunes.

Despite practical and theoretical limitations, a classification of defense mechanisms is useful in linking defense mechanisms to stages of psychosexual development, levels of adaptability, and types of psychopathology. Table 4-1 classifies the 10 defense mechanisms according to psychosexual stage, level of adaptability, and frequently-associated psychopathology. While some defense mechanisms, such as denial and projection, are often associated with severe psychopathology, and other defense mechanisms, such as sublimation, are associated with normal adult func-

Table 4-1
Classification of Defense Mechanisms*

Defense Mechanism	Developmental Stage	Level of Adaptability	Psychopathology
Denial	Oral	Narcissistic	Psychoses
Projection	Oral	Narcissistic	Psychoses
Introjection	Oral	Narcissistic	Psychoses
Regression	Oral–phallic	Immature	Psychoses, obsessions, and compulsions
Turning against the self	Oral–phallic	Immature	Depression
Reaction Formation	Anal	Neurotic	Obsessions and compulsions
Isolation	Anal	Neurotic	Obsessions and compulsions
Undoing	Anal	Neurotic	Obsessions and compulsions
Repression	Phallic	Neurotic	Hysteria
Sublimation	Latency–Adult	Mature	Normal adult

* Adapted from Kaplan HT, Freedman AF, Sadock BF: The Compressive Textbook of Psychiatry, 3rd ed, Vol 1, pp 691–692. Baltimore, Williams & Wilkins, 1980

tioning, psychotic individuals may occasionally use sublimation and normal adults may occasionally use denial and projection. A defense mechanism itself is not pathognomonic; however, observing how often, with whom, in what situation, and for what purposes a defense mechanism is used by a person greatly contributes to understanding that person's behavior.

Symptom Formation

According to psychodynamic theory, behavior is motivated by the basic biological requirements for oxygen, water, food, elimination of waste, and sexual satisfaction; as well as the emotional needs for love, approval, and success. Anxiety results when these needs are blocked, causing one to attempt to change environmental conditions. If this attempt fails, defense mechanisms are employed. If anxiety continues to persist, physical or emotional symptoms may result.

These physical and emotional symptoms differ, depending on the particular stress and environmental conditions, and one's particular character or behavior patterns. These patterns of responding to emotional conflict can be broadly separated into four areas: psychosis, personality disorders, psychosomatic disorders, and psychoneurotic disorders.

Psychosis

Psychosis is an impairment in the recognition of reality. A psychosis is understood from a psychodynamic perspective as a psychiatric disorder in which the ego is overwhelmed by the drives of the id. In persons with a psychosis, the ego uses highly unsuccessful defense mechanisms in an attempt to cope with anxiety. Psychological conflict within oneself is refuted and externalized. Persons with psychoses do not believe they are the cause of their difficulties. Instead, they are severely debilitated by their perception of society as hostile and threatening.

☐ Mr. P is a 29-year-old, single, college graduate, who works as a night shift janitor at a community college. Mr. P has had several psychiatric hospitalizations over the last 2 years and is diagnosed as having chronic paranoid schizophrenia. He is prescribed a major tranquilizer that he takes irregularly. Mr. P was brought to the emergency room by the police, who were called to the college at which he works. The police found him sitting in front of the smashed pane of a vending machine, desperately consuming candy bars. He told them that he was being attacked, and that he was defending himself by devouring his enemy's lifeblood. His enemy was a middle-aged man who tended the vending machines during the day. Mr. P was convinced that the man was plotting to take control of his mind. He became aware of the plot that day, when the candy machine had not given him change for a purchase he had made, and the vending machine operator had pretended not to notice. While working that evening, Mr. P heard a voice telling him to destroy all candy bars before the vending machine operator could destroy him. Mr. P had no knowledge of breaking into the vending machine. When asked about a cut on his hand, he stated that the vending machine operator had stabbed him.

Since his adolescence, Mr. P has been considered by others to be strange. Although others view him as isolated, as having bizarre ideas, and functioning poorly, Mr. P believes he has a special understanding of the world that is unappreciated by others. Mr. P's episode of psychosis was secondary to feelings of aggression that he was unable to control. Under the threat of being overwhelmed, his ego attempted to defend itself by use of the unsuccessful defense mechanisms of introjection, projection, and denial. By using these defense mechanisms, he was able to separate himself from any psychological conflict. In exchange, Mr. P was forced to construct an unreal, dangerous, and frightening world.

Personality Disorders

Personality consists of the habitual attitudes, affects, and mannerisms of a person. Personality includes a person's customary means of coping with sexual and aggressive drives. A personality disorder exists when a person's personality is characterized by a rigid, restrictive means of coping with sexual or aggressive drives. The same constellation of defense mechanisms is consistently used to cope with every psychological conflict.

The superego in persons with personality disorders may be prohibitive to the degree that sexual and aggressive drives are disavowed. Or, the superego may be so feeble that the drives of the id are allowed unqualified expression. In either situation, a decisive imbalance exists between the superego and the id. Instead of attempting to resolve the conflict between the superego and id, the ego completely and repetitively allies itself with one or the other. The alliance is syntonic to the ego and its id or superego ally is viewed as an acceptable part of one's personality. Defense mechanisms are used by the ego to subdue either the superego or the id. Psychological conflict is avoided and its accompanying anxiety is not experienced.

Although persons with personality disorders appear comfortable with themselves, they actually suffer; and they cause much discomfort to others. They sacrifice adaptability for a reflexive response to life's circumstances. Persons with a prohibitive superego endure an impoverished life, and persons with an uncontrolled id repeatedly clash with society. Under the pressure of certain events, the ego of a person with a personality disorder may collapse and a severe psychiatric disorder may result.

□ Miss D is a 48-year-old single woman who asked to be hospitalized because she was unable to swallow food. She also reported a decreased appetite and weight loss of 25 pounds, low energy, especially in the morning, and feelings of worthlessness. She appeared sad and tearful, protested her loss of pleasure in life, and admitted to occasionally longing to join her dead mother. Her symptoms had been present for about one month and her mother had died slightly over a year ago. For the past 30 years, she had attended to her invalid mother. She managed a small craft shop next door to her mother's home in order to be constantly near her. Over the years, she had served faithfully as her mother's companion, guardian, and nurse. Her mother was extremely weak during the last month of her life; her appetite was poor, she lost several pounds, and she complained that she did not have enough energy to chew her food. Miss D was terrified that if she forced her mother to eat, she might choke. She lamented that she had not done more for her mother.

Miss D has a dependent personality disorder. Since early childhood, she had always completely subordinated her needs to those of her mother. Never had she thought or expressed a harsh word toward her mother. Whenever her mother would criticize her, she would berate herself for the lack of consideration towards her mother. Her mother's death was extremely stressful for Miss D. She felt lost and abandoned, and developed a major depression. All of her life, she had used the defense mechanism of turning against the self in her constant effort to deny any expression of aggression. After her mother's death, she turned her anger at her mother against herself. She suffered all the symptoms her mother had previously complained of before her death.

Psychosomatic Disorders

Psychosomatic disorders are characterized by physical symptoms that result from psychological factors. The symptoms are mediated through the autonomic nervous system. Psychsomatic disorders illustrate the intrinsic relationship of mind to body. It is thought that unresolved psychological conflicts, through the use of unsuccessful defense mechanisms, result in physical symptoms in susceptible persons.

Defense mechanisms are central to how a person copes with the stress of illness. Prior to illness, certain defense mechanisms may be able to maintain a state of psychic equilibrium. But illness may increase id or superego pressures on the ego, to which the ego responds with a mobilization of defense mechanisms in an attempt to control anxiety. The use of successful defense mechanisms allows for adaptation to physical illness, while the use of unsuccessful defense mechanisms results in a worsening of physical symptoms.

☐ Mr. A is a 50-year-old, single, hard-working administrator who is always extremely calm and rational in his handling of problems at work. He rarely displays any emotional reactions to the frequent irritations of his job. Whenever problems occur within his department, he blames himself, and refuses to criticize his employees.

Mr. A was hospitalized after he experienced a myocardial infarction while he was at work. He was indifferent to his requiring hospitalization and unconcerned about his condition. He refused to believe he had suffered a heart attack, but felt he had undergone a bout of chest tightness caused by inactivity. He complied poorly with his rehabilitation program and insisted on prematurely returning to work, pressuring his physician into discharging him from the hospital. Two days later, he was rehospitalized with unstable angina.

Prior to his illness, Mr. A habitually used the defense mechanisms of isolation and turning against the self. He attempted to cope with the stress of his myocardial infarction by continuing to use these defense mechanisms. He appeared to accept his hospitalization with equanimity and blamed his condition on his not working hard enough. From the stress of his illness, he also began to use the defense mechanism of denial. He disavowed his disability and attempted to return to work. Unfortunately, his defense mechanisms were unsuccessful in coping with his illness and caused his physical symptoms to worsen, forcing him to return to the hospital.

Psychoneurotic Disorders

Pyschoneurotic disorders manifest underlying, unresolved, psychological conflicts dating from childhood, in which drives of the id that are unacceptable to the superego press for fulfillment. The ego may feel anxious if the id is constitutionally powerful, or if the superego is weak because of overly permissive parents. The ego may also feel anxious if the id is moderate, but the superego is rigid and punitive because of overly strict parents.

The id and superego must be in balance in order to allow the ego to develop successful defense mechanisms to cope with psychological conflicts. Two cases are presented to illustrate how adult anxiety disorders result from unresolved childhood conflicts. A childhood anxiety disorder is also presented.

☐ Little Hans was a 5-year-old child with a separation anxiety disorder, or a childhood phobia, who was seen in consultation by Sigmund Freud. Little Hans' psychoneurotic symptoms included a fear of horses biting him, which prevented him from leaving his home and caused him to spend his days in the company of his mother.

Several months before the first consultation, Little Hans had started to develop a type of affection for his mother in which he desired to be the only recipient of her love. He unconsciously became hostile toward his father and jealous of his father's relationship to his mother. He unwittingly desired that this father be maimed or killed, and projected his aggression toward his father by becoming afraid that harm would come to himself. He displaced the source of the potential harm to himself, from his father to horses. He then regressed by fearing that the harm that would come to him would be a horse biting him, rather than being castrated by his father because of his own affection toward his mother. He suffered from his fear of horses, but gained the constant companionship of his mother.

Over a 4-month period, with Freud's advice, Little Hans's father treated his son in psychotherapy. As Little Hans became aware of his jealousy of his father, his fear of horses disappeared. He developed successful defense mechanisms of coping with his affection toward his mother and his rivalry with his father by imagining the time when he would have a wife himself.

☐ Mr. O is a 35-year-old married accountant who consulted a psychiatrist because of exasperating rituals he had developed several weeks previously. He was compelled to check and recheck his ledger figures at work because of the recurrent, intrusive thought that if his figures were not absolutely correct, harm would come to his boss and to his own wife. He felt like a superstitious child who believes in magic. His behavior greatly disrupted his previous excellent job performance, even though he arrived at work early and left late in order to placate his boss. He doted on his wife, but refused to have intercourse with her because it might hurt her. He detailed his problems in a calm and controlled manner, frequently using stilted words and accounting terms to describe his distressing symptoms. He prided himself on being a clear thinker, and explained that his intrusive thoughts were caused by pressures at work. Although he loved his work, he felt cheated by its demand on him. His first fears for his wife and his boss occurred on the evening of an office party. His wife and his boss were dancing when suddenly he had the disturbing thought that an overhead chandelier might crash upon them. He corrected this thought by calculating that the pull of the chandelier was balanced by its supporting pins.

Mr. O was an only child of an indulgent mother. During the first 2 years of his life, his father was overseas. Upon his father's return home, he repeatedly wished that his father would disappear. When he told his father to go away, his father severely spanked him and he thereafter rarely said a harsh word toward his father. He later became an extremely conscientious and hard-working student.

Mr. O has an obsessive compulsive disorder, for which the psychoneurotic symptoms are his rituals or compulsions caused by his obsessive thoughts. His disabling symptoms defend against his anxiety over his intrusive thoughts that harm will come to his boss and to his wife. He developed his psychoneurosis because his defense mechanisms of regression, reaction formation, isolation, and undoing were unsuccessful in resolving his psychological conflict.

Since the evening of the office party when his boss and wife danced together, he has unconsciously felt extreme aggression toward them. His long workday and doting on his wife are reaction formations against his unconscious anger. His calmness and logical thinking are attempts to isolate his thoughts that harm will come to his wife and to his boss, from his anger towards them. He displaces his feelings of being cheated by them onto feeling cheated by his job, and he attempts to undo his aggressive thoughts toward them by magical rituals.

□ Mrs. H is a 32-year-old, married lawyer who is undergoing psychotherapy. She is confused by a conflict she has with a senior male colleague. She constantly argues with him over issues she cannot remember later. She describes her colleague as handsome and clever, but rejects the thought that she may be attracted to him. Sometimes she forgets he is married and frequently asks him if he is dating anyone. If he compliments her she is offended, but if he does not speak to her, she is tense and occasionally has a stomach ache.

Mrs. H's father was an often-absent businessman. When he was at home, he spent a lot of time with her on outings. She was her father's "special girl," and greatly enjoyed his company. Her parents divorced when she was six, and since then she has rarely seen her father. Now she never consciously thinks about him.

Mrs. H has a generalized anxiety disorder. Her symptoms of tenseness, stomach aches, and irritability result from repression of her feelings toward her senior male colleague. She has an intense unconscious attraction toward her colleague, who represents her father. Since she represses her powerful feelings towards her colleague, she is only aware of her unaccountable tenseness around him that results in her stomach aches and irritability. Her relationship with her father was originally one of much fulfillment. She initially felt tremendous resentment toward her father after her parents were divorced, and she seldom saw him. Gradually, she thought of him less often and tried to forget him.

Summary

The purpose of this chapter has been to introduce the concept of defense mechanisms and symptom formation, and to outline their role in psychodynamic theory. Defense mechanisms are an unavoidable result of our struggle to adapt to our internal needs and the frequently contrasting demands of our society. Defense mechanisms evolve as we develop from children to adults. They range from unsuccessful to successful in the degree to which they allow us to fulfill our needs within the limits set by our society. Psychoneurotic disorders result from the use of unsuccessful defense mechanisms retained from childhood in an attempt to resolve persisting psychological conflict. Psychosis, personality disorders, and psychosomatic disorders were also discussed.

Bibliography

Bibring GL, Dwyer TF, Huntingdon DS, Valenstein AF: A study of the psychological processes in pregnancy and of the earliest mother–child relationship, II, Methodological Considerations, Appendix B, Glossary of Defenses. Psychoanal Study Child 16:25–72, 1961

Brenner C: An Elementary Textbook of Psychoanalysis, 3rd ed. Garden City, Anchor Books, 1974

Fenichel O: The Psychoanalytic Theory of Neurosis, pp 129–192, 453–540. New York, WW Norton & Company, 1945

Freud A: The ego and the mechanisms of defense (1936). In: The Notes of the Writings of Anna Freud, Vol 2, pp 3–196. New York, International Universities Press, 1966

Freud S: Inhibitions, symptoms and anxiety (1926). In: The Standard Edition of the Complete Psychological Works of Sigmund Freud, Vol 20, pp 77–174. London, The Hogarth Press, 1981

Freud S: The ego and the id (1923). In: The Standard Edition of the Complete Psychological Works of Sigmund Freud, Vol 19, pp 3–36. London, The Hogarth Press, 1981

Freud S: Further remarks on the neuro-psychoses of defense (1896). In: The Standard Edition of the Complete Psychological Works of Sigmund Freud, Vol 3, pp 159–185. London, The Hogarth Press, 1981

Freud S: The neuro-psychoses of defense (1884). In: The Standard Edition of the Complete Psychological Works of Sigmund Freud, Vol 3, pp 43–61. London, The Hogarth Press, 1981

Kaplan HI, Freedman AM, Sadock BJ: The Comprehensive Textbook of Psychiatry, 3rd ed., Vol 1, pp 691–692. Baltimore, Williams & Wilkins, 1980

Vaillant GE: Theoretical hierarchy of adaptive ego mechanisms. Arch Gen Psychiatry 24:107–118, 1971

Roy M. Stein

5 The Psychiatric Evaluation

The physician performing a psychiatric evaluation seeks to develop a comprehensive, multidimensional assessment of the patient's illness and overall personality functioning. Such a broad-based evaluation takes into account such factors as the description of the present illness, physical problems, social and personal history, and educational, occupational, and family data. From such a data base the psychiatrist can reach a descriptive diagnosis (*e.g.*, major depression or panic disorder), and is able to develop a formulation of the psychodynamic, interpersonal, social, and physical factors that have contributed to the etiology or that have shaped the course of the illness. Factors like these, along with the primary descriptive diagnosis, are often crucial in determining the most appropriate approach to treatment. George Engel has advanced the biopsychosocial model, an integrative approach that views all illnesses as the outcome of the interplay between biological, psychological, and social factors, and moves away from the older linear cause-and-effect model of etiology. The clinician who routinely considers these three dimensions in each patient who has psychiatric illness is able to achieve the comprehensiveness and breadth required in modern practice.

The necessary data of the evaluation are obtained through several means. These include interviews of the patient and, depending on circumstances, interviews of family members, employers, teachers, or police. Old medical and psychiatric records must be reviewed. Further relevant information may be obtained from a physical examination, performed either by the psychiatrist or by a medial consultant, along with laboratory tests as indicated by the history and examination. Psychological testing, generally performed by clinical psychologists, can be helpful in certain situations. In many settings the psychiatric evaluation is conducted as a team effort, involving contributions by psychologists, psychiatric social workers and nonpsychiatric physicians. In addition to conducting a significant part of the direct evaluation of the patient, the psychiatrist plays a critical role in coordinating and planning the overall effort and in synthesizing the data into a comprehensive formulation. In this chapter the various components of the psychiatric examination are discussed.

The particular format, focus, and depth of the examination will be shaped by the setting, characteristics of the patient, resources, and time available. There are necessarily practical differences in the emergency room evaluation of the acutely psychotic patient and the office assessment of the self-referred patient with neurotic complaints. Nevertheless, the organization of the psychiatrist's thinking, his comprehensiveness, and respectful and humane attitude should not differ. Furthermore, any deviation from the complete diagnostic process as outlined here should be undertaken thoughtfully and with adequate justification, both to insure the best care of the patient, and for the physician's medicolegal protection.

The Psychiatric Interview

While the history is recognized as a major element in the diagnostic process in all areas of clinical medicine, it becomes the central instrument in psychiatric diagnosis. In addition to providing factual historical data, the interview allows the clinician to interact with the patient and to observe directly many aspects of his mental, emotional and social function. The challenge for the interviewer, then, is to observe and critically evaluate simultaneously *what* the patient says and does not say, *how* he says it, and how he *behaves* as he says it. Thus, history-taking and examination are performed simultaneously in the psychiatric evaluation.

A second notable feature of the psychiatric interview is that this diagnostic process also serves a therapeutic purpose. The opportunity for a person with emotional or mental disturbance to describe his or her difficulties to a concerned and objective listener can provide great relief, particularly when that listener has professional skill and authority. The diagnostic and therapeutic processes are very much interwoven, because as the patient experiences some relief from his anxiety and distress, he is much more able to share further information. If the physician conducts the interview in a manner that increases the patient's anxiety, that patient becomes less able to examine and discuss his difficulties.

The *physician–patient relationship,* then, is of critical importance in the psychiatric evaluation. What is most essential is that the physician convey to the patient a sense of concern, empathy, and respect, with a recognition of their common humanity. This is the foundation on which the success of any further diagnostic or therapeutic endeavors will depend. The psychiatrist should treat the patient with the same amenities and courtesies that would be afforded a distinguished visitor, starting from the time that the patient arrives at the office or clinic. Unnecessary delays in seeing the patient should be avoided, and if a delay must occur, it is incumbent on the psychiatrist to offer an explanation to the patient. In the initial encounter, the physician shakes hands with the patient, introducing himself clearly. Courtesy and respect are further communicated by taking efforts to ensure that the interview will not be interrupted by telephone calls or persons entering the room. In a teaching setting, it is important to introduce by name and role any individuals who will be observing the interview, and to respect the patient's wishes regarding their presence or absence. It is helpful to find a quiet and private location for the interview and to provide comfortable seating for the patient, preferably at the same height as the physician.

The patient is often accompanied to an initial interview by a relative or friend. The historical information that can be obtained from such individuals is often very important, especially in the case of more severely disturbed patients. As a general rule, however, it is best to see the patient alone first, and then to interview significant others after obtaining the patient's permission. This approach communicates to the patient that his relationship with the physician is primary, and that his thoughts and feelings are of foremost importance. It helps to diminish the patient's defensiveness about what others may have reported about his behavior. The interview of the significant others may be conducted either with or without the presence of the patient, depending on the particular situation. The advantage of the former approach is that the examiner has the opportunity to observe the manner of interaction between the patient and significant other persons in his life.

While emphasizing a tone of genuine human concern and respect, the psychiatrist must also work to establish the professional, therapeutic nature of the relationship with the patient. This relationship is unique because the patient is expected to discuss very intimate aspects of his life with a stranger, and the sole purpose of the interaction is to understand and alleviate the patient's difficulties. The mutual nature of ordinary social relationships is thus absent. In general, the psychiatrist shares information about himself only in regard to his professional role, rank, and level of training. Patients often ask about the physician's age, marital status, family, religion, use of alcohol, and so forth. They may do this out of a wish to put the relationship on a more social basis, thus denying that they are seeking psychiatric help for a significant problem. Attempting to shift discussion to the physician and his personal life can thus be a way for the patient to avoid the anxiety associated with talking about his own problems. The psychiatrist can respond by openly and honestly explaining that he does not typically answer such personal questions because the purpose of their meeting is to work on understanding what is troubling the patient, and that discussion of the physician's personal characteristics will only distract them from that goal. By openly establishing this ground rule, the physician begins to educate the patient about the unique aspects of the therapeutic relationship. The patient's concern or ideas about the psychiatrist can then become a meaningful topic for inquiry. The approach described here need not be applied in a rigid or mechanical fashion, but it remains critical for the psychiatrist, and especially the trainee, focus on the development of the therapeutic nature of the relationship.

The psychiatrist must not give premature, unrealistic reassurance to the patient; doing so may simply make the patient feel that the therapist does not fully appreciate the seriousness of his problems. More meaningful support is provided by the psychiatrist's reliable, attentive listening and his pursuit of an understanding of the patient's troubles. The physician's ability to listen in a calm, nonjudgmental manner, no matter how bizarre or deviant the patient's experiences or behavior may be, is another source of meaningful reassurance. It conveys to the patient that anything is acceptable to talk about, and that he will be accepted for who he is.

The psychiatrist's role with the patient has been described by Harry Stack Sullivan as that of the *participant–observer*. That is, he participates in the relationship and at the same time observes both his own and the patient's reactions and behavior. The patient's responses to the psychiatrist can be thought of as a composite of *realistic* reactions and *transference* reactions. Realistic reactions occur in response to the actual behavior of the psychiatrist, and are appropriate in their quality and intensity. For example, a patient might well express some anger and resentment at a psychiatrist who is 40 minutes late for an appointment, appears hurried and distracted, and allows the interview to be interrupted by several phone calls. On the other hand, another patient might become enraged at a therapist who is 2 minutes late, and might conclude that this is evidence that the physician is uncaring and insensitive toward his problems. This type of reaction is a reflection of transference, in which an individual carries over, or transfers, feelings onto persons in his present-day life that originated in relationships with persons that were important in his past, such as his parents. Transference is present to some degree in virtually all relationships, including those of healthy individuals, but it is especially heightened in the interactions of patients with physicians, in which they find themselves in a vulnerable, dependent position in relation to an authority figure. The examining psychiatrist can learn a great deal about the way the patient sees himself in relation to other people by being observant of transference reactions. In addition, it is critical for the psychiatrist to recognize transference reactions that may be so intense as to threaten to disrupt the diagnostic process.

Transference and realistic reactions on the part of the patient have their analogs in the reactions of the therapist, known as *counterreactions* and *countertransference*. Counterreactions are realistic, appropriately intense feelings on the part of the therapist toward the patient. Fear on the part of the psychiatrist when interviewing a large, agitated psychotic patient who has a history of assaults against physicians illustrates a realistic reaction. Countertransference refers to feelings toward the patient arising out of the therapist's past experiences, that are triggered simply by the patient's characteristics. Counterreactions can serve as useful diagnostic data because they illustrate the way other people are likely to react to the patient. Countertransference reactions, however, are more likely to hamper the clinical process because they interfere with the psychiatrist's objectivity toward the patient.

In order for the psychiatrist to deal effectively with the nuances of the physician–patient relationship by distinguishing transference and countertransference from realistic reactions, he must develop considerable awareness and understanding of his own behavior and emotional life.

Two other concepts, resistance and therapeutic alliance, are useful in assessing the physician–patient relationship. *Resistance* refers to all behaviors on the part of the patient, conscious and unconscious, that obstruct the process of diagnosis and treatment. While the patient wants relief from his distress, the actual process of working on his problems can bring up thoughts and feelings that are unpleasant and frightening to him. Resistance springs out of the patient's reluctance to face these difficult aspects of treatment. The case mentioned earlier of the patient who persists in questioning the psychiatrist about his own personal life is an example of resistance to the diagnostic and treatment process.

Therapeutic alliance is the positive working relationship that develops between the physician and the healthier aspects of the patient's personality, with the goal of dealing with the patient's problems. As this positive, realistic relationship develops, the physician and patient are able to look together at the more disturbing aspects of the patient's difficulties. With an intact therapeutic alliance, a psychotic patient could discuss with his physician his resentment at having to take medications and how this leads to his noncompliance and consequent relapse of symptoms.

To conclude this discussion of the physician–patient relationship in the psychiatric evaluation, a comment is needed on the issue of confidentiality. Physician–patient communications are privileged; that is, the physician may not share the contents of their discussion with anyone without the patient's permission. It may be helpful to point this out to the patient, who may be reluctant to discuss sensitive topics out of fear that information will be released and will damage or embarrass him. There are exceptions to the privileged nature of the patient's communications with the physician; for example, in cases in which the patient is a child, in court-ordered evaluations, and in situations in which the patient makes serious threats to harm identifiable individuals. The latter instance has been, and continued to be, a matter of great legal and ethical controversy. In general, if the situation is one in which strict rules of confidentiality do not hold, it is incumbent on the psychiatrist to inform the patient of this. Clinicians, and especially trainees for whom the experience of seeing patients is a new and exciting one, need to keep in mind the matter of confidentiality at all times, and must refrain from discussing patients with their friends and colleagues except in formal clinical conferences. Discussion of patients in hospital and clinic elevators and cafeterias is a practice that can have harmful results for patients, their families, and for the clinicians themselves.

Interviewing Technique

A number of the interpersonal aspects of the psychiatric interview have already been discussed in the context of the physician–patient relationship. The skilled psychiatrist is also aware of a number of technical considerations in carrying out the interview. The primary job of the interviewer is to listen. It should be an active and informed listening, that brings to bear the psychiatrist's knowledge of normal and pathologic behavior upon the patient's narrative. From the onset of the interview he listens for patterns and begins to generate hypotheses, which are then subject to further testing during the interview. The interviewer uses a variety of techniques to enhance the flow of relevant information, which are described below. These techniques are not employed in a rigid, standardized fashion, but are tailored to the unique aspects of each patient and his or her particular problems. An elderly patient with a history of chronic alcoholism may exhibit the difficulty in attention span, memory, and concentration that are characteristic of an organic brain syndrome. The interview in this situation will be more actively structured and directed by the psychiatrist, with more specific, directed questions than would be used with an anxious, obsessive patient who is very verbal.

The most familiar interviewing technique is the question. Questions can be classed as *directed* or *open-ended.* Directed questions ask for specific pieces of information and they generally elicit brief answers, for example, "How many children do you have?," "What medicines are you taking?," or "Do you ever hear voices when there is no one there?" Such questions obviously have an important role in bringing out necessary details and in interviewing the patient who has difficulty in fluently expressing his thoughts. The tendency to overuse this technique, however, leads to a staccato question-and-answer format in which the patient never has a chance to tell about any relevant aspects of his history that the interviewer has not asked about. In the open-ended question, the interviewer asks the patient to talk openly about a particular topic. For example, "Tell me about your family life" or "What has it been like for you, being in the hospital?". Such questions throw out a wide net, allowing much unanticipated information to be shared. They also convey to the patient the sense that whatever is on his mind is of importance to the doctor. Overuse of open-ended questions with some patients can lead to rambling, tangential talk that conveys little substance. The interviewer must then be able to redirect the patient in a respectful manner, leading the interview back to more fruitful material. A successful interview usually consists of a balance between these two types of questions, with open-ended ones predominating early, and directed questions used more heavily later in the interview to fill in and clarify details.

Facilitative communications, both comments and gestures, are used to encourage the continuing stream of talk, and to direct and focus the patient on areas the interviewer judges to be meaningful. Comments like, "Really—tell me more about that" or "I see" and gestures such as leaning forward or nodding affirmatively, and even changes in facial expression, can do much to enhance the patient's communication, if done in a natural and unforced manner. In *reflecting back,* the interviewer repeats a word or phrase just spoken by the patient in order to focus attention on it and to encourage elaboration. In *summary statements* the interviewer summarizes or paraphrases a portion of the patient's narrative. This serves both to show the patient that the doctor has been listening and comprehending what he has been saying, and to give the patient a moment to reflect further on its meaning. It also allows the patient to correct the interviewer if he has misunderstood some part of what has been said. *Silence* on the interviewer's part can be yet another facilitative behavior, allowing the patient time to reflect and to gather his thoughts. *Clarifications* go a step beyond summary statements and reflecting back because the interviewer points out patterns or interconnections between events or behaviors that the patient may not have been aware of. This may spur the patient to look for other such connections or to find additional examples relevant to the physician's hypothesis.

It is particularly important to observe the patient's emotional reactions to the content under discussion and to the interviewer's interventions. It is helpful to ask the patient who is recounting events in a factual manner about how he felt when these events occurred.

The synthesis of these techniques into an effective and natural style of interviewing takes time and experience. Trainees should take advantage of the experience of skilled clinicians, should have direct supervision of their own interviews, and should make use of videotaping facilities to observe their own performance in a critical manner.

The Psychiatric History

This section provides an outline of the information called for in the psychiatric history. It must be emphasized that this outline should not be the basis for a mechanical question-and-answer approach to the psychiatric history. It is intended as an aid in organizing the interviewer's thinking and as a format for the consistent reporting of the data, whether in written or oral form. The clinician who has such an outline in mind will be able to conduct the interview in a flexible and natural manner without missing important areas of inquiry. In essence, this outline differs little from the traditional medical history; it does place greater emphasis on social and developmental history and on emotional reactions to the events and symptoms reported by the patient.

1. *Identification.* Note the age, marital status, sex, and race of the patient as well as current residence and occupation. (It is often helpful to ask mundane questions like these at the start of the interview because they may help put the patient at ease before he is asked to discuss his problems.)
2. *Circumstances of referral.* Indicate whether the patient was referred by himself or by another physician or social agency, or is being seen at the request or insistence of an employer or family member, or is under court order. If the evaluation is being initiated by another agency or physician, carefully record the name, address, and phone number for further communication.
3. *Chief complaint.* What is the main problem for which the patient seeks help? In some cases the chief complaint will be obtainable only by those initiating the referral, as in the case of some commitment evaluations. Try to record the chief complaint in the patient's own words.
4. *History of present illness.* Focusing on the chief complaint, the interviewer seeks a detailed description of the patient's problems and symptoms. Emphasis is given to the circumstances under which the symptoms first developed, and to those circumstances that seem to aggravate or ameliorate them. It is especially important to clarify why the patient is seeking help for the problem at this particular time. The patient's own reactions to the problem, and those of important

persons in his life, are sought; as are changes in daily functioning, such as schoolwork, household duties, or outside employment.

The psychiatrist asks specifically about any major changes in the patient's life that may be associated with the illness; especially losses such as death, divorce, job loss, a child leaving home, and so forth. Changes that may not appear to be negative are also important; for example, moving to a new town or neighborhood, job promotion, or graduation. Physical illnesses and their treatments should be detailed, including specific medications.

Previous episodes of similar psychiatric problems are described, and the treatments are discussed in detail. It is important to know the duration of treatments, doses and names of drugs given, and those therapies that the patient considers to have been most beneficial. Relationships and problems encountered in dealing with previous therapists are described.

Changes in diet, appetite, and weight should be noted, along with an account of drug and alcohol use, and any association between substance use and other symptoms. Alterations in sexual desire and sexual performance are recorded. All patients should be asked about changes in sleep patterns, and the particular pattern of sleep disturbance should be described. Other generally useful questions include difficulties in thinking, concentration, and memory.

Specific lines of inquiry will be based on the diagnostic hypotheses generated by the more general questioning, and on the psychiatrist's knowledge of various psychiatric syndromes.

The patient's current living situation is described, including information on members of his household; also, his marital, economic, and legal status are determined. A thorough picture of the patient's important relationships and social supports is developed. The patient's educational background, detailed work history (including reasons for job changes), military service, marital, and sexual history are recorded. This portion of the psychiatric evaluation allows the patient's illness to be viewed in the context of his overall life history and social setting.

5. *Family history*. The diagnoses and treatment histories of family members who have had any type of psychiatric illness are recorded. It is helpful to ask specifically about cases of mental illness, alcoholism, suicide, and psychiatric hospitalization. A person who has a relative who never had psychiatric treatment but did commit suicide may not spontaneously report this as a case of psychiatric illness.

   The information in this section is useful in identifying genetic risk factors for psychiatric illness, and in revealing past experiences that the patient or his relatives may have had with mental illness. Significant medical illnesses in family members are noted as well, with particular emphasis on epilepsy and other neurologic disorders.
6. *Developmental history*. This material overlaps with that in the two

previous sections, but focuses on experiences and influences on the patient during childhood and adolescence. The patient is asked to describe each of the members of his family of origin, including the extended family, if more distant relatives had significant relationships with the patient. The patient's place in the birth order and his parent's ages and occupations are essential information. His relationship to the parents (or other primary caretakers) receives emphasis. It is useful to know about childhood illnesses and illnesses in family members. The patient may be able to give only limited information on these topics, so interviews of family members may be helpful.

The development of academic abilities and performance, peer relationships, interactions with authority figures, and early experiences with sexuality are all traced. Episodes of delinquency are noted.

A broad question such as "Tell me about your childhood" is often a good starting point. The interviewer is aware that the adult patient's accounts of childhood experiences may be distorted and skewed, especially in light of the current illness; nevertheless, the patient's memories and perceptions of his childhood are useful information in their own right, even if their historical accuracy is not completely reliable. A severely depressed patient is likely to report a picture of deprivation and neglect in childhood; there may be some truth in this account, but it also reveals something about how the patient sees himself in the world.

7. *Past medical history.* This section is identical to that in a general medical history. Types and dates of major injuries (especially head injuries) and operations are noted, along with any significant medical illnesses. Psychiatric illnesses are recorded here also. Current alcohol and drug use, current medications (both prescription and over-the-counter) and their doses are noted. Drug sensitivities and other allergies are recorded.
8. *Review of systems.* This is carried out and recorded as for medical evaluation, with attention focused on any possible problems suggested in the history.

The psychiatric history outlined above is intended to develop a broad, biopsychosocial picture of the past and present factors involved in the etiology, course, and impact of the illness. As noted earlier, this is not intended to be used in a rote, questionnaire fashion, but is a guide to and organization of relevant information. Depending on realistic time constraints, as well as the stamina of both doctor and patient, it may, and usually will, be impossible to cover all these topics in depth in an initial interview. Still, the various topics can be at least touched upon, and the clinician must make a judgment as to which areas are most pressing, and which can be deferred to subsequent interviews.

The Mental Status Examination

The purpose of the mental status examination (MSE) is to develop a cross-sectional view of the patient's mental functioning at a given moment in time. This cross-sectional view provides a complement to the longitudinal picture generated by the history. In contrast to the history, which is based primarily on the subjective report of the patient, the mental status examination is based on the physician's direct observations of the patient's behavior, speech, emotional state, and thinking. It thus seeks to complement the subjective report with objective observation. In this regard, the mental status examination is analogous to the physical examination in a medical evaluation, just as the psychiatric history is comparable to the medical history.

It is useful to separate the history from the mental status examination for purposes of discussion, as well as for written and oral case presentations, because it allows for clearer organization and analysis of the data. However, the actual processes of the mental status examination and history-taking occur simultaneously in the psychiatric interview, if performed by a skilled clinician. While actively listening to the patient's historical narrative, the psychiatrist is continually observing the features of the patient's physical appearance, motor behavior, speech, emotions, thought processes, and intellectual function. These observations constitute the bulk of the data of the mental status examination, and provide clues as to which areas require more formal inquiry. An example is the patient who, as he is giving his history, cannot remember the number of years he has been married or the ages of his children. The psychiatrist would note this and specifically ask the patient about memory problems he has experienced, and would then conduct detailed, formal memory testing. Similarly, a patient who is noted to be mumbling to himself occasionally during an interview would then be asked specific questions about hallucinations.

As emphasized earlier with regard to the history, the outline presented below is intended for use as a format for organization and to ensure completeness of information, not as a mechanical questionnaire. The interview will most likely be successful, both diagnostically and therapeutically, if the clinician listens actively to the patient's story, using questions to clarify and deepen the material. Only after the patient has had a full opportunity to present his own account is it appropriate to fill it in with questions on problem areas that the patient has not raised, and to conduct formal testing.

Appearance

Comment on overall physical appearance, clothing, grooming, facial expression, gestures, and any particularly unusual features. Try to provide a concise description that would theoretically allow the reader to select the patient from a waiting room.

Attitude

Describe the patient's attitude toward the physician, the interview situation, and his illness as being cooperative or uncooperative, submissive and compliant or angry and demanding, overtly hostile and belligerent, indifferent, evasive, or suspicious.

Motor Behavior

Describe posture and gait, as well as overall level of motor activity. Note motor manifestations of anxiety, such as fidgeting, foot-tapping, or frequent position changes. Depressed patients may exhibit either *psychomotor* retardation, an overall slowing and reduction of movement; or agitation, or elements of both. Manic patients often display marked hyperactivity, and may even pace the floor.

Note any abnormal movements such as tics, tremors, rigidity, or choreoathetoid movements. Note any focal weakness, such as hemiparesis. Schizophrenic patients occasionally display unusual stereotyped movements of bizarre postures; more commonly, they exhibit a stiffness and awkwardness of movement.

Speech

In this section the characteristics of speech are described, that is, how the patient speaks. Thought processes and content reflected in speech are discussed separately. Note, the *rate, amount,* and *tone* (*e.g.,* monotonous or sing-song). Manic patients display rapid, "pressured" speech, in which it is difficult for the interviewer to "get a word in edgewise." Depressed patients typically speak in a slow monotone. Patients with schizophrenia may exhibit a paucity of spontaneous speech or may even be mute; they may use neologisms (coining new words), string words together in nonsensical fashion (*word salad*), or display milder aberrations in syntax.

Dysarthria, a difficulty in speech production due to incoordination of the speech apparatus, suggests drug intoxication or organic brain disease, especially of the cerebellum. *Aphasia,* the impairment or absence of communication through speech, writing, or signs, is typically due to dysfunction in language centers in the dominant hemisphere. It must be differentiated from elective mutism, which may be seen in psychotic and hysterical states.

Any other uncommon speech characteristics, such as unusual dialects or accents, affectations, and the use of jargon, should be noted.

Emotions

Emotional state is characterized in terms of *mood* and *affect. Mood* refers to a pervasive and sustained emotion that tends to color one's perception of the world. It is described primarily in terms of the patient's subjective report. *Affect* is the outward manifestation of a person's feelings, emotional tone, or mood. It refers to how the patient feels at the moment, and is thus evaluated primarily in terms of the clinician's observations of the outward expression of emotions.

A patient's mood may be described in the following ways: depressed, gloomy, bored, empty, hopeless, anxious, excited, elated, hopeful, expansive, or suspicious.

Affect is described in terms of its intensity, quality, degree of variation, and appropriateness. There may be a deficiency in the expression of any emotion; this is described as flat or blunted affect, and is seen in some patients with schizophrenia or organic brain syndrome. Particular affects include anxiety, depression, fear, euphoria, elation, ecstasy, rage, anger, hostility, despondency, and worry.

Euphoria is an exaggerated feeling of physical and emotional well-being. It may be seen in manic states, organic mental disorders, and in drug-induced and toxic states. *Ecstasy* is an intense feeling of rapture and joy that may be seen in similar situations, as well as in acute psychotic exacerbations of schizophrenia.

The examiner notes the range of variation of affect over the course of the interview. Patients with labile affect exhibit sudden and marked shifts in emotional state; for example, between euphoria and tearful anguish. Lability of affect is characteristic of mania, but may be seem in a variety of psychotic states, and in organic brain syndromes. Depressed patients may show lability in the depressed end of the affective spectrum. In contrast, other patients show a *constricted* affect, with little or no shift in emotion during the interview. This is commonly seen in depressed patients, especially those with obsessive-compulsive character traits, who tend to restrain any displays of emotion.

Normally, a person would be expected to display a range or variation in emotions expressed during an in-depth interview, depending on the particular matters he is discussing at the moment. This is what is meant by the *appropriateness* of affect to the content of thought and speech. Patients with inappropriate affect, which is characteristic of schizophrenia and other psychoses, display emotions that are incongruent with the conversation's subject matter. An example is an individual who laughs to himself as he relates his history of serious medical problems.

Thought Processes

The interviewer notes the quality of associative processes, logic, and flow of ideas. In normal thought processes there is an orderly progression, so that one idea follows smoothly after another toward an identifiable goal. The interviewer is clear about what the patient is trying to say.

The terms used to describe abnormalities in thought processes refer to varying degrees of disruption and disorganization of this orderly flow of thoughts. Other terms refer to variations in the rate of thoughts and their expression.

Tangentiality refers to the patient's replying to a question in an oblique or irrelevant way. In the related phenomenon of *circumstantiality,* speech is indirect and is delayed in reaching its goal. There are many digressions regarding details that are of little significance to the point of the conversation. These disturbances can be fairly mild, occurring in persons who are especially anxious and have obsessional characteristics, but may also be seen in patients with more severe disturbances. A more severe loss in the logical flow of ideas is observed in *loose* associations in which the individual shifts from idea to idea without apparent logical connection. The interviewer may be able to surmise connecting links, but it requires considerable effort and imagination on his part to do so. The interviewer is able to follow the ideas for brief periods but many sudden shifts are encountered. *Incoherence* refers to a gross disorganization of speech and thought.

A number of particular thought disturbances have been described in schizophrenic patients, though none is pathognomic per se. *Word salad* is a mixture of words and phrases that lacks logical coherence. *Verbigeration* is the stereotyped and seemingly meaningless repetition of words and sentences, which is similar to *perseveration,* the tendency to emit the same verbal or motor response again and again to varied stimuli. *Echolalia* is the parrotlike repetition of overheard words or fragments of speech. These disturbances are seen in organic brain syndromes as well as in schizophrenia.

Another severe disturbance in the flow of thought is *blocking,* in which thought processes appear to cease entirely, as if the mind has gone blank. While this is most often described in schizophrenia, it is also observed in patients with marked anxiety, and many represent an unconscious avoidance of a distressing affect associated with a particular topic.

Flight of ideas is defined as verbal skipping from one idea to another. The ideas appear to be continuous but are fragmentary and determined by chance or temporal associations. This condition, which is characteristic of mania, seems to combine a marked acceleration of thought processes with loosening of associations. At the opposite extreme is *retardation* of thought processes, associated with slowing of speech, long pauses, and increased latency of responses. This is typical of severe depression.

Thought Content

Abnormalities of thought content include delusions, obsessions, preoccupations, and phobias. *Delusions* are false beliefs that are firmly held despite obvious evidence to the contrary. The beliefs are not consistent with the accepted beliefs of members of the individual's culture or subculture. A young man with schizophrenia was convinced that all members of the Masonic order were involved in a conspiracy to monitor his behavior and thwart his activities. This is an example of a *persecutory* or *paranoid* delusion. Others include delusions of grandeur, delusions of being controlled by an outside force, the feeling that thoughts are being inserted or withdrawn from one's mind, and *somatic delusions*.

Paranoid ideation refers to a marked suspiciousness, associated with the belief that one is being harassed or persecuted, that is not specific or intense enough to be considered delusional. Delusions are remarkable for their fixed nature and the avidity with which they are held by the individual. While common in schizophrenia, they can occur in any psychotic state, including organic brain syndromes.

In examining for delusions, the best evidence arises in the patient's own narrative. In the appropriate context, the interviewer may inquire more specifically about feelings of being controlled, harassed, and so forth. Persons without delusions will typically be puzzled by such questions, whereas those with some form of delusional thinking will often be sparked to further elaboration. Paranoid individuals, because of their suspicion and guardedness, are reluctant to reveal their paranoid delusions to the psychiatrist, and may successfully conceal them; repeated, skilled interviews will be required to elicit these ideas.

Obsessions are persistent, unwanted ideas or impulses that cannot be eliminated by logic or reason. While obsessions are generally considered to be neurotic symptoms, it is obvious that a severe obsession can border on the intensity of a psychotic delusion, and the two can be thought of as existing on a continuum. Obsessions often occur together with compulsive acts, as in obsessive–compulsive disorder. Obsession with guilt or evil may be seen in depression. Obsessive concern or preoccupation with physical health problems, out of proportion to actual physical illness, is called *hypochondriasis*. This can occur in many clinical settings, and ranges from a neurotic character trait to depression and schizophrenia. A *phobia* is an obsessive, persistent, unrealistic, intense fear of an object or situation. There are a large number of specific phobias, each with a Greek name. A few of the more common ones are *agoraphobia,* (the fear of leaving the familiar home setting), *claustrophobia* (fear of closed places), and *acrophobia* (fear of heights). It is important to note whether the patient has a single phobia or multiple ones.

It is critical to determine the presence or absence of *violent* ideation, that is, suicidal or homicidal thoughts. It is important to ask every patient about these matters, and there is no evidence to support the fear that such inquiry will suggest such an idea to a patient who had not thought of it. It is important to exercise tact and sensitivity in this area of questioning, ideally relating it to severe depressive or hostile thoughts the patient may have expressed. If the patient in any way confirms the presence of such thoughts, it is critical to explore them in depth. With respect to suicide, is there a plan? If so, what is it? Does the patient have the means to carry out the plan? Has he taken any steps toward carrying out the plan? Does he believe himself capable of such an act? Similar questioning is indicated if the patient mentions homicidal feelings; in particular, it is important to determine if there is an identifiable intended victim. These issues have major clinical and medicolegal ramifications. Any serious threat of violence on the part of the patient should be discussed immediately by the psychiatric trainee and a supervisor to determine the appropriate course of action. With respect to the impact of this type of in-depth discussion with the patient, it is likely that having the opportunity to talk about such frightening thoughts with a concerned physician will provide relief, lessen anxiety, and help the patient to arrive at a safer course of action.

Perception

An *illusion* is the misinterpretation of a real experience, typically visual, such as seeing human figures among clothes hanging in a closet at night. Illusions are common in toxic and other organic disorders and in schizophrenia. A *hallucination* is a false sensory perception in the absence of corresponding sensory stimuli. Hallucinations may involve any sensory modality: auditory, visual, olfactory, tactile, gustatory, and kinesthetic.

Auditory hallucinations, especially of voices, are common in schizophrenia, though they may occur in mania as well. Schizophrenic patients may hear voices talking about them, criticizing them, narrating their behavior, or giving them commands. Command hallucinations regarding violent acts are particularly worrisome to the patient. Hearing one's name called out loud is of limited significance as an isolated finding.

Visual hallucinations may occur in any type of psychoses, but suggest a toxic or drug-induced state. *Olfactory* (smell) and *gustatory* (taste) hallucinations may be seen in schizophrenia, but their presence should alert the clinician to possible temporal lobe disease, such as temporal lobe epilepsy. *Kinesthetic* hallucinations involve feelings of movement or altered bodily awareness.

Hallucinations of touch (tactile) occur primarily in toxic states such as delirium tremens and in cocaine and amphetamine abuse. *Formication* refers to the hallucinatory sensation of insects crawling under the skin.

The interviewer evaluates perceptual disturbances not only by asking the patient about them, but also by inferring their presence from the patient's behavior. Patients with auditory hallucinations may be noted to speak back to their "voices" or respond to them in other ways; an individual with formication may be noted to pick at his skin in an effort to remove imaginary insects.

Other perceptual disturbances include depersonalization and derealization, referring to extreme feelings of detachment from oneself or from one's environment.

In reporting perceptual disturbances, abnormalities actually present during the interview should be distinguished from previously occurring symptoms not currently present; these should be indicated in the history.

Orientation

The patient is tested for orientation to person (himself and the interviewer), place, time (month, day, year, approximate time of day), and situation (*i.e.*, the purpose and nature of the interview). This information is critical because disorientation strongly suggests organic brain dysfunction, especially of an acute nature, and its presence would influence the focus of further investigation. Even patients who are markedly psychotic as part of a schizophrenic illness will generally remain oriented to person, place, and time. The presence of disorientation to one's own identity suggests advanced neurologic dysfunction or hysteria.

Inquiry into orientation, as well as the other formal tests of cognitive function discussed below, should be conducted in a respectful but unapologetic manner. Comments like "I'm going to ask you some silly questions" are not helpful in putting the patient at ease. More useful is an introduction like "I'm going to ask you some routine questions to check out your memory and thinking." One should not hesitate to evaluate orientation and cognitive functions just because a patient is neatly dressed, articulate, or socially functional. Serious diagnostic errors can result; furthermore, a documentation of normal function at one point in time serves as a useful baseline for comparison, should cognitive problems arise later.

Cognitive or Intellectual Functions

Memory. Memory is assessed under different temporal categories, ranging from remote to immediate.

Remote memory is reflected in the patient's recall of events from years past. This function is usually preserved even when more recent memory functions are impaired, as in dementia. To assess remote and other types of memory, the interviewer needs to have information to independently corroborate the patient's report.

Recent past memory refers to events of the past few months, while *recent* memory refers to the day or two before the interview. For this category, it is useful to ask what the patient had for lunch the day before, how he came to the interview, and so forth.

Immediate retention and *recall* are tested by naming three objects and asking the patient to repeat them immediately and again after 5 minutes. The patient is also asked to repeat six digits forward and in reverse, and his responses are recorded.

Memory is typically impaired in organic brain syndromes; if orientation is intact, a diagnosis of dementia or amnestic disorder is suggested.

General Information. The general information assessment, along with vocabulary, reflects general intelligence. Much can be inferred during the general history, but standard questions are helpful for comparison. The patient is asked to list the last five presidents starting with the current one, and some basic geography questions. The patient's general information, like calculations and abstractions, is influenced by his educational and cultural background.

Calculations. The patient is asked to do basic arithmetic calculations; in performing *serial sevens,* he is asked to serially subtract sevens from 100, reporting each result; which tests concentration as well as arithmetic ability.

Abstract Thought. Here the patient is asked to describe similarities and differences between objects. A simple example is given first to illustrate the task. For example, "If red and blue are both colors, what have lions and mice in common?" The patient is asked to interpret some common proverbs, such as "Don't cry over spilled milk." A typical *concrete* response would be, "It's already spilled." Schizophrenic patients may give concrete or *bizarre* responses, such as "It might turn to blood." Concrete responses are also typical in patients with organic brain disease.

Other tasks that are sensitive to organic brain dysfunction include asking the patient to read aloud, to write down dictated material, to follow two- and three-step commands, and to draw and copy simple figures. These tests are generally employed only when the more general evaluation suggests organicity.

Insight. *Insight* refers to the patient's awareness and understanding of his difficulties. This can range from total denial of illness or problems to acknowledgment of distress but denial of the need for help, to acceptance of the need for help, all the way to an awareness of the underlying causes of the symptoms. The interviewer will get a sense of the patient's level of insight throughout the interview; it is also useful to ask specifically about his own ideas and understanding of the problem.

Judgment. *Judgment* refers to the patient's ability to evaluate new situations, anticipate consequences of actions, and to function adaptively. The most useful basis for assessing judgment is to consider the patient's recent behavior, including the circumstances under which he came in for evaluation, and how he is handling the situation. Of secondary importance in assessment of judgment is to ask the patient how he would handle various hypothetical situations, such as finding a stamped, sealed, addressed envelope in the street.

The clinical relevance of insight and judgment is highlighted by the following two cases of schizophrenia. One patient was brought to the psychiatrist at the insistence of family members because he had stopped taking his medication, was responding to auditory hallucinations, and was threatening his family because he believed that they were involved in a conspiracy against him. A second patient with the same illness came to the clinic by bus and reported that he was experiencing an increase in his auditory hallucinations, suspicious feelings, and sleep disturbance as a result of missing his last scheduled injection of depot antipsychotic drug. He requested medication to help him control his symptoms. The clinical management of these two patients would be very different, not because of any difference in symptoms or diagnosis, but because of their marked difference in insight and judgment.

In concluding the mental status examination it is worth making some judgment as to the patient's reliability as a historian.

Physical Evaluation

All patients presenting with significant psychiatric complaints should receive a thorough medical evaluation, including a review of medical history, review of systems, and complete physical examination. This is imperative for several reasons. First, physical diseases can present with psychiatric symptoms. A number of studies suggest that in roughly one fifth of psychiatric patients, a physical disorder is causal, both in typical "organic brain syndromes," such as CNS infection producing delirium and psychosis, and in "functional" psychiatric disorders without cognitive impairment, such as pancreatic cancer or endocrine diseases presenting as major depression. Thus, the absence of cognitive dysfunction does not rule out a physical causative factor. Second, physical illness can coexist with and aggravate psychiatric illness. There is a dangerous tendency on the part of medical professionals to ascribe all physical complaints to a psychogenic origin once a patient has received a psychiatric label. The stress of physical illness may be a precipitant of psychiatric illness, such as a patient who develops severe anxiety and depression as a consequence of ischemic heart disease. Third, many psychiatric patients receive physical treatments such as drugs or electroconvulsive therapy (ECT). The use of such treatments can be complicated or even contraindicated by the presence of certain physical illnesses or medical treatments. From the perspective of the biopsychosocial model, the distinction between "medical" and "psychiatric" illnesses is arbitrary and artificial, and thus any patient with significant impairment requires both thorough psychological and physical evaluation.

In some situations the psychiatrist will perform the physical examination personally. This is typically true in inpatient psychiatric units and often in emergency room settings. In other situations, particularly in general outpatient settings, the psychiatrist will obtain a consultation from a colleague in internal medicine, family medicine, or pediatrics. It is nevertheless the psychiatrist's responsibility to ensure that the medical evaluation is completed promptly and to integrate the findings into the overall assessment of the patient.

Laboratory Studies

The psychiatrist uses the laboratory in a number of ways in the evaluation of patients. First, laboratory studies may be used in a screening fashion as an aid in detecting physical abnormalities. There is no universally agreed-on set of screening studies for all newly presenting psychiatric patients, particularly in the outpatient setting. For adults requiring hospital admission, however, a typical screening admission evaluation includes a complete blood count with differential, erythrocyte sedimentation rate, electrolytes, glucose, serum creatinine, blood urea nitrogen, calcium, magnesium, total protein and albumin, liver function tests, serologic test for syphilis, chest x-ray, urinalysis, and electrocardiogram. While the measurement of serum thyroxine has been used as a screening test in the past, it has been found to yield an excessive number of false positive elevations in acutely admitted psychiatric patients, so that it is better reserved as a specific test when indicated on clinical grounds. In some settings, the drug or toxic screen (blood, urine, and gastric aspirate) may be useful in a screening approach.

A second use of laboratory studies is to investigate questions raised in the clinical evaluation. For example, when the history or mental status examination suggest a diagnosis of dementia, additional studies are indicated. These include a brain CT scan, electroencephalogram (EEG), lumbar puncture (with determination of CSF cell count, differential, protein, glucose, VDRL, cytology, cryptococcal antigen, Gram's stain, and bacterial and fungal cultures), serum B_{12} and folate, and thyroid panel (T_4, RT_3U, and TSH). When the clinical situation raises the possibility of intoxication, the drug or toxin screen is necessary. This is true in cases of psychosis, agitation, and confusion. The samples must be obtained quickly for the maximum yield, and the ordering physician should communicate directly with the laboratory personnel to see that the correct samples are obtained and to ensure that the substances in question are investigated. The blood alcohol level is useful in cases where alcohol intoxication is suspected but is not confirmed by the clinical history or examination. An EEG is essential in cases where a seizure disorder could account for the psychiatric presentation, as in the patient with episodic bizarre behavior.

The third use of the laboratory is in conjunction with the use of drugs or ECT. Baseline tests may be used to assess the capacity to metabolize or excrete a drug, as in testing of hepatic function prior to tricyclic antidepressant use, or assessment of renal function prior to administration of lithium carbonate. Baseline tests are also used to assess systems that may be adversely affected by drug administration, as in the pretricyclic baseline ECG, the prelithium thyroid panel, and the blood count obtained before starting carbamazepine. Plasma drug levels are used to monitor the adequacy of drug dosage and to avoid toxicity, as in the measurement of lithium and tricyclic levels. The specific applications of these tests are discussed in detail in connection with the specific agents (see Chapter 23).

A fourth area of laboratory studies in the psychiatric evaluation is in the use of biological markers for specific psychiatric illnesses, aside from the typical "organic" disorders. There is current interest in the use of such markers in the diagnosis of affective disorders, particularly in using neuroendocrine tests such as the dexamethasone suppression test (DST) and the thyrotropin-releasing-hormone (TRH) stimulation test, as well as the sleep EEG. The exact clinical application of these tests is under investigation (see Chapter 2).

Psychological Testing

Psychological tests are usually performed by clinical psychologists, and are used to answer the same types of questions as the clinical psychiatric interview. Psychological testing can be used to assess personality, descriptive psychopathology, emotional and thought processes, and cognitive functions. Psychodynamic conflict areas can also be studies. Because these tests are administered in a systematic format, the results can be compared and standardized for large numbers of individuals. This allows comparison of the individual patient's responses to those of populations of patients and normals, thus enhancing the value of the tests as objective measures.

Psychiatrists vary in their approach to the use of psychological testing services in the evaluation of patients. It is important for the psychiatrist to be aware of what psychological services are available and to be familiar with the particular expertise of local psychologists in order to make the best use of what they offer. Psychological testing may not add a great deal to the information gained in a skilled clinical interview in the evaluation of personality and psychopathology in a straight-forward case, but it may be very helpful in clarifying confusing situations or in providing corroborating evidence, if that is needed for some administrative or legal matter. Psychological testing is very helpful in the assessment of intelligence and in the detailed evaluation of cognitive deficits.

In most cases, psychological tests are obtained by consulting a clinical psychologist rather than ordering tests directly. It is imperative that the psychiatrist requesting testing discuss the consultation directly with the psychologist in order to clarify the specific questions being asked and to get an idea of how the psychologist will approach the problem. This helps the psychiatrist to understand what he can realistically expect from the results, and to prepare the patient appropriately for the testing; and it also helps the psychologist to focus his evaluation in order to provide the most useful information. The psychologist generally performs a *battery* of tests, and a clinical interview; in the written report he synthesizes the findings, emphasizing those points relevant to the requesting psychiatrist's questions.

While the details of testing are beyond the scope of this chapter, the psychiatrist does need to be familiar with the basic types of psychological tests and the information that they can provide. In *projective* tests, a standard series of ambiguous stimuli or tasks are presented to the patient, whose responses are then recorded. Examples include the well-known Rorschach inkblot test, in which the patient reports what he sees in a series of ambiguous visual forms; and the Thematic Apperception Test (TAT), in which the patient is asked to make up a story based on a picture shown to him. These tests, in eliciting the patient's subjective responses, reveal information about conflicts, fantasies, and fears, and are useful in developing a psychodynamic understanding of the patient, and in initiating psychotherapy. They are less useful for highly quantitative analysis, but may become more useful because there have been recent developments in the categorization and standardization of responses to the Rorschach test.

Objective tests are highly structured and standardized, and generally provide quantitative scores on a number of scales. Examples include the Minnesota Multiphasic Personality Inventory (MMPI) and the Wechsler Adult Intelligence Scale (WAIS). The MMPI is a widely used inventory or series of standardized questions. It was developed in the 1940s, and has been administered and studied extensively in the years since. It consists of several hundred questions, each calling for a *yes, no* or *cannot answer* response, which the patient records on an answer sheet. It can be scored either using a mechanical template or computer. The results are reported according to scores on nine scales: hypochondriasis, depression, hysteria, psychopathic deviate, masculinity–femininity, paranoia, psychasthenia, schizophrenia, and social introversion. There are also scales reflecting the validity of the patient's responses. The psychologist interprets the pattern of scores on these scales, as well as on a number of subscales, in comparison with previously reported standard data, to describe the overall profile, and what it suggests about the individual's personality or psychopathology.

The WAIS is an objective test of intellectual function that is divided into a verbal scale and a performance scale. The verbal scale consists of 6 subtests: information, comprehension, arithmetic, similarities, digit span, and vocabulary; while the performance scale includes digit symbol, picture completion, block design, picture arrangement, and object assembly subtests. Results are reported as *verbal IQ*, *performance IQ*, and *full scale IQ*, in which *IQ* refers to *intelligence quotient*, defined as mental age/chronological age × 100. The mean IQ is thus 100. Of particular significance to the psychiatrist is a discrepancy between *v*erbal IQ and *p*erformance IQ of greater than 10, which suggests organic brain dysfunction. IQ determinations can also be useful clinically when evaluating the degree of intellectual deficiency in a patient, or in assessing an individual's capacity of participating in psychotherapy.

Another area in which testing is clinically helpful in the psychiatric evaluation is neuropsychological assessment. Here, specialized tests are used to assess specific cognitive functions in patients with suspected or known brain damage. The most widely used neuropsychological instrument is the Halstead–Reitan Battery, which is used to assess such functions as formation and flexibility of concepts, learning and memory, and visual—motor organization. The neuropsychological evaluation, which requires consideration expertise on the part of the examiner, is useful in detecting subtle degrees of cognitive dysfunction and in assessing particular strengths and deficits in patients with known brain damage, which is helpful in planning rehabilitative programs.

The Diagnostic Formulation

In order to be clinically useful, the findings of the psychiatric history, mental status examination, physical evaluation, and specialized studies must be reported in a clear, well-organized, and legible form. The report should list the specific sources of information (*e.g.*, interviews of patient, patient's mother, teacher, review of old records) and an estimate of their reliability.

Having reported the information gained in the evaluation, the psychiatrist must then use his clinical knowledge and experience to integrate the data into a meaningful diagnostic formulation. It is important to separate clearly the observations and information, which are to be reported under History and Examination, from diagnostic impressions, which are to be discussed in the formulation. The diagnostic assessment needs to take into account the interaction of the various psychological, biological, behavioral, and social factors in the case, as advocated in the biopsychosocial model. The multiaxial diagnostic system proposed in the

American Psychiatric Association's Diagnostic and Statistical Manual, Third Edition (DSM-III) embodies this model in its five axes: Axis I is used to list major psychiatric disorders, such as schizophrenia, alcoholism, and major depression. Axis II is used to characterize personality traits or disorders; Axis III is used to list physical disorders; Axis IV is used to rate the severity of and to discuss the patient's current psychosocial stressors; and Axis V is used to estimate the patient's overall level of adaptive functioning, particularly its highest level during the preceding year. If one avoids the tendency to use the five axes simply to list diagnoses, and instead uses them as a guide to facilitate thinking about the case in a comprehensive manner, they can be of great value. The assessment, then, needs to include a written discussion in paragraph form, in addition to the enumeration of diagnoses. As in the case in general medical diagnosis, one should include a discussion of the differential diagnostic possibilities, and a rationale for the particular diagnoses reached. In using the DSM-III system, multiple diagnoses are allowed in Axes I, II, and III; although certain diagnostic combinations are not permitted, due to the hierarchy of diagnoses. It should be emphasized that, given the vagaries of psychiatric diagnosis, a definitive conclusion cannot always be reached after one or even several diagnostic interviews and examinations. The discussion will then simply have to take into account the various possibilities, and outline means for further investigation. It is only from an organized and comprehensive diagnostic assessment that a complete and meaningful treatment plan can be developed.

Bibliography

American Psychiatric Association: Diagnostic and Statistical Manual of Mental Disorders, 3rd ed. Washington, DC, 1980

American Psychiatric Association: Psychiatric Glossary, 5th ed. Boston, Little, Brown, 1980

Engel GL: The need for a new medical model: A challenge for biomedicine. Science 196:129, 1977

Hoffman RS, Koran LM: Detecting physical illness in patients with mental disorders. Psychosomatics 25:654, 1984

Kolb L, Brodie HKH: Modern Clinical Psychiatry, 10th ed. Philadelphia, WB Saunders, 1982

Leff JP, Isaacs AD: Psychiatric Examination in Clinical Practice. Oxford, Blackwell Scientific Publications, 1978

Mackinnon RA: Psychiatric interview, history and mental status examination. In Kaplan HI, Freedan AM, Sadock BJ (eds): Comprehensive Textbook of Psychiatry, 3rd ed, pp 895–919. Baltimore, Williams & Wilkins, 1980

Nicholi AM: The Harvard Guide to Modern Psychiatry, pp 3–40. Cambridge, Massacusetts, 1978

Spratt DI, Pont A, Miller MB, et al: Hyperthyroxinemia in patients with acute psychiatric disorders. Am J Med 73:41, 1982

Walker JI: Psychiatric Emergencies: Intervention and Resolution. Philadelphia, JB Lippincott, 1983

Weiss JL: The clinical use of psychological tests. In Nicholi A (ed): The Harvard Guide to Modern Psychiatry, pp 41–58. Cambridge, Massachusetts, Harvard University Press, 1978

Part II
The Clinical Syndromes

Jacqueline J. Maus

6 Schizophrenia

Schizophrenia has been described as a conglomeration of symptomatology and signs. It has vastly different manifestations, multiple considerations in etiology, and a wide variety of treatments. The following chapter will briefly discuss the history of this pervasive mental illness and discuss its epidemiology. The clinical manifestations of the various types of schizophrenia will be described, with diagnostic protocols and differential diagnoses provided. The hypothesized etiologies will be covered, concluding with the prescribed treatment modalities available today.

History

Schizophrenia has been described throughout the ages, with the interpretation and acceptance of the disease varying markedly. As early as 1400 BC, Hindu authors wrote of their mentally ill population as being gluttonous, filthy, and wild. The next 2500 years demonstrated a perpetuation of the superstitious tales regarding schizophrenics. Portrayed as evil souls, the schizophrenics were embued with incredible powers and were worshipped; or considered consorts of the devil, and tortured and murdered. The witch hunts that occurred during the Renaissance were postulated to be triggered by fear and loathing of the mentally ill. It was not until the early 1500s with Pinel and Weyer that schizophrenia was widely considered anything beyond the deranged soul, meriting at best life-long imprisonment under unspeakable conditions. Weyer and Pinel were the primary investigators for progressive social reform and "moral treatment" of the mentally ill, recommending improved maintenance facilities and less decadent modes of treatment.

In the early 1800s, neurology, as a subspecialty of medicine, moved to the forefront in its description and treatment of the mentally ill. It was a time of focusing on scientific observation, systematization, and classification. Neurological symptoms were grouped into syndromes, and neurological lesions were postulated as being etiologic in schizophrenia.

Morel first coined the phrase *dementia praecox* in 1857 to describe those psychoses with a poor prognosis, terminating in incurable deterioration; *praecox* referred to the early onset of the disorder. Kraepelin expanded on the systematization of descriptive psychiatry, focusing also on dementia praecox; he posited an organic basis for schizophrenia, speculating that an unknown metabolite leads to brain damage, and hence schizophrenia. He accurately described the progressive deterioration in the life of a schizophrenic. Consideration of schizophrenia as a medical disease was also emphasized, with a concomitant physical syndrome and defective course. He considered dementia praecox to be a disease of the cerebral cortex, with a tendency for deterioration, associated with physical stigmata. He described people with "mental illness from youth," with clear consciousness, developmental delay, problems with memory, loss of goal directedness, inappropriate affect, and physical stigmata such as choreic movements, smacking lips, and athetoid motions. He was one of the first to divide schizophrenia into subtypes: hebephrenic (characterized by an inappropriate affect), catatonic (often manifested with psychomotor retardation), paranoid (feelings that others are out to harm or discredit one) and simple (psychoses without the aforementioned overlays).

Bleuler first introduced the term *schizophrenia* in 1921, to replace the phrase *dementia praecox,* because he had observed that not all psychoses terminate in dementia, and not all initiate in early childhood. Under the influence of Freud, and subscribing to the power of the unconscious, Bleuler focused on the unconscious bizarre symbolic ideation often demonstrated by schizophrenics. He felt that schizophrenia is manifested with the "four A's": loose associations, blunted affect, ambivalence, and autism. More recently, Kurt Schneider delineated his first-rank symptoms of schizophrenia, which focused more on hallucinations, delusions, and thought disorganization.

Since the 1920s, the focus of the study of schizophrenia has vascillated between environmental or biological etiologies, with most of the genetic and family studies performed in the 1970s, and biochemical neurotransmitter studies that are continuing to date. The inevitable pendulum in psychiatry has most recently swung to biological descriptions and explanations of schizophrenia; but pendula are not stationary, and someday the focus may swing to a more intermediate position that incorporates both environmental and biological input.

Epidemiology

The *incidence* of a disease is the number of new cases discovered or manifested within a given time frame. The *prevalence* of a disease is the total number of existing cases within a given population. The incidence of schizophrenia in the United

States is 0.05%, or approximately 100,000 new cases a year. The prevalence of schizophrenia in the United States is about 1%, or close to 2 million people (not including those people with schizophrenia spectrum disease). No statistically significant sex differences have been noted, but there have been noted increases in the number of schizophrenics in the lower socioeconomic status (SES) populations, with considerable controversy surrounding the explanation for these differences. There are more nonwhites than white patients with schizophrenia. Transculturally, the figures vary dramatically, undoubtedly depending on diagnostic criteria, acceptability of schizophrenia traits within a given culture, extant support systems, and availability of treatment facilities.

Manifestations

As noted above, the first systematic descriptions of schizophrenia were offered by Bleuler and Kraepelin. Bleuer elucidated the four A's:

Association: looseness in the thought process with bizarre symbolism attached to the phrases, characterized by illogical thoughts. The thinking is without goals or purpose. For example, in response to the question, "How are north and west alike?" (correct answer—they are both directions), one schizophrenic patient answered, "All of north and half of west are moving in the same direction. Go west, young man, go west."
Autistic thinking: self-centered, regressive thinking coupled with withdrawal from reality. Frequently, schizophrenics are noted to live socially isolated lives, with very poor social skills and interpersonal relationships characterized by coldness and aloofness.
Affect: inappropriate affect, where the affect is incongruent with the emotional state of the patient. For example, Mr. H, a 49-year-old paranoid schizophrenic, laughingly reporting his desire to strangle his neighbor.
Ambivilence: contradictions in the thoughts of the patient

Bleuler also focused on other peculiarities in the looseness of association of schizophrenics, including irregularities in the association of time, stereotype (perseverating ideas), echolalia (the patient echoes what is said to him), poverty of ideas, bizarre associations, exaggerations, and flight of ideas. He also described thought deprivation, thought withdrawal (believing that someone is able to remove one's own thoughts), and thought blockage, where the flow of thoughts is disrupted. Bleuler attached much less importance to the occurrence of hallucinations and delusions.

Since Bleuler's time, the overriding descriptions of schizophrenia identify certain common subjective experiences, including the difficulty the patient has in maintaining organized thinking (with blockage or flooding of the thought processes), the patient's inability to organize sensory or emotional input or output, and his problems integrating perceptions with ideation.

Schneider described his first-rank symptoms to include:

Audible thoughts
Voices disagreeing or debating over the patient
Voices commenting on the patient's actions

Sensations being imposed on the patient's body by outside forces
Thought withdrawal
Thought insertion
Thought broadcasting (the ability to project one's thoughts into another's mind)
"Made" feelings
"Made" impulses
"Made" acts (All three deal with the perception that his own feelings, impulses, and actions are not his; that they are being imposed on him.)
Delusional perceptions

It should be noted that according to one study using Schneiderian criteria, 57% of those patients with a diagnosis of schizophrenia had one or more of the criteria (40% did not); Schneider's criteria hence are considered to have general diagnostic applicability, but are not pathnognomonic for schizophrenia.

More recently, the constructs of Bleuler, Kraepelin, and Schneider have been consolidated into the DSM-III (*Diagnostic and Statistical Manual of Mental Disorders,* 3rd ed, of American Psychiatric Association), which list the following criteria that are thought to be more descriptive than Schneider's elucidation of schizophrenia:

Diagnostic Criteria for a Schizophrenia Disorder[1]

A. At least one of the following during a phase of the illness:
   1. Bizarre delusions (content is patently absurd and has no possible basis in fact), such as delusions of being controlled, thought broadcasting, though insertion, or thought withdrawal
   2. Somatic, grandiose, religious, nihilistic, or other delusions without persecutory or jealous content
   3. Delusions with persecutory or jealous content if accompanied by hallucinations of any type
   4. Auditory hallucinations in which either one voice maintains a running commentary on the individual's behavior or thoughts, or two or more voices converse with each other
   5. Auditory hallucinations on several occasions with content of more than one or two words, having no apparent relation to depression or elation
   6. Incoherence, marked loosening of associations, markedly illogical thinking, or marked poverty of content of speech if associated with at least one of the following: (a) blunted, flat, or inappropriate affect, (b) delusions or hallucination, (c) catatonic or other grossly disorganized behavior
B. Deterioration from a previous level of functioning in such areas as work, social relations, and self-care
C. Duration: continuous signs of the illness for at least six months at some time during the person's life, with some signs of the illness at present. The six-months period must include an active phase during which there were symptoms from A, with or without a prodromal or residual phase, as defined below.

Residual Phase: persistence, following the active phase of the illness, of at least two of the symptoms noted below, not due to a disturbance in mood or to a substance use disorder

Prodromal or Residual Symptoms: (1) Social isolation or withdrawal; (2) marked impairment in role functioning as wage-earner, student, or homemaker; (3) markedly peculiar behavior (*e.g.*, collecting garbage, talking to self in public, or hoarding food); (4) marked impairment in personal hygiene and grooming: (5) blunted, flat or inappropriate affect; (6) digressive, vague, over-elaborate, circumstantial, or metaphorical speech; (7) odd or bizarre ideation, or magical thinking (*e.g.*, superstitiousness, clairvoyance, telepathy, "sixth sense," "Others can feel my feelings," overvalued ideas, ideas of reference)

D. The full depressive or manic syndrome (criteria *A* and *B* of major depressive or manic episode), if present, developed after any psychotic symptoms, or was brief in duration relative to the duration of the psychotic symptoms in *A*.
E. Onset of prodromal or active phase of the illness before age 45
F. Not due to any organic mental disorder or mental retardation

Diagnostic criteria have also been determined for several different types of schizophrenia:

Disorganized Type: A type of schizophrenia in which there is (1) frequent incoherence, (2) absence of systematized delusions, (3) blunted, inappropriate, or silly affect.

Catatonic Type: A type of schizophrenia dominated by any of the following: (1) catatonic stupor (marked decrease in reactivity to environment or reduction of spontaneous movements and activity) or mutism, (2) catatonic negativism (an apparently motiveless resistence to all instructions or attempts to be moved), (3) catatonic rigidity (maintenance of a rigid position against efforts to be moved), (4) catatonic excitement (excited motor activity, apparently purposeless and not influenced by external stimuli), (5) catatonic posturing (voluntary assumption of inappropriate or bizarre posture)

Paranoid Type: A type of schizophrenia dominated by one or more of the following: (1) persecutory delusions, (2) grandiose delusions, (3) delusional jealousy, (4) hallucinations with persecutory or grandiose content

Undifferentiated Type: A type of schizophrenia in which: (1) there are prominent delusions, hallucinations, incoherence, or grossly disorganized behavior; or (2) the illness does not meet the criteria for any of the previously listed types, or meets the criteria for more than one

Recently, a select group of investigators has divided schizophrenia into different types of subgroups: those with *positive* symptoms, or with hallucinations and delusions, and those with *negative* symptoms, including a lack of goal-directedness, blunted affect, and a longer duration of illness. It is hoped that by focusing on the positive and negative manifestations as target symptoms for treatment, we might be better able to discuss those symptoms that are best treated biologically with medications, and those more aptly suited for treatment with therapy (individual, group, and milieu).

It might prove helpful at this time to present some typical (albeit by no means standard) findings in the mental status exam, to elaborate on the aforementioned criteria. Let us demonstrate with Mr. Smith, who is presenting with his first psychotic break:

> ☐ Mr. Smith is a 28-year-old white man who requested to see the psychiatrist in the emergency room. His clothes were disheveled, his hair was askew, and he admitted to "living on the streets" for about four weeks prior to admission.
> *Cooperation:* He was shy, noncommunicative, and hesitant; and had poor eye contact.
> *Speech:* Although rate and rhythm were normal, speech was rarely spontaneous.
> *Motor:* Some psychomotor agitation was noted, particularly when he described his voices.
> *Mood:* "I'm OK; I'm a bit scared, but I'm OK."
> *Affect:* Constricted
> *Thought process:* No tangentiality, circumstantiality, or flight of ideas (FOI) was noted. Looseness of associations (LOA) was present (*e.g.*, "You know, there I was under the bridge . . . ridge . . . midge . . . Madge, my wife, left about two years ago; then I turned left. No, wait! It was right; right, it's OK by me.")
> *Thought content:* No suicidal or homicidal ideation was present, except that he was very angry with his voices: "If I could kill them, I would." He denied neurovegetative signs of depression, except that he was afraid to sleep. He denied manic symptoms. He did report feeling anxious much of the time, particularly regarding the voices and being with other people: "I'm no good with people, we can't seem to get along, not even my family." He did report auditory hallucinations, with two or three voices that were constantly commenting on his behavior, occasionally criticizing and debating his actions. He denied thought blockage, but believed that others could push thoughts into his brain or pull them out. "My mind is like taffy, push and pull, push and pull, bull, full, I am full . . ." He had fleeting paranoid ideation: "Sometimes I'm afraid of others on the streets; no, no one specific."
> *Cognitive functioning:* He was awake, alert, and oriented to person, place, and time. His sensorium was clear; and he was able to spell *world* forward and backwards. He was unable to perform serial sevens, but he had only completed the seventh grade. Slow, accurate serial threes and simple calculations were performed. He expressed very concrete thoughts: ("Grass" proverb: "Grass is greener on the other side? Well, that means that you walk to the fence, crawl over, and look at the grass there."). His judgment was intact, but insight poor: "My worst problem is I don't have anywhere to sleep."

Be aware that the case of Mr. Smith is but one of many scenarios that could present with the initial mental status exam of a schizophrenic. They are often typified as being shy and retiring, but they may be outgoing and gregarious or outraged and thundering. They may either demonstrate catatonia (significantly decreased motor activity), or uncontrolled agitation. Their speech may flow fluently, or it may manifest their social ineptness. Typically, their affect is thought to be constricted (many speak of flattened, immobile facies), but agitated schizophrenics can have extraordinarily labile affects. Thought processes are most frequently laden with loose association, and thought content may represent a spectrum, including auditory and visual hallucinations, delusions, thought insertion (TI), thought withdrawal (TW), and thought blockage (TB). Cognitive functioning is usually relatively intact, unless the patient is grossly psychotic, distorting orientation. Memory and calculation performances may be slowed, but are generally accurate. Proverbs are frequently concrete or bizarre, with the patient demonstrating impaired judgment. Insight might be well-worded but often has no impact on the patient's behavior or prognosis.

Course

Studies have shown that a statistically significant proportion of schizophrenics are born in the late winter and early spring months. There is no predominantly "typical" child that eventually becomes a schizophrenic, but it has been noted that many children that ultimately become schizophrenic often manifest schizotypal or schizoidal premorbid personality characteristics. Patients will initially present any time from their late teens to their sixties, but most commonly presenting in their early twenties. Occasionally there will be only one psychotic episode, but most schizophrenics experience multiple psychotic episodes in their lives. It has been postulated that this frequency makes it difficult for them to maintain satisfactory interpersonal relationships, and exacerbates work problems, leading to "downward mobilization," a drifting into the lower socioeconomic sector. There are, however, a significant portion of schizophrenics who respond well to medication, are compliant, and are able to lead relatively happy, healthy lives.

The prognosis of schizophrenia can be grim. Many become progressively worse and disabled, with more intense and frequent episodes occurring as they age. A "burned out" schizophrenic is hypothesized to be one who often demonstrates several schizotypal and schizoidal tendencies, with no acute exacerbations of previously expressed first-rank symptoms. The best prognostic signs include acute onset of the disease, married status, well-preserved affect, relative youth, and short duration of illness. More malignant prognostic signs include self-mutilation, total loss of affect, olfactory hallucinations (particularly if genital in nature), gustatory hallucinations, chronic onset, middle or old age, and gross distortion of thought organization.

The case examples that follow illustrate the different types of schizophrenia possible, while delineating common threads, such as the predominance of early onset, the oft-cited premorbid personality (personality structure of the patient prior to the first outright psychotic episode), the infrequent occurrence of complete remission, and the inevitable progressive deterioration of the schizophrenic's life.

☐ *Undifferentiated schizophrenia.* Mr. P is a 28-year-old black man undergoing his fifth psychiatric admission in 10 years. His family reported that he had never moved beyond the confines of the family unit's physical environs, remaining isolated from any friendships and relatives more distant than the nuclear family. He had performed adequately in high school, with the exception of some magical thinking, feeling occasionally as if others were placing thoughts in his head, and that he could read other people's minds. He suffered his first psychotic break in his first year of military service, which was immediately after high school. He characterized this as a time during which he felt distant from everyone. It was during this time period that he noted the beginning of his auditory hallucinations, which consisted of two or three people talking about him, commenting on his work. He was discharged from the army and treated intermittently at Veterans Administration hospitals, but continued to remain socially isolated, worked odd jobs, and occasionally heard voices. His chief complaint at the last admission was, "The voices are telling me I'm doing everything wrong."

Paranoid schizophrenia. Mr. Z is a 38-year-old white man who was brought to the emergency room. He s a tall, lanky man, with bright eyes that darted from the interviewer to his sister and back. He perched on his chair, and alternated between belligerence and hesitance in his answers. He reported anger at his family for bringing him in, and said that they were planning to take his home away. This has been validated by the voices he heard, taunting him outside his home. He had felt that everyone on the street was talking about him, and heard messages from the phone wires and trees confirming this. His family had brought him in after they broke through the barricade Mr. Z had placed in front of his living-room door. This was Mr. Z's eighth admission since his first paranoid presentation (with very similar symptoms) at age 20. He had stopped taking his medications approximately two months prior to admission.

Disorganized schizophrenia. Ms. A is a 47-year-old white woman brought in from the local indigent halfway house, where she had become progressively more agitated and incoherent. The administrator reported that she had had to be restrained when they found her babbling in the bathroom, and scratching figures of hearts on the wall and herself. When asked why she had been brought to the emergency room, she began to laugh and rock while she described her fantasies of killing her six beloved cats. She then jumped from the chair and skipped around the room, singing "A tisket, a tasket," flinging her arms as if she were distributing flowers.

Catatonic schizophrenia. A 28-year-old male has maintained an uncomfortable crouched position in the corner of his hospital room for several years, except for a brief daily walk.

Differential Diagnoses

In psychiatry, as in every other specialty of medicine, it is imperative to approach a patient while keeping in mind a framework for differential diagnoses. Of course, prior to speculation of diagnosis, the patient must receive a thorough, complete history and physical, including a mental status exam, and routing labs. Information regarding family history of psychiatric illness and the patient's past hospitalizations and response to prior medications are important data to obtain.

There are a vast number of possibilities to explain a patient's psychotic behaviors. For ease and efficiency consider the following differential of etiologies, that can easily be applied to any psychiatric disorder: (1) organic disorders, (2) other functional psychotic disorders, (3) affective disorders, (4) personality disorders, (5) neurotic disorders, and (6) adjustment (or acute situational) disorders.

Organic Disorders

Possible Organic Bases for Psychotic Behavior briefly outlines a differential diagnosis of schizophrenia in terms of possible organic disorders. If there is any suspected organic basis for psychotic behavior, further evaluation beyond routine admission labs and radiographic studies is imperative. For example, beyond the routine complete blood count (CBC) and chemistry panel (SMA-20), one might want to include thyroid function tests, heavy metals screen, drug urine screen, blood screen (for magnesium, zinc, and copper), B_{12} and folate levels, arterial blood gases, blood cultures, computed tomography (CT) scans, electroencephalogram (EEG), and lumbar puncture

Possible Organic Bases for Psychotic Behavior

Drugs: cocaine, amphetamines, psychomimetics, alcohol, barbiturates, steroids, anticholinergics

Deficiencies or Metabolic Problems: deficiencies in B_{12}, folate, thiamine, and niacin; decreased O_2, hyperthyroid, hypothyroid, Cushing's disease, Addison's disease, porphyria, abnormal electrolyte levels

Vascular: collagen vascular diseases, atrioventricular malformations, intracranial hemorrhages

Infections: encephalitis, meningitis, SBE, kuru, Jakob-Creutzfeldt disease

Neoplasm/space-occupying lesion: tumor, (primary or secondary), abscess

Trauma: Subdural hematoma

Miscellaneous: Alzheimer's disease, seizure disorders, normopressure hydrocephalus

If one is concerned about an anticholinergic delirium, IV physostigmine salicylate can be administered; IV thiamine can be given for Wernick's encephalopathy.

Other Functional Psychotic Disorders

Other functional psychotic disorders should be included in the differential with the aforementioned criteria. One should be aware that brief psychotic reactions may fit the criteria for schizophrenia, but not those reactions that last less than two weeks. Schizophreniform disorders usually last longer than two weeks, but less than six months. Note that these disorders are indistinguishable from schizophrenia with the exception of the duration of the illness. According to DSM III, *paranoia* occurs with persecutory delusions or jealousy that is of delusional proportions, but without any other Schneiderian first-rank symptoms.

Affective Disorders

It is often difficult to distinguish an acute manic patient (see Chapter 7) from an acutely schizophrenic patient on the clinical presentation alone. This is when background information, family pedigree history, and family corroboration can aid in the differential.

One must ascertain the occurrence of any previous psychiatric history, past psychiatric diagnoses, results of psychological testing, and response to medication. It is also important to distinguish any first- or second-degree relatives with affective, suicidal, drug abuse, or schizophrenic tendencies. The life history of the patient may elucidate the diagnosis. What was the patient's premorbid personality (*e.g.*, schizoidal, schizotypal)? When was the patient's first psychotic break? Did the patient appear to remit back to baseline and continue with only occasional psychotic breaks, always returning to baseline, or did his life demonstrate a progressive, chronic deterioration in work, leisure, and interpersonal relating, with a rare return to baseline functioning? The latter is often common in schizophrenics. If the clinician is unable to adequately differentiate between an affective and schizophrenic disorder, *Schizoaffective disorder* is the diagnosis often given.

Personality Disorders

Delineated in the DSM-III manual are several types of personality disorders that should be in the differential for schizophrenia. The *schizoid* personality is characterized by aloofness and an inability to form close, warm, lasting relationships. The *schizotypal* personality disorder, in addition to aloofness, will also manifest magical thinking. *Paranoid* personality disorder is often manifested by unwarranted distrust of others, hypersensitivity, and constricted affect. *Borderline* personality disorder with impulsivity, unstable interpersonal relationships, inappropriate unstable affect, identity disturbance, and often self-damaging acts might also be misdiagnosed as schizophrenia.

Neurotic Disorders

Some neuroses can be characterized by feelings of aloofness and aloneness, distancing from others, with occasional magical and/or paranoid thinking. These are, however, usually without severe thought disorder or first-rank symptoms; they are also usually ego-dystonic (the patient is uncomfortable with these symptoms).

Adjustment Disorders

Patients with adjustment disorders respond to a situation in a way that may appear psychotic. For example, someone in the normal grieving process may have auditory or visual hallucination of the loved one; this occurs in 50% to 60% of those in the process of grieving over a loss. Note, however, that these are not accompanied by thought disorganization or the more severe Schneiderian criteria.

Etiology

Consideration of the etiology for schizophrenia has as long a history as the disorder itself. As noted at the beginning of this chapter, schizophrenia has been considered to be caused by demons and witchcraft, focal brain lesions, unknown metabolites, family dynamics, and, at present, varying levels of neurotransmitters.

Genetics

There is an undeniable biological component to schizophrenia, which has been most clearly delineated in the study of the genetics of schizophrenia, focusing on three areas: studies of consanguinity, twin studies, and adoption studies.

Recall that the prevalence of schizophrenia in the general population is 1%. If a genetic factor is operating in the transmission of a disorder, the prevalence rate for the disorder will be increased in family members, compared to the general population rate. The higher the degree of consanguinity (or relatedness), the higher the prevalence rate. An increased prevalence rate of schizophrenia has been noted in the biological relatives of schizophrenics; first-degree relatives (siblings, children, and parents) of schizophrenics have a 10% to 15% prevalence rate for schizophrenia.

The twin method hypothesizes that if a disorder has a genetic component, then the concordance (or occurrence of the same or similar condition) of that disorder should be greater in monozygotic twins (MZ—with identical genetic makeup) than in dizygotic twins (DZ—sharing, on the average, only half the genetic makeup). The concordance rate for schizophrenia, age-corrected, in MZ twins is significantly higher than in DZ twins. Studies demonstrate that the concordance rate in MZ twins ranges from 35% to 58%, averaging 48%, with no difference in the concordance rate of DZ twins and the prevalence rate of siblings, which is approximately 15%. Interestingly, however, it has been noted that twins of schizophrenics who are free of schizophrenia themselves are just as likely to produce schizophrenic children as the schizophrenic member of the pair.

Criticisms of these studies abound. Many complain about the diagnostic criteria of schizophrenia (vs schizophrenic spectrum disorders), and the determination of zygosity in MZ and DZ twins. Many of these complaints have been addressed with suggestions for improvement in interrater reliability, use of strict diagnostic criteria, double blind studies, and biological tests to assess zygosity. Criticisms of the consanquinity studies comment that many characteristics that "run" in families may not be determined genetically; instead they manifest themselves secondary to shared experiences of close family members.

The adoption studies, predominantly performed in the Scandinavian countries, addressed this last issue using several methods. Initially, investigators observed the prevalence rate of schizophrenia in offspring of schizophrenic mothers who were raised by adoptive parents with no known mental illness; the prevalence rate was significantly increased over the general population. Next, biological families of adopted schizophrenics were located, and noted to have a higher prevalence of schizophrenia spectrum illness. It was then demonstrated that the adopted children (with presumed-normal biological parents) of schizophrenic adoptive parents had no significant increase in schizophrenia. Lastly, there has not been any difference noted in the prevalence rate in schizophrenic offspring, that depends on the sex of the schizophrenic parent.

A consensus has been reached that a genetic factor does operate in the transmission of the disorder. Many clinicians support the diathesis stress model, in which the schizophrenic individual is considered to have a genetic predisposition or vulnerability (diathesis); the degree of schizophrenia that is manifested depends on the patient's response to variable degrees of stressors in the environment.

Social Influences

Other investigators have focused on social impact in the etiology of schizophrenia. Social and environmental factors have been postulated to play a role in the initial psychotic break, its perpetuation, the response of the patient to treatment, and his adaptation to the symptoms. Several lines of evidence have been highlighted to demonstrate these factors.

Class

It has been reported that more schizophrenia exists in the lower socioeconomic classes. It was initially hypothesized that this occurred solely because of the vast social stressors, isolation, and deprivation noted in these classes. Reconsideration of the situation has led investigators to believe that this increased prevalence is secondary to selection, or a downward drift. For example, the patient has a poor premorbid personality, is socially withdrawn, and is isolated from family and friends. He quits school, and has increasing difficulty in obtaining and keeping a job. He becomes more socially impaired, withdrawn, and is unable to work altogether. He spends most of his time at the downtown mission center, waiting for his meals and lodging. Of course, not all schizophrenics manifest downward mobility; many are able to maintain responsible positions, and some obtain only less than expected upward mobility.

In addition to poor premorbid functioning and impaired abilities to attain work and education, there is also differential access to quality health care in the lower socioeconomic classes. These individuals are known to be less likely to pursue health care; it has also been speculated that health care workers and the patients within the lower socioeconomic classes might be less willing to attempt rehabilitation.

Culture

It has been noted that diagnosed schizophrenics remain longer in remission if they come from developing countries (*e.g.*, India as opposed to Denmark). Investigators are uncertain if there is some difference in the genetic and biological backgrounds of these people, or if the culture itself sustains the remissions: For example, is rural life less stressful? Are families more supportive or more structured within a rural context?

Stress

Several studies have demonstrated that schizophrenics have usually had a high number of abrupt changes in their social environment within the three weeks prior to admission.

Family Supports

The stereotype of the cold, aloof "schizophrenogenic" mother has fallen by the wayside, with the focus of research instead being placed on the entire family constellation. There are no apparent consistent psychological frameworks that will inevitably lead to schizophrenia. It has been noted, however, that the interpersonal processing within the family has a great predictive value in terms of the rate of relapse of the patient. Families with high emotional overinvolvement were found four times more frequently in the background of schizophrenics who had relapsed. There was an even greater relapse rate if the patient was situated within a high-expressed-emotion family *and* sustained an undesirable or stressful life event. It has also been noted that schizophrenics have fewer relapses if provided with structured environments and a low level of change, and are administered by competent, caring individuals.

Biological Factors

Many biological hypotheses have been postulated as the basis for schizophrenia. Inconclusive data has been offered regarding abnormal immune mechanisms in schizophrenics. Alleged schizophrenic "factors" have been isolated, but have not yet been conclusively linked to the etiology of schizophrenia. Speculation regarding a slow virus has intrigued the scientific world, particularly given the fact that a significantly high percentage of schizophrenics are born in late winter and early spring. Morphological changes have been chronicled with CT scans in schizophrenic patients, demonstrating a relationship between cerebral atrophy and enlarged lateral ventricles and the aforementioned "negative" symptoms.

Perhaps on the forefront of biological investigation is the research into biochemical changes in the brains of schizophrenics. Research on megavitamins, gluten, prostaglandins, prolactin, growth hormone, and gamma-aminobutyric acid (GABA) have been performed, with only inconclusive evidence found concerning their role in the etiology of schizophrenia. Enzymatic changes have been elucidated (Fig. 6-1). Lower levels of monoamine oxidase (MAO, which metabolizes dopamine by transmethylation) in the platelets of patients with schizophrenia have been demonstrated; hence it is postulated that if the MAO is low, that dopamine levels will be higher in these schizophrenic patients. Decreased levels of dopamine-β-hydroxylase have been observed in the postmortems of schizophrenics, also leading to the speculation of increased levels of dopamine in these patients.

At the neurotransmitter level, several hypotheses have been postulated: decreased serotonin, increased norepinephrine (with increased plasma levels of norepinephrine noted in schizophrenics), and the most accepted hypothesis to date, increased levels of dopamine.

A vast amount of literature dealing with these enzymatic modifications and neurotransmitters exists, making it impossible to review it extensively. A broad distillation reveals several hypotheses. The current predominant hypothesis concerns a change in the turnover in dopamine (with postulated changes in synthesis, transport, and reuptake), concomitant with an alteration in receptor sensitivity. Evidence revealing that antipsychotic drugs block dopamine, that dopamine ago-

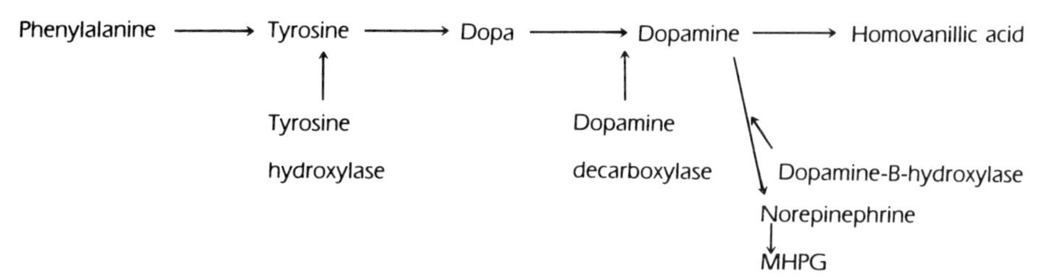

Figure 6-1. Enzymatic changes in patients with schizophrenia.

nists worsen schizophrenia, and that hallucinogens that exacerbate the production of dopamine also exacerbate or impersonate schizophrenia, all tend to strengthen the dopamine hypothesis.

Endogenous opiates (endorphins, enkephalins) have been noted to be located in increased densities in regions of dopamine receptors; attempts have been made to use the endorphins to improve schizophrenic symptomatology with variable success. It is felt that these polypeptides may play a major role in neurobiological functioning.

As of yet, no single biochemical factor has been determined solely as the etiological basis of schizophrenia; however, evidence strongly points to the dopamine hypothesis at this time.

Treatment

Several avenues of treatment are available for schizophrenia disorders. Some facilities favor a more psychodynamic therapeutic design, while others support more psychopharmaceutical treatment regimens. It is probably a more balanced approach to incorporate a biopsychosocial model when designing treatment programs for schizophrenics.

Biological Treatment

Antipsychotic agents have proven effective in ameliorating acute psychotic episodes (see Chapter 23). Choice and dosage of a particular agent may depend on the patient's past response to medication, and any anticipated side effects. The method of introduction of the medication into the patient is also a consideration. Intramuscular (IM) use of neuroleptics results in faster onset of action, and is often used with agitated patients (for example, the use of 2–5 mg of Haldol). Orally administered (PO) liquid concentrate can also be used if patients are thought to be "cheeking" their medications or destroying them in other ways.

The low-potency neuroleptics, such as chlorpromazine (Thorazine) and thioridazine (Mellaril), are much more sedating, and also have the anticholinergic side effects of dry mouth, blurred vision, urinary retention, and decreased gastric motility. Orthostatic hypotension is also a side effect, making it a less than optimal choice for elderly patients who might be prone to hypotension, poor vascular tone, and falling. One must also be wary of cholestatic jaundice, agranulocytosis, breast enlargement, and galactorrhea.

High-potency neuroleptics such as haloperidol (Haldol), trifluoperazine (Stelazine), and thiothixene (Navane) are much more likely to demonstrate extrapyramidal symptoms (EPS). One of these symptoms is *acute dystonias,* manifested by an abrupt onset of tonic contractures of the neck muscles (torticullis), eyes (oculogyric crisis), and back (opisthotonos). These contractures can be relieved with IM or intravenous (IV) Benadryl (25–59 mg) or 1 mg to 2 mg of Cogentin IM. *Parkinson symptoms* may also occur, including rigidity (cogwheeling), akathisia (motor restlessness), tremor, salivation, masked facies, and shuffling gait. These symptoms can be relieved with the following anticholinergic agents: Cogentin (1–

4 mg a day), Benadryl (35–100 mg a day), Artane (1–4 mg a day), or Symmetrel (100–300 mg a day).

More serious side effects of the neuroleptics are tardive dyskinesia and neuroleptic malignant syndrome (NMS). Tardive dyskinesia usually occurs a significant amount of time after starting the drug; it is characterized by oral buccal movements, fasciculations of the tongue, and choreathetoid (writhing) movements of the extremities. It is uncertain as to whether this side effect is reversible if the drug is discontinued. NMS is manifested with rigidity, fever, autonomic changes, and an alteration in mental status. It can occur abruptly, and can be fatal. Treatment entails discontinuation of the medication, with supportive monitoring. Bromocriptine has been used recently as a possible antidote.

Other pharmaceutical agents have been used to treat schizophrenia. Barbiturates have been prescribed for sleeping aids; lithium carbonate has been used if there appears to be an effective component to the psychotic episode; beta blockers have been tried as an adjunct to neuroleptic therapy. Electroconvulsive therapy (ECT) is never used as a treatment of choice for schizophrenia unless the patient is having a life-threatening catatonia, and possibly if there is no response to therapeutic trails of neuroleptics.

Psychosocial Treatment

Individual, family, and milieu therapy have all been attempted with schizophrenics with variable success. It is imperative that the psychotic patient be dealt with in a warm, compassionate, empathic manner, regardless of treatment modality. Attempts at ego-strengthening and encouragement in the growth of a separate self are difficult; this is particularly true within the context of a reality-oriented therapy in which the psychiatrist is aware of the magical thinking and social withdrawal of the schizophrenic patient.

Family therapy can play an important role in terms of remission (see Family Support under Etiology). Therapy is often initially crisis-oriented (*e.g.*, dealing with the acute disruption in the home), but should also focus on long-term conflicts and affects held within the family.

There is no prominent evidence that milieu therapy by itself is effective; however, when performed within the context of psychopharmacologic treatment, there is some evidence of improvement. The milieu should be structured and very concrete, with attention given to the safety of the patient, other patients, and staff; with a limited setting as a basic part of the milieu. Grossly psychotic patients may need one-on-one supervision, seclusion, or restraints. The psychotic patient will often need help with reality testing and reorientation.

The course of schizophrenia can be modified somewhat, depending on a number of variables. Treatment with neuroleptics does not guarantee a cure; approximately 50% of those treated with neuroleptics relapse within a year. Only about 15% of those receiving all the aforementioned treatment modalities remain functioning within society without a relapse. It is necessary, therefore, to be aware of the prognosis for schizophrenia, and to prepare the patient, the family, and oneself for the moderate response to any treatment. Perhaps the ongoing advances in research related to both biological and psychosocial aspects of schizophrenia will lead to improved diagnosis and treatment of this pervasive, disabling disease.

Conclusion

Schizophrenia has been described throughout the ages, with more recent systematic observation and description culminating in the DSM-III criteria presently in use. Various theories on the etiology of this disorder that affects approximately one percent of our population have been offered, with apparent evidence of a strong biological component. The leading neurotransmitter hypothesis postulates an increase in the level of dopamine in schizophrenics. This is not to discount social, psychological, or cultural impacts on the development of schizophrenia. Indeed, a diathesis/stress model seems to best explain the development of schizophrenia, its perpetuation, the patient's response to treatment, and the relapse rate. It is imperative to view each patient within a biopsychosocial context, considering not only biological predispositions, but also individual stressors and precipitants, family structure, and support systems. Given this approach, the best prognosis is probably attained by those who are treated with antipsychotic medications and live in structured supportive environments with families who are educated regarding the schizophrenic process.

Reference

1. American Psychiatric Association: Diagnostic and Statistical Manual of Mental Disorders, 3rd ed, p 188. Washington, DC, American Psychiatric Association, 1980

Bibliography

Alexander FG, Selesnick ST: The History of Psychiatry. New York, Harper & Row, 1966

Bleuler E: Dementia Praecox or the Group of Schizophrenias (1908). J. Zinkin (trans): New York, International Universities Press, 1950

Cancro R: The role of genetic factors in the etiology of the schizophrenic disorders. In Grinspoon L (ed): Psychiatry 1982 Annual Review, Chapter 10, pp 92–97. Washington, DC, American Psychiatry Press, 1982

Davis, JM, Janicak P, Chang S, et al: Recent advances in the pharmacologic treatment of the schizophrenic disorders. In Grinspoon L (ed): Psychiatry 1982 Annual Review, Chapter 15. Washington, DC, American Psychiatry Press, 1982

Kraepelin E: Dementia Praecox. London, Livingston, 1918

Liberman RP: Social factors in the etiology of the schizophrenic disorders. In Grinspoon L (ed): Psychiatry 1982 Annual Review, Chapter 11, pp 112–153. Washington, DC, American Psychiatry Press, 1982

Schneider K: Clinical Psychopathology. New York, Grune & Stratton, 1959

Will OA: Schizophrenia: Psychological treatment. In Kaplan HI, Freedman AM, Sadock BJ (eds): Comprehensive Textbook of Psychiatry/III, Vol 2, 3rd ed, Chapter 15, pp 1217–1240. Baltimore, Williams & Wilkins, 1980

Wyatt RJ, Culter NR, DeLisi LE, et al: Biochemical and morphological factors in the etiology of the schizophrenic disorders. In Grinspoon L (ed): Psychiatry 1982 Annual Review, Chapter 12, pp 112–153. Washington, DC, American Psychiatry Press, 1982

Susan R. Levy

7 Affective Disorders

Affective disorders, characterized by a disturbance of mood, embrace two emotions, depression and mania. Some patients will suffer from both depression and mania at different times in their life. These patients are said to have *bipolar* illness, also called *manic–depressive* illness. A patient who describes only manic episodes is classified in the bipolar category because it is believed that such a patient will eventually experience a depressive episode. Other patients may suffer only depressive episodes, and these patients are said to have *unipolar* depressions; they may have single or recurrent episodes.

Depression

Depression, a word with many meanings, describes a mood in which an individual feels blue, sad, low in spirits, or down in the dumps. There are several types of depression: major depression with melancholia, major depression with mood-congruent psychotic features, major depression with mood-incongruent psychotic features, dysthymia, cyclothymia, bipolar disorder with depressed mood, and atypical depression.

Major Depression

Major depression describes a clinical syndrome in which a dysphoric (or depressed) mood is accompanied by certain specific somatic signs and symptoms, psychomotor changes, and a diminished ability to experience pleasure. Depression is common; the current point prevalence of major depression is 3% to 5%. The diagnostic criteria for a major depressive episode, as established by the American Psychiatric Association (1980) include:

1. A relatively persistent dysphoric mood–described as feeling blue, down in the dumps, depressed, sad, low in spirits—leading to loss of pleasure in usual activities
2. Four or more of the following symptoms, lasting at least two weeks:
   - Change in appetite or weight
   - Hypersomnia or insomnia
   - Psychomotor agitation or retardation
   - Decreased sexual drive
   - Decreased energy
   - Feelings of worthlessness
   - Diminished concentration
   - Suicidal ideation
3. The symptoms are not secondary to a paranoid disorder, uncomplicated bereavement, organic brain syndrome, schizophrenia, or any other psychiatric illness.

☐ A 36-year-old woman came to her family physician complaining of fatigue and low energy. Further questioning revealed that for several months she had for no apparent reason been feeling "down in the dumps." She also reported poor appetite, trouble falling asleep, and a diminished interest in sex; these symptoms had been progressive over the month prior to her visit. Physical examination and laboratory evaluation were normal. A diagnosis of major depression was made, and the patient responded to a tricyclic antidepressant.

Major Depression with Melancholia

To merit the diagnosis of major depression with melancholia, an especially severe form of depression, the patient must demonstrate anhedonia (the total inability to experience pleasure) and mood nonreactivity (the inability to respond to pleasurable stimuli). According to the Diagnostic and Statistical Manual of Mental Disorders (DSM-III), at least three of the following symptoms must also be present:

- A depressed mood that is so different from bereavement that the patient has difficulty explaining the feeling
- The depression is more severe in the morning
- Awakening at least two hours earlier than normal
- Extreme psychomotor retardation or agitation
- Significant weight loss or severe anorexia
- Overwhelming guilt

☐ A 57-year-old farmer was brought to the emergency room by his family, who stated that for the past 6 months he had "not been himself." The patient was of frail appearance; he sat with downcast eyes, wringing his hands. His speech was low in volume and halting, with long pauses between phrases. He admitted that for the past year he had been feeling increasingly sad and despondent, and found that he was no longer able to cheer up or enjoy himself. His appetite was poor and he reported a 30-pound weight loss over the preceding six months. He had difficulty sleeping: it often took him several hours to fall asleep and then he would awaken frequently throughout the night. He was often not able to return to sleep and would lie awake for several hours before getting out of bed in the morning. He described fatigue, low energy, trouble concentrating, and loss of interest in his work. His family confirmed that he was no longer functioning effectively as a farmer. The patient felt that he was a burden on his family and revealed that he had contemplated suicide. A diagnosis of major depression with melancholia was made.

Major Depression With Mood-Congruent Psychotic Features

Some depressed patients may manifest psychotic features (*i.e.*, their contact with reality is impaired). Often psychotic symptoms are comprehensible in relation to depression; if so, they are considered ***mood-congruent psychotic features***. Examples include delusions of guilt and delusions of poverty. Somatic delusions (*e.g.*, of body rotting, of having a terminal illness) are often mood-congruent. The following case illustrates a mood-congruent psychotic depression.

☐ Although never employed outside the home, Mrs. A, a 56-year-old married woman and mother of two adult children, had been long active in family and community activities. For the past year she had gradually withdrawn from her usual social activities. Initially she had maintained her involvement, even though she had to push herself to participate. Slowly she lost interest entirely and began to stay home.

Soon she began to have difficulty getting out of bed in the morning. Usual household chores became an immense effort. Not only did she feel tired and lack energy, but she found she had trouble concentrating and felt blue and down in the dumps. Mornings were the worst time; frequently she wondered how she would get through the day. Mrs. A also complained of trouble sleeping. She would be awake at night unable to fall asleep; when she finally dozed off she would reawaken several times during the night and be unable to return to sleep. Often she was awake at 3 AM and could not fall back asleep. Mrs. A's appetite was also poor. Although she tried to push herself to eat, she found that food had little taste and she continued to lose weight. Her thoughts turned increasingly inward, and she began to brood about past errors and developed the delusion that she was an inadequate wife and mother. She ruminated on having cheated on her income tax many years before, and became convinced that she would be jailed. No such cheating was ever corroborated by her husband. Mrs. A was diagnosed as having major depression with mood-congruent psychotic features.

Major Depression With Mood-Incongruent Psychotic Features

Rarely, depression may have associated mood-incongruent psychotic features, which are delusions or hallucinations that do not focus on themes of guilt, personal inadequacy, or nihilism. Examples include delusions of passivity, persecutory delusions, and auditory hallucinations with commentary content.

☐ A 22-year-old woman was brought to a psychiatrist by her parents. Since graduating from college 3 months before, she had become increasingly withdrawn and socially isolated. She admitted to feeling low in spirits, often cried, had little energy and had lost interest in old friends and hobbies. She attributed a 20-pound weight loss to fear of eating, stating that the food had been poisoned by the grocer. The diagnosis was major depression with mood-incongruent psychotic features. Treatment with a combination of an antipsychotic agent and a tricyclic antidepressant resulted in a marked improvement.

Dysthymic Disorder

Some patients describe long periods of depressed mood, accompanied by symptoms such as poor sleep or low energy, but the intensity and number of symptoms are insufficient to make a diagnosis of major depression. These patients would be diagnosed as suffering *dysthymic disorder,* also called *depressive neurosis.* Because some of these patients show a few of the biological abnormalities characteristic of major depression (*e.g.,* decreased rapid eye movement (REM) latency), they may represent an attenuated form of major depression, dysthymic disorder. DSM-III criteria for a dysthymic disorder follow.

1. The patient goes through a 2-year period during which, for the majority of the time, he suffers depressive symptoms. There may be periods of normal mood that separate the periods of depression, but such euthymic periods do not last more than a few months at a time. The depressive symptoms are neither of sufficient severity nor duration to meet diagnostic criteria for major depression.
2. During periods of depression, the mood is depressed, sad, or low; or there is a marked loss of interest or pleasure in most usual activities.
3. Three of the following symptoms are present:
   Insomnia or hypersomnia
   Low energy or chronic fatigue
   Feelings of inadequacy
   Diminished performance at work or home
   Poor attention or concentration
   Social withdrawal
   Anhedonia
   Anger or irritability
   Lack of pleasure in response to rewards or praise
   Decreased activity, less talkative, feeling slowed down or restless
   Pessimism or brooding over the past
   Crying or tearfulness
   Frequent thoughts of death or suicide

☐ Mr. B was a 47-year-old man who presented to his family physician complaining of chronic fatigue. At work he found that his job performance had deteriorated. He described his mood as "generally low," but did recall several enjoyable vacations. He dated the onset of his symptoms to financial difficulties five years earlier. Medical evaluation was negative. A diagnosis of dysthymic disorder was made.

Cyclothymic Disorder

Cyclothymic disorder is a disorder in which depressive periods alternate with periods of hypomania. There may be intervening periods of normal mood. During the affective episodes, the symptoms are not of sufficient number, intensity, or duration to meet diagnostic criteria for major depression or mania. As in dysthymic disorder, the duration of symptoms is two years.

☐ Miss C was a 33-year-old advertising executive. She complained of "unstable mood—highs and lows". At times she felt "on top of the world," had more than her usual energy, needed only a few hours of sleep, found herself enormously creative and productive at work and unusually gregarious. Such episodes might last from days to weeks. At other times she found herself in low spirits, with little energy, poor concentration at work, and socially withdrawn. She dated this pattern to college years. The diagnosis was cyclothymic disorder.

Atypical Depression

The term *atypical depression* is used in a variety of ways. As defined by DSM-III, atypical depression is a residual category without specified diagnostic criteria, and is used for individuals with depressive symptoms who do not fit another specific affective syndrome. For example, a brief episode of depression that does not meet diagnostic criteria for major depression and is not an adjustment disorder would be considered an atypical depression. Another example would be a patient with residual schizophrenia who then develops a major depressive episode.

Atypical depression has historically been used in another way; to designate a patient with depressed mood, prominent anxiety or phobias, hysterical features, and the atypical vegetative symptoms of hypersomnia, increased appetite and weight gain (rather than the more typical insomnia, poor appetite, and weight loss). Such patients have been observed to show little benefit from electroconvulsive therapy (ECT). It is likely that such a group of atypical depressives is diagnostically heterogeneous by current diagnostic criteria, combining both depressive and anxiety disorders.

More recently, some investigators (see Leibowitz) have developed operational criteria for atypical depression. They define atypical depressives as patients who meet research diagnostic criteria for major, minor, or intermittent depression, demonstrate mood reactivity even when depressed, and exhibit two or more of the following symptoms: overeating, oversleeping, extreme lethargy or fatigue, and extreme sensitivity to rejection. Their data showed better response to a monoamine oxidase inhibitor (MAOI) (phenelzine) than to placebo, but a nonstatistically significant advantage over imipramine.

Differential Diagnosis of Depression

The evaluation of a patient with depression should focus on the psychiatric and medical history, mental status examination, physical examination, and pertinent laboratory tests. To avoid failing to diagnose depression, the clinician must remember that many depressed patients may not initially describe their mood as depressed; instead, they may focus on feeling tired and run-down, or on vague physical complaints. On the other hand, but equally important, many patients with primarily organic illness will present with symptoms of depression.

Organic Affective Syndrome

Perhaps the most important part of the evaluation of a patient with depression is to rule out possible medical conditions that may cause depressive symptoms. Organic affective syndrome is characterized by symptoms of mania or depression that are caused by a specific physical condition. Medical conditions that may present with, or aggravate psychiatric conditions include: endocrine disorders (most commonly thyroid dysfunction, adrenal dysfunction, and diabetes), cardiovascular disease, infectious disease (including syphilis), pulmonary disease, gastrointestinal disease, hematopoietic disease, neurologic illness, malignancy (pancreatic cancer is often described as presenting with depression, but other neoplasms may also present this way), inflammatory and collagen vascular disease, fluid and electrolyte imbalances, and nutritional deficiencies. Depressive symptoms can often be caused by a wide variety of medications (reserpine, methyldopa, and oral contraceptives are just a few among many); as well as drug intoxication, including alcohol. The following case represents an example of organic affective syndrome:

☐ A 42-year-old woman sought psychiatric treatment for "depression." She described several months of low spirits, fatigue, little energy, poor concentration, and diminished interest in previously enjoyed activities. The physical examination was notable for hyporeflexia, and laboratory evaluation revealed both low T_3 and elevated TSH. Her symptoms cleared following correction of her hypothyroid status.

Organic brain syndrome and depression are often mistaken for each other. Such a diagnostic error is most common in the elderly, where depression may be mistakenly diagnosed as dementia. For this reason, a retarded depression in the elderly is sometimes called *pseudodementia* (Table 7-1).

☐ An 82-year-old man, previously active and living alone in his apartment, was brought by his daughter to the doctor. She stated that the patient was "becoming senile" and she felt he needed nursing home placement. She described her father as forgetful, inattentive, and no longer able to take care of himself. He was listless and uninterested in activities and previous hobbies. Over the past 4 months he had lost 20 pounds; he also had a marked sleep disturbance. Cognitive testing was remarkable for poor attention and concentration, and minimal effort at responding to test questions. Many questions were answered with an immediate "I don't know." The patient, with much encouragement, revealed himself to be fully oriented, but his calculations were poor.

A diagnosis of major depression was made, and the patient was treated with a tricyclic antidepressant. He showed substantial improvement in mood, interests and activity level returned to previous levels, and cognitive deficits cleared. He was able to continue living in his apartment without assistance.

☐ Mrs. D, a 73-year-old retired accountant, was found wandering along a highway and brought to the emergency room of the local hospital. When her

Table 7-1
Depression (Pseudodementia) *vs* Dementia

	Depression (Pseudodementia)	Dementia
Onset	Discrete	Insidious
Course	Depressed mood generally precedes cognitive changes. Rapid progression of symptoms	Depressed mood, if present, follows cognitive losses. Slow progression of symptoms
Chief complaint	Patient complains of cognitive dysfunction, highlights disability.	Patient denies cognitive dysfunction, conceals failures.
Mood	Sadness or apathy	Labile affect, often shallow
Motivation	Patient gives up easily, typically makes "I don't know" answers.	Patient struggles to accomplish task.
Diurnal change	Often worse in morning	Worse at night
Other symptoms	Frequent sleep and appetite disturbances, guilt, low self-esteem, fatigue, anhedonia	Generally not present
Behavior	Cognitive losses often inconsistent across different tasks.	Consistent loss
Past or family history	Affective disorder	No association with previous psychiatric illness
Response to treatment	Responds well to antidepressant treatment	Irreversible, poor response to treatment

distraught husband was contacted, he revealed that they had become separated on a shopping trip earlier that day. Mrs. D denied being lost, stating that she had gone "window shopping." Further history revealed that over the past several years Mrs. D had been misplacing items and having difficulty maintaining the household and balancing the checkbook. Mental status examination was notable for memory impairment and poor abstraction and calculating ability. Medical evaluation was unremarkable. A diagnosis of senile dementia of the Alzheimer's type was made.

Bereavement

Major depression must be distinguished from bereavement. A sad mood and the associated vegetative symptoms of sleep and appetite disturbance, loss of energy and libido, and diminished interest in usual activities are commonly seen in persons who are mourning the death of a loved one. Such a response is a normal human response to a loss.

☐ Mrs. H was a 53-year-old woman who came to the emergency room stating, "Life isn't worth living anymore." Mrs. H's husband had been killed in an automobile accident three weeks earlier. Since his death Mrs. H had been despondent, crying and often wishing that she too would die. She was unable to sleep at night. She had no appetite for food and had lost ten pounds since the accident. Concentration was markedly impaired and she was unable to take care of household responsibilities.

Mrs. H was treated with brief, crisis-oriented psychotherapy. Over the next two months her depressive symptoms lifted and she was able to resume previous activities.

The grief response will gradually diminish over time, and psychiatric treatment is not generally indicated. If, however, the mourning is unduly prolonged (greater than several months), then the illness would be classified as a major depression and psychiatric treatment (either medication, ECT, psychotherapy, or a combination of therapies) may be needed.

☐ A 47-year-old man was hospitalized following an overdose of medication. History revealed that his wife had died one and a half years earlier of metastatic carcinoma. Since then the patient had become progressively more sad, hopeless, and withdrawn. He lost interest in work and previous hobbies, and "longed to join his wife in heaven." He described both initial and terminal insomnia, had little appetite for food, and had lost 15 pounds over the past six months, and had little energy. A diagnosis of major depression was made. The patient responded well to antidepressant medication.

Etiology of Depression

Many theories have been proposed for the etiology of depression. Although there is no conclusive evidence for one particular cause for depression, patients with affective disorders do manifest various, often subtle, biological abnormalities. Whether such defects are sufficient to cause affective illness is as yet unknown. An important question that remains to be answered is the extent to which the biological abnormality represents a *state* phenomenon (only found in the individual when he is depressed) or a *trait* phenomenon (if it exists in the individual before, during, and after the depressive episode). In addition, it is likely that depression is heterogeneous, and that subgroups of depressed patients may have different etiologies, including different neurochemical abnormalities.

Genetic Factors

Some of the most compelling evidence for a biological basis of affective illness comes from epidemiologic studies. Important findings include the following:[1]

First-degree relatives of patients with unipolar depression have an increased risk of major depression. (Weismann and colleagues in 1981 demonstrated a 17% risk of unipolar depression in first-degree relatives of unipolar probands. The risk for first-degree relatives of normal probands was 6%.)

First-degree relatives of bipolar probands have an increased risk of both bipolar illness and unipolar depression. (Gershon and colleagues in 1981 and 1982 showed an 80% risk of bipolar disorder and a 15% risk of unipolar depression in first-degree relatives of bipolar patients. For first-degree relatives of normal probands, the risk of bipolar disorder was less than 1%, and the risk of unipolar depression was 6%.)

Twin studies show an increased concordance rate for affective disorder in monozygotic over dizygotic twins. For bipolar disorder, monozygotic twins showed 79% concordance, and dizygotic twins showed 24% concordance. For unipolar probands, the concordance rate for monozygotic twins was 54% and for dizygotic twins 19%. (Bertelson et al. 1977, 1979 in a study using the Danish Twin Register)[4]

Neuroendocrine Factors

There is increasing evidence that neurotransmitters and hormones are important in the etiology of depression. Schildkraut, in 1956, proposed one of the first biological theories of depression, the cathecholamine hypothesis: this theory, subsequently extended to include indoleamines and renamed the *biogenic amine hypothesis,* states that depression is due to a deficiency in central nervous system catecholamines. To prove this theory, the quantity and functional activity of neurotransmitter at the synaptic level must be known. Technical limitations, however, have limited work to the examination of norepinephrine (NE) and NE metabolites, such as 3-methoxy-4-hydroxyphenolglycol (MHPG) in the urine and cerebrospinal fluid. At this time, the catecholamine hypothesis remains unproved.

The extension of the catecholamine hypothesis to include indoleamines (*e.g.,* serotonin) postulates that some depressions are due to decreased NE, and some to decreased serotonin. This theory, too, remains speculative at this time.

Janowsky and colleagues have hypothesized a "cholinergic–adrenergic balance hypothesis of mania and depression." They propose that a relative increase in central cholinergic activity is associated with depression and that a relative increase in central nonadrenergic activity is associated with mania. Some findings support this theory (*e.g.,* physostigmine, a centrally acting acetylcholinesterase inhibitor, can transiently reverse mania), but this theory too remains speculative.

More recently, evidence has accumulated that suggests that neuroendocrine regulation is altered in patients with affective disorder. Depressed patients appear to have a defect in the hypothalamic–pituitary–end organ axis (in particular, the adrenal or thyroid gland).

Let us briefly review the pertinent neuroanatomy. In the hypothalamic–neurohypophysial (posterior pituitary) system, axons that originate in hypothalamic nuclei (the supraoptic and paraventricular tracts) terminate on blood vessels in the posterior pituitary and thereby regulate secretion of vasopressin and oxytocin. In the hypothalamic–adenohypophysial (anterior pituitary system) tuberoinfundibular neurons terminate on blood vessels of the portal system, where they release hypothalamic hormones and other neurotransmitters. The portal vessels drain into the anterior pituitary. Hypothalamic hormones (also called *releasing factors*) are carried in the portal system and reach the anterior pituitary, where they regulate the release of anterior pituitary hormones (thyroid-stimulating hormone (TSH), growth hormone (GH), luteinizing hormone (LH), follicle-stimulating hormone (FSH), TSH, prolactin). Many other neurotransmitters may be involved in neuroendocrine regulation at various levels in the brain. Limbic pathways appear particularly important. Neurotransmitters that appear important in neuroendocrine regulation include norepinephrine, epinephrine, dopamine, serotonin, acetylcholine, histamine, and various peptides such as enkephalins, endorphins, substance-P, neurotensin, gastrin, cholecystokinin and vasoactive intestinal protein.

Key findings suggesting that neuroendocrine abnormalities exist in patients with affective disorder include the following:

- Approximately 50% of patients with major depression show hypersecretion of cortisol and an altered diurnal variation in the pattern of secretion. Depressed patients show excessive secretion in the afternoon, evening, and early morning; times when cortisol secretion is normally low. They thus show "flattening" of the normal circadian curve of cortisol secretion.
- Depressed patients have an unusually high rate of escape from dexamethasone suppression (see below). Dexamethasone suppression test (DST) nonsuppression occurs in 40% to 60% of depressed patients.
- Depressed patients have an unusually high incidence of blunted TRH response to DST. The incidence of blunted TRH response in depressed patients is approximately 25% and is not related to alteration in baseline TSH or thyroid hormone levels.
- Depressed patients have a diminished growth hormone response to insulin-induced hypoglycemia.

Psychodynamic Theory

In *Mourning and Melancholia* (1917) Freud observed that both the states of mourning (grief, bereavement) and melancholia (depression) are responses to the loss of a loved object. This object may be a real person lost by death or rejection, or may instead be an abstraction such as an ideal or value. Freud postulated that by a mechanism of introjection the lost object becomes identified with the ego. The hostility that was directed toward the lost object thus becomes directed inwardly toward the ego. A key element of this conceptualization is that the relationship with the lost loved object is ambivalent: The relationship has hostile as well as positive components. The hostile components, when directed toward the ego, result in self-reproach and guilt (hallmarks of depression). Thus, in this view, depression results from the transformation of hostility.

This classic psychoanalytic view of depression has undergone major modifications. One important revision is that depression has come to be seen as an affective state characterized by loss of self-esteem. Bibring proposed that self-esteem can be reduced in a variety of ways, including the frustration of narcissistic aspirations as well as the loss of love. Failure to meet these goals would result in feelings of helplessness and diminished self-esteem, and would cause depression. Bibring's contribution was to emphasize depression as an ego state, and he focused on the importance of self-esteem in the development of depression. Jacobson, reflecting the influence of ego psychology, expanded the theory of depression to include more recent concepts of the self and object relations. She too postulated that loss of self-esteem was central to depression, and proposed factors that could contribute to this loss of self-esteem (for example, pathologic self-representations, an unrealistic or grandiose ego-ideal, an overly strict and critical superego). Many current theories about psychological predisposition to depression focus on disturbances in object relations between the child and its primary love objects at an early stage of development.

Cognitive Theory

The cognitive theory of depression, as elaborated by Beck, postulates that an individual tends to structure his interpretation of the world in stable ways; these cognitive patterns determine emotions and behavior. Depressed individuals are felt to have distorted views of themselves, their experiences, and the future. Beck uses the term *cognitive triad* to express this concept. The cognitive triad consists of the individual's negative view of himself (defective, worthless); negative misinterpretation of events (all his efforts are seen as failures); and negative view of the future (expects failure and suffering).

These cognitive errors are felt to be due to faulty information processing: Despite evidence to the contrary, the individual continues to maintain an inaccurate view of himself and his experiences. These negative thoughts (or cognitions) precede the depressed mood and behavior. A patient who incorrectly thinks he has failed will respond with the same feelings (perhaps sadness or guilt) that he would have toward real failure. When a patient expects to fail, he may develop despondency, dependency, and loss of motivation, even if in reality failure is unlikely. Thus, cognitive theory postulates a theory of depression in which the primary pathology is in information processing (resulting in negative cognitions), while the depressed affect and behavior are regarded as secondary features. Cognitive therapy focuses on correction of the primary cognitive defect: identification of these cognitive distortions (also called dysfunctional beliefs), logical analysis of the negative thoughts, and substitution of more reality-based interpretations.

Laboratory Aids in the Diagnosis of Depression

The DST is a helpful diagnostic aid in depression. Sixty percent of patients with endogenous depression demonstrate abnormal dexamethasone suppression.

The DST is performed in the following way. Dexamethasone 1 mg is administered orally at 11 PM. Serum cortisol is assayed at 4 PM and 11 PM the next day. The normal response is for serum cortisol to fall following dexamethasone administration. Patients with depression often have an abnormal response, in which they show nonsuppression of cortisol. Nonsuppression is defined as serum cortisol greater than 5 μg per dl. With this cut-off value, in an inpatient population of melancholic patients, Carroll and colleagues found a sensitivity of 67% and a specificity of 96%. Another way of expressing this is that 67% of patients with depression showed nonsuppression, and 96% of patients with nonsuppression were depressed. The diagnostic confidence (predictive value) was 92%. High specificity (low incidence of false positive results) means that nonsuppression strongly supports a diagnosis of depression. However, only moderate sensitivity (substantial incidence of false negative results) means that normal suppression cannot be used to rule out a diagnosis of depression.

The TRH stimulation test is another neuroendocrine challenge test, and is currently used as a research tool. In this test, protirelin (TRH) 500 mcg is administered intravenously at 9 AM; serum TSH is measured at baseline and at intervals for 90 minutes following TRH. An abnormal response (also known as a blunted response) is defined as a rise in TSH of less than 5 μU per ml over baseline levels following TRH infusion. Peak serum TSH usually occurs at 30 minutes after TRH administration. Approximately 25% of depressed patients will show a blunted response to TRH .

The usefulness of these neuroendocrine tests in clinical psychiatry is being actively investigated. One important question is whether the abnormality is a state or trait phenomenon: Does the abnormality exist only when the patient is suffering from a clinical depression, or does it precede the episode or persist during clinical remission? Greden and colleagues found that in melancholic patients who were DST nonsuppressors, normalization of DST preceded or coincided with clinical improvement. These data suggest a role for DST in monitoring treatment response and possibly in predicting relapse.

Electroencephalogram (EEG) sleep studies are also helpful in diagnosing depression. These studies have shown that patients with major depression demonstrate consistent and specific changes in sleep architecture. The most prominent change is decreased REM latency (shorter time from sleep onset to REM sleep). Normal REM latency is 90 minutes, whereas endogenously depressed patients have an REM latency of 40 to 50 minutes. Other EEG sleep abnormalities commonly seen in depression include increased REM activity and REM density for the total night, and a shifting of REM activity to the first half of the night (in normal sleep, REM activity is greatest during the second half of the night). There does not seem to be a significant difference in the REM latency, REM density, or distribution of REM sleep between unipolar and bipolar depressives.

EEG sleep studies show fairly high sensitivity (61% to 90%), specificity (80 to 100%), and diagnostic confidence (83% to 100%) in several studies that attempted to discriminate endogenous or primary depression from other psychiatric disorders (see Kupfer). Sleep studies may be particularly useful in difficult diagnostic questions, such as the diagnosis of pseudodementia or depression in a medically ill patient. Thus, sleep studies appear to be a potentially useful laboratory aid in the diagnosis of depression. Sleep study data may also have utility in the prediction of treatment response; this area is one under current investigation.

Treatment of Depression

Major depression is one of the psychiatric disorders most responsive to treatment. Treatment can be divided into two categories, somatic and psychotherapeutic. There is little controversy over the efficacy of somatic treatment for major depression. Psychotherapy augments somatic treatment for major depression; on the other hand, psychotherapy is the treatment of choice for dysthymic disorder because drug therapy may be of very little help.

Medications

Medication is the most common somatic treatment of major depression, of which there are several classes available.

Tricyclic Antidepressants (TCA). TCAs were the first effective medication treatment for depression, and still remain the preferred treatment by many physicians. Double-blind placebo controlled studies have demonstrated a 70% response to TCA, *vs* a 40% placebo response. The TCAs include such drugs as amitriptyline, imipramine, desipramine, nortriptyline, doxepin and others (see Chapter 23). The mechanism of action is postulated to work through their increasing concentrations of biogenic amines (norepinephrine, serotonin) at the synaptic level. TCAs inhibit reuptake of certain neurotransmitters, resulting in higher functional levels of neurotransmitter at the synapse. The TCAs are both noradrenergic and serotonergic, although certain TCAs are more serotonergic (*e.g.*, amitriptyline), while other TCAs are more noradrenergic (*e.g.*, desipramine).

TCAs do not show immediate therapeutic efficacy. Often, three to four weeks of treatment at therapeutic doses is needed before clinical response is seen. One acceptable method of administration is to initiate treatment at a dose of 50 mg to 75 mg by mouth qhs, and increase the dose over the next week to 150 mg to 300 mg. Although serum levels of several TCAs are available, at the current time the relationship of serum TCA level to clinical response remains unknown. Clinical monitoring and adjustment of drug and dose is thus recommended. The only current exception to this rule of thumb is in the case of nortriptyline, where serum levels should be maintained within the "therapeutic windows" of 50 ng/ml to 150 ng/ml (usual dose requirement is 75 mg to 150 mg daily).

The most common side effects of TCAs are due to their anticholinergic properties. Autonomic side effects include: dry mouth, constipation (and, at times, paralytic ileus), blurry vision (due to decreased visual accommodation), urinary retention, tachycardia, sweating, orthostatic hypotension (at times with dizziness and fainting), and aggravation of narrow angle glaucoma. Cardiovascular effects include conduction disturbances (both atrioventricular nodal time and ventricular conduction may be prolonged) and tachycardia. Agranulocytosis is a rare but serious complication. Sedation may be a problem with the more serotonergic drugs, such as amitriptyline; paradoxical agitation may occur with imipramine. Exogenous norepinephrine is potentiated by TCAs and is therefore contraindicated. Some, although not all, of the side effects are dose-related, but there are wide variations among patients in their sensitivity to side effects. Amoxapine (a dibenzoxazepine) is a newer tricyclic antidepressant that has noradrenergic, serotonergic, and dopaminergic effects. Because of its dopamine-receptor blocking properties, amoxapine may have the additional side effects of extrapyramidal symptoms, and may have the potential to cause tardive dyskinesia.

Suicide attempts with TCAs are common and overdose should be considered a medical emergency. Signs and symptoms include peripheral anticholinergic effects, central nervous system effects (initially manifested by agitation but progressing to loss of consciousness and coma), hypotension and cardiac conduction disturbances, and arrhythmias. Gastric lavage and supportive treatment, observation in an intensive care unit, and specific treatment of cardiac complications are indicated.

Tetracyclic Antidepressants. The tetracyclic antidepressants appear to be similar in mechanism of action to the TCAs, because they increase effective levels of neurotransmitter at the synaptic cleft. It is possible that the latency of action of the tetracyclic compounds is a bit shorter than for the TCAs. Maprotilene, a tetracyclic antidepressant, is primarily noradrenergic. Side effects are similar to those of the TCAs.

Trazodone. Chemically unrelated to the tricyclic and other known antidepressants, trazodone selectively inhibits serotonin uptake. Its mechanism of antidepressant action, however, is still not fully understood. The most common side effects include drowsiness, dizziness and light-headedness, fatigue, gastrointestinal distress, headache, nervousness, and autonomic symptoms (dry mouth, constipation, blurred vision). Hypotension, arrhythmias, and priapism have been associated with use of trazodone.

Monoamine Oxidase Inhibitors (MAOI). Monoamine oxidase (MAO) is an enzyme that is found in the nervous system and the blood. It is one of the principal enzymes involved in metabolism of biogenic amines; it catalyzes the oxidative deamination of monoamines (including norepinephrine, serotonin, dopamine, and tyramine). Inhibition of MAO causes decreased degradation of biogenic amines and results in increased levels of neurotransmitter at the synapse, as well as increased levels of monoamines throughout the body.

Clinically available MAOIs are divided into two groups: hydrazines, which have predominant hepatic toxicity; and nonhydrazines, which have more potential for hypertensive reactions. The most commonly used MAOIs in psychiatric practice include phenelzine and isocarboxazid (both hydrazines), and tranylcypromine (nonhydrazine).

Side effects of the MAOIs include orthostatic hypotension, dizziness, constipation, delayed micturition, sexual dysfunction, fluid retention, weight gain, and insomnia. Rarely, a peripheral neuropathy secondary to pyridoxine deficiency can occur; however, the most dangerous side effect is the hypertensive crisis that results from interaction of MAOIs with foods containing tyramine, or other medications containing sympathomimetics. Tyramine is an amino acid found in many foods, including hard cheeses, beer and red wine, and pickled products. Inhibition of MAO results in the inability to degrade tyramine (a precursor of norepinephrine) and results in hypertension. Other interactions with MAOIs may occur with over-the-counter medications (especially cold preparations and nasal decongestants), anesthetics (*e.g.,* in dental visits, the use of epinephrine in local anesthetics), as well as with amphetamines, methylphenidate, asthma medications, and dopamine. Hypertensive crises are not common, but they are potentially serious. They can be managed with several agents, including phentolamine, which is an alpha-adrenergic blocker.

In addition, it should be remembered that MAOIs may potentiate other drugs: A partial list includes opiates, anticholinergic drugs (including TCAs), antihypertensive agents, barbiturates, insulin (MAO may lower serum glucose), and antiparkinsonian drugs. Finally, liver function should be assessed.

In initiating treatment with MAOIs, the appropriate low-tyramine diet should begin at least 24 hours before the drug is started. Dosage differs with the various drugs. Platelet MAO levels may provide an indication of the extent of central MAO inhibition, with current research suggesting that at least 80% platelet MAOI inhibition should be attained. As with TCAs, it may take several weeks for a clinical effect to appear. Upon discontinuing an MAOI, the patient should remain on a low-tyramine diet for at least two weeks (which is most important for hydrazines), so that MAO can be synthesized and lost stores replenished. Current evidence supports the use of MAOIs in patients with atypical depression, as well as major depression that fails to respond to other antidepressants.

Lithium. More and more evidence suggests that lithium is an effective treatment in major depression. Although not used as a first-line treatment, lithium may be quite effective in patients who are unresponsive to other medications, or in those bipolar patients who become manic on TCAs. In addition, the combination of lithium and a TCA may be effective in patients refractory to TCAs alone. Lithium is not currently FDA-approved for treatment of depression.

Electroconvulsive Therapy. Electroconvulsive therapy (ECT) is the oldest effective treatment for depression. Patients who fail to respond to antidepressant drugs (TCAs, MAOIs) will often respond to ECT. Likewise, patients refractory to ECT may respond to medication.

The most common side effects of ECT are transient memory deficit, confusion, and headache. Modified ECT, using anesthesia and muscle relaxants, has made bone fracture a rare complication. Both unilateral and bilateral ECT is currently practiced. Side effects appear to be decreased with unilateral electrode placement, although bilateral ECT may give a somewhat better antidepressant effect. Although many people worry about a permanent organic brain syndrome following ECT, there is little data to support this contention.

It is important to remember that, following the completion of ECT, maintenance treatment with antidepressant medications should be continued for at least 6 months, in order to prevent the reemergence of depressive symptoms.

Psychotherapy

The treatment of acute depressive episodes is probably most commonly managed with a combination of medication and psychotherapy. Different psychotherapeutic techniques are used, and include psychoanalysis and psychodynamically oriented individual psychotherapy, cognitive therapy, group therapy, family therapy, and behavior therapy. Goals of treatment during the acute depressive episode are often quite different from the goals later in treatment. Once acute symptoms have subsided, psychotherapy may then focus on such issues as problems of self-esteem, difficulties in interpersonal relations, and intrapsychic conflicts; often with a developmental perspective.

Maintenance Treatment

The optimal maintenance treatment for patients who are in remission following a major depressive episode is as yet unknown. Available data suggests that patients in remission following either medication or ECT should be maintained on medication for at least six months. TCAs have been most commonly used and studied as maintenance medication. Recent studies suggest that lithium is also effective in prophylaxis of recurrent unipolar depression (as well as for bipolar disease, discussed below). The dexamethasone suppression test and other biological markers may prove useful in indicating the length of an effective episode, and as a marker of the need for continued treatment.

Hospitalization vs Outpatient Treatment

In psychiatry, a particular diagnosis is rarely an indication for hospitalization in itself. Affective disorders (both depression and mania) can often be treated on an outpatient basis. Indications for psychiatric hospitalization include:

- Potential danger to self or others (*e.g.*, suicidal behavior in a depressed patient)
- Impaired reality testing with behavioral disturbances (*e.g.*, sexual promiscuity and public disrobing in a manic patient with mood-congruent psychotic features)
- Need for continued skilled observation for diagnostic assessment
- Need for intensive observation during ECT or chemotherapy (including monitoring for or treating complications of treatment)
- Failure of outpatient treatment program and need for more intensive treatment setting
- Lack of family or social supports needed to maintain outpatient treatment program
- Impaired cognition or judgment (often with behavioral implications such as the inability to comply with outpatient treatment regimen, or difficulty taking care of self)
- Medical illness requiring hospitalization, but psychiatric problems cannot be managed on a medical unit

Bipolar Disorder

A proportion of patients with bipolar affective disorder will show alteration between manic and depressive states, generally with an intervening euthymic period. Some patients will switch between mania and depression without intervening periods of normal mood; this pattern, however, is uncommon. Rarely, a patient may switch very rapidly (within 24 hours). At times, a patient may show a mixed syndrome, exhibiting both manic and depressive features at the same time.

The clinical features of the manic syndrome can be viewed as the opposite of depressive symptomatology. As in depression, the essential feature of mania is a disturbance of mood. In mania, the predominant mood has classically been described as elevated or euphoric; it may, instead, be irritable and angry. Often the manic patient has an extremely labile mood, with rapid shifts between euphoria, sadness, and irritability. A key symptom is psychomotor acceleration, often manifested by hyperactivity, decreased need for sleep, racing thoughts, and talkativeness. In contrast to the depressed patient, the manic patient may show an enormous increase of self-esteem, at times to the point of delusional grandiosity, and unwarranted optimism. Judgment is often impaired, and the manic patient may enthusiastically engage in buying sprees, embark on foolish business ventures, and exhibit flamboyant sexual indiscretion.

The DSM-III diagnostic criteria for mania include:

1. Elevated or irritable mood
2. Three of the following symptoms, lasting at least one week:
   Hyperactivity
   Pressured speech
   Racing thoughts
   Grandiosity
   Decreased sleep
   Distractibility
   Overinvolvement in activities that may lead to undesirable consequences, such as foolish business investments, reckless driving, buying sprees, or sexual indiscretions
3. The symptoms are not secondary to schizophrenia, paranoid disorder, or any other psychiatric illness.

☐ Miss T was a 36-year-old investment banker who reluctantly saw a psychiatrist at the insistence of her fiancé. He stated that for the past two weeks this normally quiet and conservative woman had been wearing unusually revealing clothing to work, had been talking constantly, and had initiated several risky business ventures. Rather than "waste time sleeping" she stayed up all night, working out her business deals on the telephone. He was concerned about her judgment in financial matters at work, but especially worried about her sexually provocative clothing and behavior, in a traditional work environment. Miss T insisted that she felt "1000% on top of the world" and defended her recent purchase of ten pairs of metallic red shoes as a need to "brighten up my image." A diagnosis of bipolar disorder, manic episode was made. Miss T responded well to lithium.

Some manic patients will demonstrate psychotic features, such as delusions, hallucinations, or extraordinarily bizarre behavior. Psychotic features are considered mood-congruent when they are consistent with themes of increased self-worth, power, and specialness (*e.g.*, delusions of grandeur).

☐ Mr. B was a 19-year-old college junior home for Christmas vacation. His family had first noticed that he seemed especially full of "Christmas cheer": he was unusually gregarious and talkative, as well as extraordinarily energetic and active. After several days in which Mr. B did not sleep, made numerous long-distance phone calls (to wish distant acquaintances "Merry Christmas" in the middle of the night), and made extravagant purchases for Christmas gifts, his family began to be concerned. It was only after Mr. B revealed that he had a special mission from God to bring about world peace by opening an international food store selling "foods of all nations," that he was brought to medical attention.

In retrospect, Mr. B had enjoyed an unusually active college semester. Not only had he headed several campus organizations, spearheaded a local political campaign, and made many new friends including several girlfriends, but he had also carried extra college courses. He slept only 2 to 3 hours a night. It was only shortly before hospital admission that his system began to fall apart. His plans became more unrealistic and as he became increasingly disorganized, he could no longer focus attention on completion of a project.

Mr. B was hospitalized, and treated initially with an antipsychotic agent. His symptoms subsided and he was then started on lithium, and the antipsychotic agent was discontinued. Once Mr. B was clinically improved, he was able to recall a similar but milder episode two years earlier. Family history revealed a paternal history of depression. The discharge diagnosis was bipolar disorder, manic episode with mood-congruent psychotic features.

When psychotic features are not consistent with such themes, they are described as mood-incongruent—examples of mood-incongruent psychotic features include persecutory delusions and delusions of being controlled.

☐ Mr. K was a 38-year-old bus driver with a past history of alcohol abuse and a hospitalization for major depressive episode one year earlier. Over several months prior to this admission Mr. K had become increasingly irritable. He slept only 2 to 3 hours a night, yet appeared to have superabundant energy. Recently, several passengers had lodged formal complaints that Mr. K was overly talkative, at times made inappropriate sexual advances, and consistently demonstrated reckless driving. When confronted by his supervisors, Mr. K accused them of eavesdropping through his television and devices planted in the bus tires; and he thought they were agents of the devil. The diagnosis was bipolar disorder, manic episode, with mood-incongruent psychotic features

Attenuated forms of mania are called *hypomania,* as in the following case:

☐ A 23-year-old woman hospitalized for depression gave the following history. Two years earlier she experienced a 2 to 3 month period of time during which she felt elated, had limitless energy, and was exceptionally creative and productive at work. She also recalled being more socially outgoing and sexually active than usual. Friends had commented on her good spirits and excellent sense of humor. Retrospective diagnosis of the earlier episode was hypomania.

Evaluation

Evaluation of a patient who presents with a manic syndrome must first focus on etiology. The possibility of an organic affective syndrome (mania that is secondary to other medical or pharmacological conditions) must also be carefully considered. A maniclike syndrome can result from drug intoxication (especially amphetamine and cocaine), endocrine disturbances (steroid psychosis, Cushing's syndrome, thyrotoxicosis), infection (*e.g.*, encephalitis), metabolic disturbances, and neoplasm. These syndromes may be difficult to distinguish from a "functional psychosis" in the mental status examination. A careful examination of physical and mental status, as well as a thorough laboratory evaluation, are therefore of critical importance. In addition, it is often difficult to distinguish an acute manic episode from an acute schizophrenic episode.

Treatment

Treatment of mania can be divided into two phases: treatment of the acute manic episode, and long-term maintenance therapy (continuation or prophylactic treatment).

Two classes of drugs are most commonly used in treating an acutely manic patient: antipsychotic agents (*e.g.*, phenothiazines, butyrophenones) and lithium. Both classes of drugs appear to be effective. Antipsychotic agents have the advantage of more rapid onset of action, and this is often critical when treating an acutely activated patient. It should be noted that acutely manic patients often require large doses of antipsychotics (at times up to the equivalent of several grams of chlorpromazine daily). For this reason, high-potency neuroleptics, which are less likely to cause oversedation or significant orthostatic hypotension, are most useful.

Acutely manic patients can also be treated with lithium alone. The disadvantage of such an approach is that it often takes at least 6 to 10 days for an antimanic effect to become apparent. If quick control of mania is necessary, then lithium is generally not the treatment of choice. However, if the patient is only mildly manic, lithium can be an effective treatment for the acute episode.

Some clinicians prefer to initiate treatment with a combination of antipsychotic medication and lithium. The reasoning behind this regimen is that the antipsychotic agent will control symptoms rapidly in the period before the lithium effect appears. A preferable regimen is to treat the acutely manic patient initially with an antipsychotic alone; once the patient is almost in remission, lithium can be begun, and the dose of antipsychotic decreased and then discontinued. The advantages of this approach are several: fewer side effects, better precision in attributing adverse reactions to the appropriate drug, and less risk of neurotoxicity (should this indeed turn out to be increased with a combination regimen). Few data are available on optimal lithium blood levels, but current recommendations are to use serum levels of 0.8 mEq/L to 1.2 mEq/L (measured 12 hours after last dose). Levels should be carefully monitored as the acute episode remits.

Carbamazepine has been reported to be effective in some manic patients refractory to standard treatment; this approach remains investigative at this time. ECT has also been used as treatment of acute mania; studies are suggestive that it is an effective treatment, but no well-controlled studies are available.

For long-term maintenance treatment of the bipolar patient, lithium is the drug of choice. Lithium appears to be effective both in preventing full-blown manic episodes, and in decreasing the severity of episodes. Determining which patient should receive maintenance therapy is a complex decision, and involves evaluation of the likelihood of a recurrence (which is more likely after two episodes), the psychosocial impact of a recurrence, medical factors, and the patient's ability to commit himself to maintenance treatment. At the present time, little is known about what lithium levels are required for the most effective maintenance treatment, or about how long treatment need be continued.

Lithium is generally administered in divided doses, and the blood level of lithium monitored at regular intervals. Generally, one aims for a level of 0.6 mEq/L to 1.2 mEq/L, although both the therapeutic and toxic levels may vary for different individuals.

Common side effects of lithium include nausea, diarrhea, fine tremor, weight gain, polyuria, polydipsia, ataxia, lethargy, and dermatologic reactions. In addition, there are several more-serious side effects:

Thyroid: Hypothyroidism may develop. Thyroid function should be regularly assessed (TSH, TRH stimulation test).

Renal: Lithium has both renal tubular and renal glomerular effects. Renal tubular effect is manifested by nephrogenic diabetes insipidus. Whether lithium damages glomerular function is still unclear.

Cardiovascular: Lithium is occasionally associated with cardiac rhythm and conduction disturbances.

Lithium toxicity must be carefully distinguished from lithium side effects. Toxicity results from lithium levels that are too high, and requires dose adjustment. Unfortunately, toxic and therapeutic lithium levels may not be far apart. It is important to remember that salt restriction, diuretics, and intercurrent illness (often with decreased fluid intake) may alter lithium levels. Early symptoms of toxicity include anorexia, vomiting, diarrhea, abdominal pain, muscle weakness or hyperirritability, polydipsia or polyuria, lethargy and confusion, and ataxia. These symptoms may progress to more severe mental and neuromuscular changes, seizures, and eventually coma and death. Lithium intoxication is treated by measures that promote removal of lithium (gastric lavage, or hemodialysis in a severely toxic patient) and supportive treatment.

Summary

Both depression and mania can present in a variety of ways. Often the patient will focus on the physical symptoms. An astute clinician will keep in mind the diagnostic criteria for the affective disorders: only then can he make an accurate diagnosis and recommend appropriate treatment.

Reference

1. Gershon E: The genetics of affective disorders. In: Grinspoon L (ed): Psychiatry Update, Vol II, pp 434–456. American Psychiatric Press, 1983

Bibliography

American Psychiatric Association: Diagnostic and Statistical Manual of Mental Disorders, 3rd ed. Washington, DC, 1980

Beck AT, Rush AJ, Shaw BF, Emergy G: Cognitive Therapy of Depression. New York, The Guilford Press, 1979

Carroll BJ, Feinberg M, Greden JF, et al: A specific laboratory test for the diagnosis of melancholia. Arch Gen Psychiatry 38:15–22, 1981

Greden JG, Gardner R, King D, et al: Dexamethasone suppression test in antidepressant treatment of melancholia. Arch Gen Psychiatry 40(5):493–500, 1983
Janowsky DS, El-Yousef MK, Davis JM, Sekerke HJ: A cholinergic-adrenergic hypothesis of mania and depression. Lancet 2:632–635, 1972
Klein DF, Gittelman R, Quitkin F, Rifkin A: Diagnosis and Drug Treatment of Psychiatric Disorders: Adults and Children, 2nd ed, Williams & Wilkins, 1980
Kupfer DJ, Thase ME: The use of the sleep laboratory in the diagnosis of affective disorders. In Akiskal HS (ed): Diagnosis and Treatment of Affective Disorders. Psychiatr Clin North Am 6(1), 1983
Leibowitz MR, Quitkin FM, Stewart JW, et al: Phenelzine *vs* imipramine in atypical depression. Arch Gen Psychiatry 41(7):669–677, 1984
Loosen PT, Kistler K, Prange AJ: Use of TSH response to TRH as an independent variable. Am J Psychiatry 140(6):700–703, 1983
Paykel ES (ed): Handbook of Affective Disorders. The Guilford Press, 1982
Rifkin A (ed): Schizophrenia and Affective Disorders: Biology and Treatment. John Wright, PSG Inc, 1983
Sachar EJ (ed): Advances in Psychoneuroendocrinology. Psychiatr Clin North Am 3(2), 1980
Schildkraut JJ: The catecholamine hypothesis of affective disorders: A review of supporting evidence. Am J Psychiatry 122(2):509–522, 1965
Wells CE: Pseudodementia. Am J Psychiatry 136(7):895–900, 1979
Weissman MM, Boyd JH: The epidemiology of affective disorders. In Grinspoon L (ed): Psychiatry Update, Vol II, pp 406–427. American Psychiatric Press, 1983

Michael R. Volow

8 Organic Mental Disorders

Impaired brain function commonly causes psychiatric disorders known as *organic brain syndromes* or *organic mental syndromes*. Such syndromes are found not only in psychiatric settings; they frequently occur in all types of medical and surgical settings in as much as 15% to 30% of patients.[1] For example, organic mental syndromes are seen in medical patients with hepatic encephalopathy, in neurology patients with stroke or encephalitis, in neurosurgical patients after head injury, in patients recovering from general surgery, and in demented patients on psychiatry wards and in nursing homes. Such syndromes can be caused either by direct involvement of the brain such as in Alzheimer's disease, in encephalitis, or more frequently by peripheral medical illness indirectly acting on the brain, as in uremia, B_{12} deficiency, or other metabolic problems.

Organic brain syndromes can be both fascinating and frustrating to the physician. Evaluation of typical organic symptoms such as confusion, memory loss, and cognitive disturbance is straightforward; however, evaluation of associated psychiatric symptoms such as hallucinations, delusions, depressive affect, or personality change may be more challenging and may mislead the nonpsychiatrist into a diagnosis of nonorganic psychiatric illness. For example, medical staff may sometimes misdiagnose the medical patient in a quiet, hypoaroused confusional state as having a depression.

Nomenclature applied to organic mental syndromes has often created misunderstanding for most physicians. *Altered mental status, acute organic brain syndrome, chronic organic brain syndrome, acute confusional state, global confusional state, toxic psychosis, clouding of consciousness, delirium,* and *dementia* have all been used to label organic mental syndromes, with varying degrees of precision. The most recent psychiatric diagnostic nomenclature, DSM-III, attempts to clear up some of this misunderstanding by proposing the following classification of organic mental disorders. In addition to the more diffuse and global changes of delirium or dementia, the nomenclature now recognizes five selective organic mental syndromes with symptoms limited exclusively to memory loss, personality change, affect change, hallucinations, or delusions.

DSM-III Classification of Organic Mental Syndromes

Organic Mental Syndromes (With Diffuse or Global Dysfunction)

Delirium (acute confusional state)

Dementia (primary dementia and secondary dementia)

Organic Mental Syndromes (With Selective Dysfunction)

Organic amnestic syndrome

Organic personality syndrome

Organic delusional syndrome

Organic hallucinosis

Organic affective syndrome

This chapter will discuss the categories of organic mental syndromes as outlined above. We will try to present a sufficiently representative selection of disorders to help the student obtain some depth of understanding, without attempting to be encyclopedic. Case examples will be presented for the main categories. The chapter will end with a discussion of the many neuropsychiatric aspects of epilepsy that are of interest to psychiatrists, neurologists, internists, and family physicians alike.

Delirium

Clinical Features

In the course of serious medical illness the mental state of many patients may change abruptly to a condition known as *delirium* or *acute confusional state.* As mentioned previously, this condition occurs widely. Delirious patients all have problems with intellect and memory, as well as *clouding of consciousness.* Clouding of consciousness is defined as "a reduction in the clarity of awareness of the environment",[2] and usually encompasses poorly sustained attention, a fragmented stream of thought, and misperception of the environment; in some mixture that may vary from patient to patient. The patient's speech is often frequently reduced or fragmented. The symptoms typically wax and wane during the course of the day, and there is often nocturnal agitation and daytime drowsiness. Perceptual disturbances may also occur, such as illusions in mild cases, paranoid delusions in moderate cases, and hallucinations in severe cases. Psychomotor activity in delirium frequently increases, as in the "anxious, panicky patient," or the "muttering, incoherent patient," or the "hallucinating patient." Sometimes, though, psychomotor activity actually decreases, as in "the quiet torpid patient" and the "blandly confused patient."[3] Quiet forms of delirium may easily (and sometimes tragically) go unnoticed by busy medical staff.

Disorientation and memory impairment are almost always present in delirium, and are detected by the usual mental status exam. The memory impairment is global and affects all aspects of memory including immediate memory, recent memory, and remote memory. Having the patient demonstrate his inability to perform complex or three-step commands is particularly helpful in confirming clouding of consciousness.

☐ A 58-year-old man in the medical intensive care unit (ICU) became paranoid and developed the delusion that some of the nursing staff were Nazis. He showed only occasional disorientation, mild euphoria, mild agitation and tachypnea, slightly illogical speech, and difficulty in concentrating and sustaining attention. Memory testing showed poor immediate, recent, and remote memory. The neurological exam was nonfocal, and an electroencephalogram (EEG) showed periods of near-normal activity alternating with generalized slowing, intermixed with triphasic waves. Concurrent medical problems included possible myocardial infarction, mild renal failure (creatinine 2 mg/dl), obstructive pulmonary disease, the possible mental effect from treatment with prednisone (20 mg/day for a vague connective tissue illness), and mild salicylate intoxication (a level of 35 mg/dl). The medical staff had initially misdiagnosed the mental condition as a psychosis or a depression because of treatment with amitriptyline before admission. Eventual background information disclosed recent unusual behavior including some mild paranoid ideation and hallucinations of barking dogs, probably related to a remote history of heavy alcohol intake until 2 years previously. The eventual diagnosis was mild underlying dementia, currently with a superimposed delirium. The etiology was felt to be multifactorial, and the symptoms of delirium responded to low doses of haloperidol, improved hydration, and reduction of the salicylate level.

This case represents the typical variety of delirium cases seen on medical wards, presenting common problems in differentiating delirium from functional psychosis, and the typically frustrating search for a single cause.

Causes of Delirium

Because many factors may cause delirium, only a few of its most important causes will be discussed.

In congestive heart failure, hypotension, and pneumonia, patients commonly experience anoxia, which is a common cause for delirium.

In patients with alcohol problems there are many causes for delirium. Delirium tremens commonly occurs 3 to 10 days after ceasing heavy use of alcohol. Symptoms include global confusion, agitation, and fear; visual and tactile hallucinations (such as rats and spiders), and autonomic release signs of slight fever and tachycardia. On the other hand, quiet confusion and sleepiness, along with a flappy tremor (asterixis), are seen in hepatic encephalopathy, a condition caused by liver failure. Sleepiness together with cerebellar ataxia and brain stem signs such as nystagmus and transitory ophthalmoplegia, are seen in Wernicke's encephalopathy, a condition caused by thiamine deficiency.

In patients with uremia, the most common cause of delirium is the direct neurologic effect of the renal failure, usually seen with blood urea nitrogen (BUN) levels of above 70 mg/dl. Agitated delirium and seizures used to be seen in the dialysis disequilibrium syndrome, a now-infrequent mental condition that commonly occurred following very brisk dialyses of severely uremic patients.[4]

Other metabolic or endocrine conditions causing delirium include: hypoglycemia, severe thyrotoxicosis, myxedema, acute intermittent porphyria, and cation deficiencies including calcium, potassium, and magnesium.

Toxic agents and drugs may cause delirium, but they may also cause other types of organic mental syndromes.[5] Bromides may cause delirium as well as dementia-like or schizophrenia-like states. Simple intoxication with alcohol may cause delirium, but much more commonly causes simple reduction in the level of consciousness. Acute exposure to heavy metals, which is rare, may cause confusion. Deliria with anticholinergic features, such as dry mouth, flushed skin, mydriasis, and tachycardia, may be caused by atropine-like agents, tricyclic antidepressants, or antiparkinsonian drugs. Psychedelic drugs such as lysergic acid diethylamide (LSD), euphoretics such as marihuana, and sympathomimetics such as amphetamines, are less likely to produce delirium but more likely to cause organic hallucinosis, organic delusional syndrome, or organic affective syndrome. Phencyclidine ("angel dust") produces a variety of psychopathologic states including delirium, schizophreniform psychosis, and organic affective or organic delusional syndromes, which include amphetamine-like syndromes with elevated blood pressure, paranoia, and posturing. Results of phencyclidine use include homicidal and suicidal behavior, hypertension, stupor, coma, and death.

In spite of the widespread use of antibiotics, systemic infections such as pneumonia, malaria, and typhoid may still occasionally cause delirium. For example, a young, recently-arrived Indian student saw an emergency room psychiatrist for confusion and an unusual delusional state in which the student believed himself to have died and to have assumed his brother's identity. His illness eventually turned out to be typhoid, which cleared completely with antibiotics.[5] Infections of the central nervous system such as acute bacterial meningitis or viral encephalitis may present as a delirium associated with fever and headache; psychotic features may be present, especially in herpes simplex encephalitis,[5] probably because of temporal lobe involvement.

Any condition of the brain acutely causing mild bilateral cerebral dysfunction may cause delirium, including increased intracranial pressure of any cause, hydrocephalus, and ictal states such as petit mal status or psychomotor status epilepticus. Focal lesions occasionally cause delirium, particularly if the lesion is associated with edema or hemorrhage, or if the focal lesion specifically involves infarction of the right parietal or inferomedial occipital lobes.[6]

Environmental factors such as sensory isolation, sensory overload, and sensory monotony may contribute to insomnia and delirium in critical care units such as ICUs and CCUs. In one variety of postoperative delirium (lucid-interval type), the patient's mind is clear for a few days after surgery and then becomes confused; this type of delirium is related to multiple factors, including age, preoperative anxiety, sleep deprivation, anesthesia and other medications, bypass pump time (in cardiac cases), the intensive care environment, and unsuspected mild dimentia. Intraoperative anoxia and hypotension have been implicated as factors in a type of postoperative delirium occurring immediately after surgery (nonlucid-interval type) and in these cases, recovery is poorer.[5]

Differential Diagnosis

The term *delirium* should be applied to states of waking confusion; if consciousness is both reduced and clouded, then the diagnosis of stupor, semicoma, or coma should be made instead, as appropriate. Delirium is a temporary condition that is often misdiagnosed as a permanent dementia. Despite altered intellectual function in both conditions, hallucinations and delusions are much more characteristic of delirium than of dementia, and disturbances of orientation and attention are usually more severe in delirium than in dementia, except in end-stage dementia. However, delirium may sometimes be superimposed on underlying dementia, a state called *beclouded dementia.*[5]

Physicians also frequently confuse delirium with a functional psychosis such as schizophrenia, or with depression. The main differential points favoring delirium are: the suddenness of onset and clear association with medical illness, the "organic" memory and cognitive symptoms rarely found in schizophrenia, and the absence of previous mental illness. Compared to the psychotic features of true schizophrenia (elaborate and bizarre auditory hallucinations, flattened affect, and thought disorder), the psychotic features of delirium are quite different (simple and fragmented illusions and visual hallucinations).

Organic hallucinosis, organic delusional syndrome, and organic affective syndrome may at times resemble delirium but are without disturbance of consciousness, memory, or cognition.

Clinical Management of Delirium

A useful approach in managing delirium is to search first for the most obvious medical cause(s), because delirium is usually secondary to a physical illness. The history and physical exam have great importance here. Instead of a single cause, there is often a combination of two or three mild metabolic causes, as in the case example, such as major pulmonary or cardiac illness, renal disease, toxicity of medications such as salicylates and steroids, as well as traces of low-grade dementia. Because of the many causes of delirium, the first laboratory tests should include routine tests as well as tests indicated by the clinical picture; this approach should help reduce unnecessary expense and effort. Straightforward examination is often sufficient, including complete blood count (CBC), routine chemistries, electrolytes, arterial blood gases, and chest film to rule out pneumonia. Blood and urine cultures are often useful in revealing unsuspected infection. A spinal tap should be considered if a cause for the delirium is not found quickly, and is most specific for suspected central nervous system (CNS) infection (as suggested by fever, headache, and somnolence) or subarachnoid hemorrhage. Computerized tomography is useful if focal neurologic features suggest structural neurologic disease. Generalized slowing of the EEG may be somewhat useful in deciding between a mild organic delirium and a nonorganic psychiatric illness; and patterns such as triphasic waves may help in other situations; such as deciding between delirium tremens and hepatic encephalopathy.[5]

Delirium often carries with it increased medical morbidity such as pneumonia or septicemia. Because many deliria are easily reversible they should receive appropriate medical treatment, which will restore cognitive functioning. It is best to treat the disease in question specifically, if possible. When delirium results from a combination of multiple mild metabolic imbalances, however, simple correction of these imbalances is frequently insufficient, with improvement in mental state often lagging several days behind improvement in the laboratory values. Therefore, physicians should not be timid about treating such deliria with modest antipsychotic regimens (if not contraindicated) such as haloperidol in the range of 5 mg to 20 mg per day. Because of the difficulty of estimating the correct dose, a useful titration procedure is to give 1 mg to 2 mg by mouth every 2 hours, stopping at an end point of decreased agitation (for agitated deliria) or of slight sleepiness (for quiet deliria). Milder deliria due to suspected sensory isolation may respond merely to improving the offending environment (night light, video monitors removed from patient's view, increased human contact, reassurance) and safe bedtime sedatives to counteract sleep deprivation (such as chloral hydrate 1–2 g, diphenhydramine 25–50 mg, or flurazepam 15–30 mg).

DSM-III Criteria for Delirium[2]

1. Clouding of consciousness
2. At least two of the following:
   - Perceptual disturbance (illusions, delusions, hallucinations)
   - Speech incoherent at times
   - Nocturnal agitation and daytime drowsiness
   - Increased or decreased psychomotor activity
3. Disorientation and global memory impairment (immediate, recent, and remote)
4. Abrupt onset and fluctuating symptoms
5. Presumed organic cause

Dementia

We define dementia as a general loss of intellectual functioning that is sufficient to cause social or occupational disability, and which arises from a definite or presumed organic etiology.[2] Most cases of dementia involve impairment of several mental functions, but the symptom common to all dementias is disturbance of memory function, especially recent memory. Most types of dementia also affect specific cognitive functions such as calculation, abstraction, reading, and spelling. With more advanced dementing illness, orientation, affect, and judgment are also affected. Some dementias are reversible and some are not; but in all dementias, either subacute or chronic, the course is protracted, compared to the brief course of delirium.

Dementia is also a widespread public health problem. Many epidemiologic surveys in the United States estimate that 10% to 15% of people over the age of 65 have some degree of dementia, and that about one third of these dementias are severe. In addition, estimates indicate that one million people in the United States are presently institutionalized for dementia.[7] Even when the demented patient can be taken care of at home, his care represents so great an economic and interpersonal burden that families often require support groups to help manage and tolerate the demented patient.

Types of Dementias

At one time there was little hope for the patient with dementia; all such patients were seen as having irreversible, untreatable, progressive, primary degenerative dementia—such as Alzheimer's disease. Research studies have shown that in heterogenous groups of dementias, often at least 10% to 15% of cases are due to reversible or treatable causes.[7] Some authorities therefore divide dementia into (1) primary dementias, usually untreatable, degenerative conditions such as Alzheimer's; and (2) secondary dementias,[6] potentially treatable conditions secondarily causing dementia, including metabolic, endocrine, neoplastic, infectious, or hydrocephalic etiologies. Although this is not a universally accepted classification, we shall see that it is a useful one.

DSM-III Criteria for Dementia[2]

1. Loss of intellectual abilities of sufficient severity to interfere with social or occupational functioning
2. Memory impairment
3. At least one of the following:
   - Impaired abstraction, difficulty in defining words and concepts
   - Impaired judgment
   - Other higher cortical function disturbances: aphasia, apraxia, agnosia, constructional apraxia
   - Personality change, including alteration or accentuation of premorbid traits
4. Consciousness not clouded
5. Definite or presumptive organic cause

Many different types of dementia exist and the next portion of this chapter will present the clinical features of the most important conditions. DSM-III labels most of these dementias as *organic mental syndromes;* however, following tradition, it labels Alzheimer's disease and multi-infarct dementia as *organic mental disorders,* and this chapter will follow the same convention.

Primary Dementias

Alzheimer's Disease (Presenile dementia, Alzheimer's type)

Degenerative disease of unknown etiology is one of the most common types of dementia, comprising roughly 50% of several heterogeneous series of dementias. The most common type of degenerative dementia is Alzheimer's disease. When the onset occurs before the age of 65, the illness is called *Alzheimer's disease* or *presenile dementia;* and when the onset occurs after 65 it is called *senile dementia of the Alzheimer's type.*

The course of Alzheimer's disease is often divided into three stages:[8] an early stage with primarily behavioral symptoms, a middle stage with familiar memory and cognitive symptoms, and a later stage with predominantly neurologic symptoms, although the clinical picture can be quite variable. In the first stage the clinical features are vague and ill-defined, often resembling functional psychiatric illness. The changes are subtle and are noticed more by the family than the patient. The patient shows decreased energy and drive, requires more effort to do previously easy tasks, and may be able to do customary tasks one at a time, but can no longer keep track of multiple tasks. At this stage mild memory disturbance may be apparent to relatives but not to the patient. Mild depression is also frequent at this point.

The more classical intellectual deterioration occurs in the middle phase of Alzheimer's, including disturbance of orientation, memory, and calculation. Comprehension of spoken language becomes less efficient and more concrete, with the patient mildly misinterpreting conversations or plots of television shows. The patient, embarrassed, may become withdrawn, shying away from old friends. Previously existing personality traits such as obsessiveness may be exaggerated, or out-of-character behavior may be released, such as irascibility in a previously mild-mannered patient. Often the patient exhibits poor judgment.

The late phase of Alzheimer's is marked by more profound psychological and behavioral deterioration, such as apathy, loss of the personality, severe disorientation, and inability to remember. Frank neurologic signs, too, are much more apparent, including gait and coordination disturbance, aphasia, apraxia, and agnosia and even cortical blindness in some patients. The late phase results in severe impairments in self-care, dressing, ambulation, and the ability to recognize close relatives.

The duration of the disease is variable but averages 2 to 5 years, often resulting in institutionalization in the later stages, with death frequently occurring from intercurrent infection.

Alzheimer's disease is considered to be a diffuse degenerative brain disease, most prominently involving gray matter. The gross neuropathologic appearance of the brain consists of reduced size and increased prominence of sulci due to atrophy of cortical gray matter, and classic, light, microscopic lesions that include numerous senile plaques and neurofibrillary tangles. Atrophy is often most prominent in the frontal lobes and hippocampi.[7] Recent studies have shown altered enzymatic activity in two subcortical nuclei, decreased dopamine β-hydroxylase in the nucleus locus ceruleus of the brain stem, and decreased choline acetyltransferase in the nucleus basalis of the forebrain. Both nuclei are thought to extrude neurotransmitters through axons into other brain regions, the ceruleus extruding dopamine and norepinephrine, and the basalis extruding acetylcholine, especially to the cortex. Therapy that is based on these deficits, however, such as the giving of choline, has been only minimally successful in treating Alzheimer's.

Senile Dementia, Alzheimer's Type

Aging is not the same thing as dementia, and not all elderly become demented. Such common misconceptions arise from uncritical observation of elderly people that are physically ill, rather than from systematic study of healthy, elderly, nonpatient volunteers. The effects of normal aging in the elderly, such as mild memory inefficiency, gait awkwardness, and slight slowing of motor and perceptual speed, may also be misinterpreted as dementia. In follow-up aging studies of healthy, elderly volunteers, some go on to develop senile dementia, some show slight mental decline, and still others remain surprisingly intact mentally.[7]

Classical descriptions of the variations of senile dementia depict several types of clinical presentation: the confusional and delirious type, the agitated and depressed type, the paranoid type, and the amnesic (Korsakoff-like) type.[7] In spite of these clinical differences between senile dementia and Alzheimer's disease, neuropathologic studies show that microscopic brain changes in senile dementia are similar to, but less numerous than, the microscopic changes in Alzheimer's disease, suggesting that they are the same disease.[7] It has been suggested that the varying clinical presentation reflects interaction of a unitary organic process with personality and other psychosocial variables.

☐ A 73-year-old woman, Mrs. E, began in 1980 to have symptoms of crying, forgetfulness, confusion, and increased fear of being domineered by her sister. She developed trouble in dressing and cooking, burned papers, and forgot to pay bills. She was angrily impatient with herself when making errors. The examination showed a calm, alert, neatly dressed woman, who was disoriented to time and only roughly oriented to place; she could do only simple calculations; immediate memory by digit span was fair, and recent memory was poor. She thought she was in the hospital "for a job" and showed concreteness on similarities and differences. Her understanding of language and of situations was only approximate. She had normal laboratory tests, including hematocrit, thyroid, folic acid, B_{12}, and calcium. Her EEG was slightly slowed and a computed tomography (CT) scan showed bilateral atrophy.

Pick's Disease[7]

Pick's disease is another degenerative disease causing dementia that bears some clinical resemblence to Alzheimer's disease, but is much rarer and has a different neuropathologic identity, which is characterized by "ballooning" of nerve cell bodies. In contrast with the diffuse atrophy of Alzheimer's, atrophy in Pick's tends to concentrate in more of a "lobar" fashion, especially in the frontal and temporal regions. Therefore, isolated focal syndromes such as frontal lobe syndromes or aphasia may appear much earlier during the course of Pick's, and may even be the earliest symptoms. The frontal symptoms include apathy, bradykinesia, episodic irritability, impulsiveness, and poor judgment.

Huntington's Disease

Huntington's disease, a relatively rare neurologic disorder, is characterized by choreiform movement and dementia. Huntington's has achieved unfortunate notoriety because of the tales of suicide, impulsiveness, the "tainted" heredity that accompanies it, and because of the very prolonged period (10–30 years) over which drastic and tragic personality disintegration occurs. Symptoms of Huntington's fall into three groups: (1) cognitive symptoms or dementia, (2) behavioral symptoms, and (3) movement disorder symptoms.[7,9] Cognitive or behavioral symptoms in many instances precede the symptoms of movement disorder, but the tendency to conceal the family history of Huntington's sometimes makes statistics difficult to obtain.

The cognitive symptoms develop insidiously: Memory function begins to deteriorate and becomes more obvious after 3 to 5 years, and the patient has trouble keeping track of more than one task or plan at one time. Personality deterioration begins with progressive apathy and motor slowing (bradykinesia), reduced quantity of speech and thought, and lessened interest and drive. In some cases, episodic behavior disturbances may be superimposed, including irritability, anxiety, sadness, euphoria, emotional storms, poor judgment, misperception of social situations, and aggressive outbursts toward the family. Although the apathetic-dementia pattern occurs most commonly, full-blown psychiatric disorders are sometimes seen, including suicidal depressions, manic-like states, paranoid syndromes, and delusional, schizophrenia-like states; and these probably give the disease its notoriety.

The movement disorder of Huntington's often, but not always, begins after the onset of the cognitive-behavioral symptoms. Initially, the patient makes inconspicuous choreic movements sometimes disguised as voluntary mannerisms, initially involving the face and trunk, but eventually extending to respiration, speech, and gait. Particularly characteristic are facial grimaces and awkward explosive speech that increase with emotion and cease during sleep.

The disease is genetic and is generally inherited as an autosomal dominant trait. Pathologic brain changes are classically reported as atrophy in the caudate nucleus and enlarged ventricles. Except for symptomatic treatment of the psychiatric complications, no definitive treatment exists.

Secondary Dementias

Secondary dementias, as previously explained, are those dementias not due primary degenerative etiologies, and are often reversible or at least potentially treatable.

Vascular Dementia[10]

After Alzheimer's disease, the second most common cause of dementia in adults is currently thought to be vascular dementia, and this represents 8% of all dementias.

The cortical form of vascular dementia, known as *multi-infarct dementia,* is characterized by focal neurologic features such as hemiparesis, aphasia, or apraxia; which are due to repeated, multiple, small strokes, eventually leading to demented cortical function. The clinical exam reveals patchy neurologic signs, and the course of the illness shows the well-known, stepwise progression due to the multiple strokes. Another pattern of vascular dementia is known as *lacunar state,* and is characterized by different patterns of motor and sensory deficits, movement disorders and bradykinesia, and disturbances of arousal and activation. The mental state shows wide fluctuations with episodic confusion and sleepiness; and in some cases, a frontal-lobe-like picture with apathy and emotional lability. The clinical picture varies, depending on which subcortical regions are damaged. The symptoms are due to multiple, small, crescent-shaped infarcts called *lacunes,* located in subcortical white or subcortical gray matter. The penetrating blood vessels serving the subcortical regions are particularly vulnerable to lacune formation because of their greater length. Although sometimes resembling the stepwise course of multi-infarct dementia, the course of lacunar state may at other times resemble the insidious course of Alzheimer's, because the small, lacunar episodes are not obvious clinically or on a CT scan. In very severe cases of subcortical white matter involvement due to vascular disease, the name *Binswanger's disease* is often applied.

In the patient with vascular dementia there is usually some predisposing medical condition, frequently hypertension or diabetes, hyperlipidemia, history of myocardial infarct, hypotensive episode or hypoxic episode, or blood dyscrasia or collagen disease in rare cases. Multiple emboli have been implicated in multi-infarct dementia. Because of the clinical variability of multi-infarct and related dementias, diagnosis is often confusing and difficult. In our experience, some cases are diagnosed at first as Alzheimer's but afterward turn out to be static, arrested, vascular dementias with superimposed depressive pseudodementia. These patients sometimes show surprising and occasionally shocking improvement after two or three years of their "progressive dementia."

Metabolic Dementias

Metabolic etiologies frequently cause altered mental status, most commonly delirium or stupor; but some metabolic etiologies lead instead to potentially reversible or potentially treatable dementias that mimic degenerative brain disease such as Alzheimer's disease. Chronic uremia, vitamin B_{12} deficiency, hypothyroidism, and thiamine deficiency are among the most frequent metabolic causes of reversible dementia.

Renal Disease.[4,5]

If chronic uremia progresses undetected until the BUN approximates the 70-mg/dl range, *uremic encephalopathy,* a dementia-like mental condition, may develop with slowing in all areas of memory and cognition, but without other distinctive psychiatric features. If untreated, it eventually progresses toward further neurologic deterioration with stupor, asterixis, myoclonus, and multifocal cortical signs such as seizures and mild aphasia. Hemodialysis treatment of uremia may produce two additional types of organic mental state disturbance: the dialysis disequilibrium syndrome, discussed in the Delirium section; and dialysis dementia, a late complication of chronic hemodialysis treatment. Dialysis dementia usually starts after months to years of uneventful, successful hemodialysis, and begins with the sudden onset of recurrent episodes of neurologic symptoms that occur soon after completing a dialysis session. The symptoms include halting, nonfluent speech, myoclonic jerks, or seizure activity. Progressive cognitive disturbance accompanies these neurologic features, and the course is usually fatal. The EEG is somewhat helpful diagnostically and shows bursts of generalized, rhythmic, sharp- and slow-wave complexes over the frontal midline. Other causes of dementia-like states in chronic renal disease include covert subdural hematoma and hypercalcemia, both of which are discussed later in this chapter.

Vitamin B_{12}. Deficiency of vitamin B_{12} commonly causes pernicious anemia, and may also cause central nervous system disorders such as the well-known spinal condition, subacute combined degeneration. Sometimes B_{12} deficiency instead causes a true dementia, even without the neurologic features of subacute combined degeneration except for positive plantar reflexes. The symptoms include nondistinctive cognitive and memory disturbance, as well as psychiatric symptoms including paranoia, irritability, confusion, and agitation. There are even rare reports of B_{12} dementia occurring without overt anemia or peripheral blood smear changes.[15] Even with B_{12} treatment, cognitive improvement is often slower than hematologic improvement.

Thyroid Disease. Hypothyroidism, a common metabolic cause of organic mental disorder, may produce a number of clinically distinct conditions. A true dementia may sometimes occur with hypothyroidism, with nonspecific memory and cognitive features similar to other metabolic dementias. More commonly, mild hypothyroidism in adults causes instead an organic affective syndrome closely resembling depression. A schizophrenic-like psychotic state may also occur in the severe, myxedematous form of hypothyroidism, and symptoms may include slowing of speech, thinking, and memory; irritability, listlessness, and apathy; and even paranoia, delusions, and hallucinations. In hypothyroid mental states, signs such as cold intolerance and diminished reflexes may serve as clues to the diagnosis; however, peripheral clinical signs of hypothyroidism may sometimes be absent. The EEG often shows generalized slowing. Laboratory documentation of low thyroid function is essential for diagnosis and follow-up. With thyroid hormone replacement the mental symptoms are completely or partially reversible, depending on the severity and duration of the preceding thyroid deficiency.

Hyperthyroidism also produces several clinical syndromes. Mild or moderate hyperthyroidism commonly produces some type of organic affective syndrome that mimicks either a chronic anxiety disorder, a hypomanic affective disorder, or occasionally a depressive disorder. Another variation of this syndrome is apathetic hyperthyroidism, which is characterized by symptoms of apathy and helplessness, and is found most frequently in the elderly. Any of these syndromes have the potential to resemble a dementia-like syndrome because memory and concentration function poorly in these hypermetabolic states. Clinical signs such as tachycardia, systolic hypertension, heat intolerance, and warm skin would normally aid diagnosis; but as described above, in some hyperthyroid mental states hypermetabolic and autonomic peripheral signs may occasionally be minimal. Acute thyrotoxicosis is associated with more serious mental and physical malfunction, and is therefore more likely to produce a severe delirium than a dementia would be.

Thiamine Deficiency. Deficiency of the vitamin thiamine,[5] often due to alcoholic malnutrition, may lead to an organic mental disorder known as Korsakoff's disease. The essential clinical feature in Korsakoff's is a profound memory disturbance known as the *amnestic syndrome,* a state in which the patient is unable to make any new memories whatsoever (anterograde amnesia), has some difficulty in retrieving old memories (retrograde amnesia), and tends to place old memories in the wrong context (confabulation); but retains some recall for ultra-remote memories. The clinical features are described in more detail under Selective Organic Mental Syndromes, Amnestic Syndrome. Because of the severe memory disturbance, Korsakoff's patients show disorientation and poor judgment, and sometimes confabulate (probably less often than described). Early treatment with thiamine may lead to improvement; but treatment later on does not lead to improvement. Amnestic syndrome may also be due to other causes, such as cerebral anoxia or bilateral temporal lobe damage from trauma or encephalitis; and to these cases we apply the term *Korsakoff's syndrome* rather than *Korsakoff's disease.*

Other causes for dementia-like syndromes include disturbances of the metabolism of calcium, glucocorticoids, glucose, hepatic detoxification, nicotinic acid, and oxygen supply. Some of these conditions have peripheral medical and biochemical signs that are diagnostically helpful; but many of their organic mental symptoms, such as confusion, irritability, and memory loss, tend to be nonspecific and not diagnostic.

Calcium.[5] Moderate elevations of serum calcium (12–14 mg/dl) may cause mild symptoms such as lassitude, depression, and irritability; but higher elevations in calcium (14–16 mg/dl) cause a more "organic" picture, with confusional or delirious states occurring more frequently then dementia, sometimes with psychotic accessory symptoms like paranoid ideation and hallucinations. In addition to hyperparathyroidism as a cause for elevated serum calcium, there are many other medical causes, including malignancy, multiple myeloma, and advanced renal disease. Low-serum calcium occurs less frequently than high-serum calcium, but is more potent in producing mental symptoms. Sometimes a dementia-like picture occurs, but other syndromes are more common, such as delirium, tetany, and seizures in full-grown individuals, or mental retardation in the developmental period. Hypoparathyroidism is more likely to be associated with mental symptoms than hyperparathyroidism.

Anoxia.[5] Residual anoxic brain injury may sometimes cause permanent dementia, although reversible confusional or delirious states may result when anoxia is partial. Although anoxia theoretically affects the brain diffusely, anoxic damage often represents a mixture of localized damage and diffuse damage. This is probably due to varying collateral circulation and preexisting localized ischemia, as well as the special vulnerability to anoxia of the cortex, hippocampus, basal ganglia, reticular activating system, and cerebellum. Reduced oxygen tension may be caused by poor pulmonary ventilation (anoxia) or by poor brain perfusion (ischemia) from conditions such as hypotension, congestive heart failure, or cardiac arrest.

Steroids. Disorders of adrenal steroids may be endogenous, as in Cushing's disease (excess) or Addison's disease (deficiency); or they may be exogenous, as in steroid treatment of medical conditions such as lupus or sarcoid. Exogenous steroids are widely used, and many persons receiving them have unusual mental experiences varying from mild to severe, depending on the dose. Although steroid excess may occasionally produce a dementia-like apathy (especially in Cushing's), it more frequently causes organic affective states of depression, irritability, or euphoria; and occasionally causes organic hallucinosis, paranoia, or psychosis. Addison's may mimic severe depression.

Liver disease. In two types of chronic liver disease, Wilson's disease and chronic hepatic encephalopathy, dementia may be a prominent symptom, but in Wilson's there are often (but not always) prominent neurologic features of the extrapyramidal type.[7]

Niacin Deficiency (Pellagra). Although rare, pellagra occasionally occurs in psychiatric patients whose suspiciousness of food or idiosyncratic diet produces selective niacin deficiency. The insidious onset of progressive cognitive changes generally precedes the well-known peripheral signs of dermatitis, stomatitis, and diarrhea.[5]

Toxic Dementias

Toxic agents may cause a variety of different organic mental syndromes, including simple intoxication, addiction; selective syndromes such as hallucinosis, or withdrawal seizures and withdrawal deliria as discussed earlier in the chapter. Some toxic agents do cause dementia, however, especially with secretive and chronic use of these agents. All kinds of sedative-hypnotic drugs, such as barbiturates, minor tranquilizers, bromides, and alcohol, are among the most frequent offenders, and all may produce a dementia-like state that improves after discontinuation of the agent. Chronic use of short-acting barbiturates such as secobarbital or pentobarbital in amounts greater than 500 mg to 800 mg per day frequently produces all signs of dementia, including blunted affect and defects in concentration, memory, calculation, and abstraction. Chronic abuse of many other sedative-hypnotics or benzodiazapines may produce the same symptom picture, as may chronic abuse of the older tranquilizing drugs like meprobamate and bromides. Clinical syndromes with any of these drugs tend to resemble each other except that bromides may produce a wider variety of mental syndromes, including delirium, dementia, organic delusional syndrome, and organic hallucinosis; an acneiform rash may alert suspicion to the possibility of bromism.

Diphenylhydantoin (Dilantin) toxicity may cause a reversible dementia syndrome with cognitive symptoms of slow thinking and memory impairment, neurologic symptoms of mumbling dysarthric speech, a broad-based gait, a fine rest tremor, and sometimes a worsening or change in the patient's seizures. Sometimes there are psychiatric symptoms such as paranoia, irritability, apathy, euphoria, or hallucinations. The EEG is diffusely slowed. Because the nystagmus and intention tremor of acute Dilantin toxicity are often absent, recognition of this type of subacute toxicity is often delayed. One important clue is the occurrence of nausea after each Dilantin dose. Another anticonvulsant, carbamazepine, also seems capable of occasionally causing a subacute dementia-like syndrome.

Chronic exposure to many toxic physical agents such as heavy metals may cause dementia, which is well known, and examples include lead, mercury, arsenic, manganese, and thallium, to name just a few. Because the possible physical agents are so numerous, the discussion of specific syndromes is best left to toxicology textbooks, but the specialized neurologic and medical features such as neuropathy or anemia, in addition to cognitive dysfunction, should raise the physician's suspicion about physical agent toxicity.

The psychedelic and "recreational" drugs available today, when used chronically, produce many kinds of organic mental syndromes, but do not commonly cause dementia-like states.

Causes of dementia in alcoholics have well-known nutritional causes (*e.g.*, Korsakoff's disease and chronic hepatic encephalopathy), and some authorities now believe that also there exists a different type of dementia due to direct alcohol toxicity to the brain, independent of nutrition.[16] This somewhat controversial syndrome is now called *dementia due to alcoholism* in DSM-III and had been called *alcoholic deterioration* in the older nomenclature. As opposed to the older Korsakoff patient, dementia due to alcoholism is said to occur in younger patients and is associated with high rates of consumption of very large quantities of alcohol. Reversible memory disturbance and reversible cerebral atrophy have been described in this condition, but further confirmation of this syndrome is needed.

Neoplasms

Some neoplastic lesions within the brain may simulate a progressive degenerative dementia and may lead to misdiagnosis and delayed treatment.[9] Tumors producing obvious neurologic features such as aphasia, seizures, or elemental sensory or motor disturbance, are unlikely to be misdiagnosed as progressive degenerative dementia. Deep tumors of the hemispheres or diencephalon, however, may produce dementia without focal neurologic signs, especially when accompanied by increased intracranial pressure, edema, or hydrocephalus; and such lesions include tumors of the basal ganglia and thalamus, butterfly tumors of the corpus callosum, and tumors of the ventricular system. Tumors of the neurologically silent higher cortical association areas, such as the frontal and anterior temporal regions, rather than producing dementia, are most likely to produce organic personality syndromes such as frontal lobe syndromes. Other tumors that may cause dementia include posterior fossa tumors such as acoustic neuromas, which have a very slow growth rate.

Head Trauma[5]

Trauma to the head is a fairly frequent cause of dementia. In a fairly typical sequence, the patient has an episode of head trauma and is unconscious for a variable period, from hours to days or weeks; and upon awakening is often delirious and confused for another variable period lasting from hours to weeks. As the patient's confusion resolves, the severity of the patient's residual cognitive deficits can be evaluated, with most of these deficits stabilizing within two years or sooner. There is no single characteristic pattern of deficit following closed head injury, but many patients have a dementia due to diffuse cortical involvement, often with some focal damage. Common types of focal involvement include hemiparesis, organic personality syndromes such as frontal lobe syndrome, parietotemporal lobe syndromes with language dysfunction, or bitemporal syndromes with temporary amnestic features. The patient's functioning eventually becomes more or less stable around these fixed deficits; but sometimes unexpected improvement occurs later than the 2-year period, due to better compensation for deficits, relief of accompanying depression, or for unknown reasons. In other cases of supposedly fixed deficits there is unexpected late worsening of function, at times possibly due to post-traumatic seizures or hydrocephalus, but at other times it is unexplainable.

If the head trauma is recent, the possibility of progressive dementia due to *chronic subdural hematoma* should be kept in mind, because of its reversibility. The clinical picture is variable, with nonspecific cognitive features in chronic cases, and greater neurologic dysfunction with headache, hemiparesis, and fluctuating level of consciousness in subacute cases. As a cause of dementia particularly in the elderly, chronic subdural hematoma should often be considered even in the absence of trauma.

In progressive traumatic encephalopathy of boxers (*dementia pugilistica*), repeated head trauma is said to lead to a progressive dementia by the mechanism of progressive demyelination.

Infectious Causes

Infectious and inflammatory conditions of the central nervous system are important to diagnose because some are potentially treatable. Some of these conditions may cause dementia, and some may cause other organic mental syndromes, including delirium, organic delusional syndrome, and organic personality syndrome. Dementia may be associated with the following conditions: chronic leptomeningitis, chronic residua of acute viral encephalitis or bacterial meningitis, acute focal encephalitis, and slow virus encephalitis.

Progressive dementia may be due to subacute or chronic leptomeningitis. The leptomeninges are thickened and inflamed, and one typical presentation is the picture of basilar meningitis with neurologic involvement of the optic, facial, extraocular nerves, or hypothalamus by thick exudate. Mental symptoms include headache, irritability, apathy, and sometimes stupor and confusion if the illness is more acute. Organisms such as Cryptococcus or Aspergillus are primarily responsible for leptomeningitis today, especially in immunocompromised individuals; but in the past tuberculosis or syphilis were often responsible. Other causes of a similar leptomeningitis syndrome include sarcoidosis and metastatic carcinomatous meningitis. Cryptococcal infections may be present for several years before being diagnosed and may truly imitate degenerative dementia.

Generalized viral encephalitis in its acute phase is likely to lead to a delirium or stupor; but during the recovery phase the residual damage may take the form of a dementia. Severe bacterial meningitis may also lead to a residual dementia.

Encephalitis due to herpes simplex virus, while diffusely involving the cortex, tends to show focal necrotic involvement, especially in the temporal regions. This leads to mental symptoms of delirium, sometimes with psychotic ideation in the acute phase, and to a dementia with severe amnestic features in the residual or chronic phase.

Progressive dementia may also be due to infection by slow viruses. This type of infection is represented in adults by Jakob–Creutzfeldt disease, which presents with early and very prominent neurologic symptoms as well as dementia, including cerebellar ataxia, extrapyramidal movement disorder, seizures, and myoclonus. The dementia may at times briefly precede the motor symptoms, but the entire course is short (2–18 months) and is almost always fatal. Transmission by tissue contact has been documented, including corneal transplant, so that premortem diagnosis by biopsy can be hazardous. Subacute sclerosing panencephalitis (SSPE), a childhood slow virus infection, seems to represent some form of subacute CNS infection by measles virus. Initially the patient experiences gradual loss of the ability to do schoolwork, followed by clumsiness, ataxia, myoclonic jerks, and eventually dementia and loss of speech. Elevated levels of measles antibody are detectable in the serum and spinal fluid. The EEG is known to be helpful diagnostically in both of these slow virus conditions. In the middle course of either illness, the EEG shows an unusual and semicharacteristic pattern of steady periodic discharges, periodic, triphasic, sharp-wave complexes at one per second in Jakob–Creutzfeldt, and periodic, sharp-wave or polyphasic slow-wave complexes at the rate of one every 3 to 8 seconds in SSPE.[7]

Normal-Pressure Hydrocephalus[7]

In this syndrome, the mental symptoms of dementia and the neurologic symptoms of gait disturbance are thought to be due to a low-pressure, communicating hydrocephalus, and are sometimes potentially surgically reversible by a shunting operation. The symptoms consist of a mild to moderate dementia, sometimes with frontal-lobe-like features. Of importance is the early development of some type of lower extremity neurologic disturbance, including hyperreflexia of the legs more than the arms, ankle clonus and spasticity, and extensor plantars. There are any one of several types of gait disturbance, including spastic gait, unsteady gait, nonspecific ataxias with short, shuffling steps on a broad base, or full-blown, "glued-to-the-floor" frontal gait apraxias. Urinary incontinence may develop.

Current pathophysiological theory suggests that in normal-pressure hydrocephalus there is defective reabsorption of cerebrospinal fluid, with atrophy of the white matter around the ventricles, due to the increased volume of the cerebrospinal fluid (CSF). The defective reabsorption of cerebrospinal fluid is thought to be due to such causes as old subarachnoid hemorrhage, trauma, chronic meningitis, or to unknown causes. Diagnostic confirmation is currently by CT scan showing ventricular dilatation, and by isotope cisternography showing failure of the isotope to flow from the ventricle into the subarachnoid space. The ventricular distention and white matter atrophy of normal-pressure hydrocephalus should not be confused with the passive dilatation *ex vacuo* due to gray matter atrophy in degenerative disease. Because of the possibility of surgical reversal, physicians should be alert for the unique syndrome of lower-extremity signs in demented patients.

Pseudodementia

Clinicians have begun to apply the term *pseudodementia* to functional psychiatric disease that closely imitates progressive degenerative dementia. It is extremely important to diagnose pseudodementia because appropriate treatment may reverse the condition, with the most frequent underlying psychiatric state being depression. Pseudodementia has been estimated to account for 4% of patients in an unselected series of mixed dementias[10]; and in a 5- to 15-year follow-up of a group carefully screened for so-called primary degenerative disease only, 13% were eventually found to have pseudodementia.[11]

Pseudodementia resembles dementia clinically, but has a more acute onset and a course measured in months. It is associated with much more distress and affect, more painful awareness of disability, poor effort and variability on testing, and remote as well as recent memory disturbance. Additional features are described in Table 8-1. The diagnosis may be confirmed by improvement following antidepressant therapy.

Recently, cases have been encountered that contain a confusing overlap of the pseudodementia pattern and "organic" dementia patterns, and that improve only incompletely on antidepressants. Some of these cases seem in retrospect to be nonprogressive "organic" dementias due to subcortical vascular disease with superimposed depression mimicking progressive illness.

Although the most common cause of pseudodementia is depression, hysterical conditions also cause pseudodementia, most typically the approximate-answer prison psychosis (Ganser's syndrome) or post-traumatic dissociative states such as occur after motor vehicle accidents.

Diagnosis of Delirium and Dementia

Accurate diagnosis of organic mental disorders is often crucial because such disorders may represent the signs of serious underlying medical illness. The diagnostic process tries to answer many important medical questions: Is the disorder temporary and short-lived, permanent and fixed, or progressive? What are the exact etiologic causes and indicated treatment? Can treatment reverse the disorder and can it be done in time? As far as prognosis is concerned, does the disorder moderately or severely degrade the quality of life, does it shorten lifespan, or does it lead to a vegetative state or death? Patients may suffer long-term institutionalization for misdiagnosis of "organic brain syndrome" or "Alzheimer's," when some of these patients may actually have treatable, reversible deliria, treatable secondary dementias, or pseudodementias responding to antidepressants; and a few may have rapidly fatal slow virus infections with unknown potential for contagion.

Delirium

The diagnosis of delirium depends on the presence of clouded consciousness or disturbed attention in the presence of disorientation, global cognitive dysfunction,

Table 8-1
Clinical Features Differentiating Pseudodementia From Dementia

Pseudodementia	Dementia
Symptoms are of short duration.	Symptoms are of long duration.
Patient emphasizes cognitive loss:	Patient minimizes cognitive loss:
Very distressed by it	Inappropriate lack of concern
Detailed complaints about poor memory and inability to function	Vague about poor memory and inability to function (relatives complain instead)
Memory loss	Memory loss
Both remote and recent	Recent more than remote
Circumscribed gaps	Circumscribed gaps unusual*
Good attention and concentration	Mediocre attention and concentration
Doesn't try to "keep up"	"Keep up" with notes, calendars
Motivation during testing	Motivation during testing
"Don't know" answers	"Near miss" answers
Little effort, "gives up"	Struggles to perform
Patient highlights failures	Highlights even trivial successes
Emphasizes disability	Tries to conceal disability
Performance variability	Performance loss consistent
Affect change pervasive	Affect mildly depressed or labile
Early loss of social skills	Social skills preserved
Rarely more confused at night	Often more confused at night
Behavior more adaptive than expected for degree of cognitive loss	Behavior consistent with degree of cognitive loss
Often previous history of psychiatric disorder	Previous psychiatric history uncommon

* Except when due to delirium, trauma, and seizures
(Modified from Wells CE, Duncan GW: Neurology of Psychiatrists, pp 92–95. Philadelphia, FA Davis, 1977)

and global memory disturbance. Delirium is most frequently confused with functional psychosis, especially schizophrenia, to which it bears a superficial resemblance because of the common presence of hallucinations and delusions. The main differential points favoring delirium are (1) abrupt onset, (2) coexisting medical disease, (3) "organic" mental features rarely found in schizophrenia, including disorientation, memory disturbance, and cognitive disturbance; and (4) absence of past or family history of functional psychiatric disease. Additional features of delirium include visual hallucinations and illusions that are disorganized, rather than elaborate and bizarre auditory hallucinations; and the absence of definite symptoms of schizophrenia such as flattened or inappropriate affect. Many of the same delirious features also help to rule out psychotic depression, and in addition, there is often absence of depressed content and depressed affect in delirium. Delirium of the hypoactive type is frequently confused with dysthymic disorder (mild depression).

Selective organic mental syndromes such as amnestic syndrome, organic hallucinosis, organic delusional syndrome, and organic affective syndrome resemble delirium at times but are without disturbances of consciousness, orientation, and cognition.

Delirium is often confused with dementia because of the altered intellectual function that occurs in both. Points favoring dementia include absence of psychotic ideation, less severe disorientation, and greater clarity of consciousness (except in end-state dementia). However, delirium may sometimes be found superimposed on underlying dementia, a state called *beclouded dementia.*

Because delirium is very common and due to a large number of possible causes, the most rational approach is to look first for an obvious medical cause within the history, physical examination, and basic laboratory values. Instead of a single cause, sometimes there are two or three mild metabolic causes in combination, such as the hypoxic, renal, and toxic causes presented in the case example. Straightforward laboratory profiles are often sufficient, including CBC, full chemistries, arterial blood gases, and chest film and urine studies to rule out infection. The possibility of some substance causing or contributing to the patient's confusion should be actively considered and biochemically screened for, if indicated. This should include medical drugs with CNS side effects, such as steroids, as well as covert exposure to other drugs or toxic substances. Delirium may often be caused not only by CNS infection, but by peripheral infection as well, and blood cultures should be performed if infection is even a slight possibility.

A head CT scan should be obtained if the suspected cause is neurologic rather than systemic, especially if there are focal neurologic features. A spinal tap should be performed right away if there is clinical suspicion of subarachnoid hemorrhage or CNS infection; in other cases a tap should be performed without delay if other tests do not quickly lead to a diagnosis. Fundi should of course be checked before all taps.

Dementia

Diagnosis of dementia should be considered when there is broad loss of intellectual abilities leading to prolonged social and occupational dysfunction. In dementia, consciousness is not clouded, intellectual dysfunction is less dramatic than in delirium, recent memory is affected more than remote memory, and the course is more prolonged than in delirium.

As can be seen in Table 8-2, the most common cause for dementia is presenile and senile degenerative disease of the Alzheimer's type. Vascular disease, intracranial masses, and alcoholism are the next most common causes. Pseudodementia is the next most frequent cause of apparent dementia.

Three issues regarding the diagnosis of dementia remain important: (1) distinguishing treatable from untreatable causes of dementia; (2) detection of dementia in the very early stages; and (3) distinguishing dementia-like psychogenic states (pseudodementia) from dementia. The etiologic diagnosis of dementia is often a complex and cumbersome process, with data drawn from numerous sources to screen many etiologic possibilities. This tends to favor a "laundry list" approach to diagnosis rather than a rational strategy.

The following strategy is often helpful in etiologic diagnosis of patients with dementia-like states. First, screen for dementias that are accompanied by highly distinctive neurologic features such as hemiparesis, movement disorders, seizures, myoclonus, and so forth. Second, screen for reversible secondary dementias with laboratory tests because there are few distinctive clinical patterns in this group

Table 8-2
Statistical Summary of Reported Series of Demented Patients Studied

Established Diagnosis	Number	Percent
Atrophy of unknown cause (largely Alzheimer's type, presenile and senile dementia)	113	50.9
Intracranial masses	12	5.4
Dementia due to vascular disease	17	7.7
Dementia in alcoholics	13	5.9
Normal pressure hydrocephalus	14	6.3
Creutzfeldt–Jakob syndrome	3	1.4
Huntington's chorea	10	4.5
Post-traumatic dementia	2	<1
Postsubarachnoid hemorrhage	1	<1
Postencephalitic dementia	2	<1
Neurosyphilis	1	<1
Dementia with amyotrophic lateral sclerosis	1	<1
Dementia with Parkinson's disease	1	<1
Thyroid disease (hypofunction or hyperfunction)	2	<1
Pernicious anemia	1	<1
Hepatic failure	1	<1
Drug toxicity	7	3.2
Epilepsy	1	<1
Depression	9	4.1
Other psychiatric disease	2	<1
Not demented (no definite diagnosis)	2	<1
Dementia uncertain	7	3.2
Total	222	

(Modified from Wells CE: Diagnostic evaluation and treatment in dementia. In Wells CE (ed): Dementia, pp 247–277. Philadelphia, FA Davis, 1977)

(except in conditions such as deficiency of B_{12} or folate. See Mnemonic For Etiology of Altered Mental Status.

Mnemonic for Etiology of Altered Mental Status

M D–IV–TENTH

M Metabolic: endocrine, biochemical, anoxia
D Degenerative
I Inflammatory: infectious, autoimmune
V Vascular
T Trauma
E Epilepsy
N Neoplasm
T Toxic
H Hydrocephalus

Use the same general laboratory approach as in delirium, expanding the range of studies to include such tests as thyroid panel, calcium, vitamins, drugs and toxic substances as appropriate, EEG, head CT scan, and spinal tap if appropriate, as outlined in Laboratory Evaluation of Organic Mental Disorders.

Laboratory Evaluation of Organic Mental Disorders

Hematology—CBC, differential, B_{12}, folic acid

Chemistries—Electrolytes, Ca^{++}, PO_4, liver and renal chemistries, blood gases and pH

Endocrine—Thyroid panel, TSH, others as clinically indicated

CNS—EEG (awake), CT scan, spinal tap (if no obvious metabolic cause), skull films for sella if indicated

Toxic—Heavy metals, drug levels, other levels if indicated

Suspected normal pressure hydrocephalus requires radionuclide cisternography. After screening out the first and second group of etiologies, the third and remaining group consists of true degenerative dementias as well as subtle pseudodementias, and these are the most difficult etiologies to sort out clinically. As discussed earlier, patients with pseudodementia tend to have a subtle but fairly distinctive onset and behavioral pattern (mentioned earlier in this chapter), which is useful in identifying the condition much of the time.

Attempting to diagnose dementia in its early stages is frustrating. Many types of direct evaluation of the patient may not be revealing, including the clinical office interview, neurologic examination, and psychological testing. Mild cognitive deficits can be covered up in the structured office setting, low-normal vs mildly demented cognitive function may be hard to distinguish, or the problem may seem to be primarily emotional. Therefore, history from relatives may be the only clue to a possible early dementia. Relatives often confirm various degrees of social withdrawal, occupational inefficiency, decreased frustration tolerance, and mild memory disturbance. There may also be changes in personality that are diagnostically helpful, such as exaggeration of previous personality characteristics like obsessiveness, or release of out-of-character behavior like impulsiveness, or depressive mood as a reaction to subtle changes in mental function. Some patients with early dementia even have a frontal-lobe-like picture with apathy, irritability, and memory problems, rather than typical cognitive deficits.

Electroencephalogram.[5] Compared to tests such as the CT scan, the EEG has less anatomical specificity, but can be helpful in certain situations when evaluating organic mental syndromes:

1. The EEG can reduce skepticism that a mild delirium is in fact present (EEG slow) rather than functional psychosis (EEG normal).
2. In clearly delirious alcoholics the EEG can help distinguish delirium

tremens (DTs) (EEG normal or diffusely fast) from hepatic encephalopathy (EEG slow plus triphasic waves), from other encephalopathies, including Wernicke's (EEG slow).

3. In dementia, a diffusely slow EEG in the early stage suggests either a treatable secondary dementia or a rapidly progressive type of dementia (such as severe Alzheimer's or early Jakob–Creutzfeldt). On the other hand, a normal EEG in the early stage suggests a slow degenerative state, and tends to exclude many treatable etiologies, except pseudodementia. Serial EEG tracings over time are also useful in tracking decline in progressive dementia; as small a drop as 2 Hz in waking EEG background frequency (if consistent and not due to drowsiness or drugs) may help corroborate dementia.
4. Fairly characteristic EEG changes can be seen in the following organic mental disorders (as described earlier in the chapter): Jakob–Creutzfeldt disease, SSPE, herpes simplex encephalitis, dialysis dementia, progressive myoclonic epilepsy, and confusional states due to spike-wave stupor.

Head CT Scan. This is a remarkable, new, computer-based, neuroradiologic technique, showing the brain and skull in great anatomical detail, at several different anatomic levels. The procedure is excellent for ruling in or ruling out many structural causes of dementia such as tumors, subdural hematoma, hydrocephalus; however, use of the CT scan is controversial in the diagnosis of degenerative dementia. Although cortical atrophy on the CT scan crudely correlates with degenerative dementia, there is too much overlap, with some demented patients not having atrophy on CT scan, and some normal patients without dementia having definite atrophy on the CT scan. Overreliance on the CT-scan findings can therefore lead to overdiagnosis of dementia.[12]

Psychological Testing. Organic psychological testing is traditionally thought of as a technique for obtaining a rough, numerical guide to the level of intellectual functioning of a patient with a potential case of organic mental syndrome, and of following this level serially over time. The physician should understand at least two of the many tests available, the Wechsler Adult Intelligence Scale (WAIS) and the Wechsler Memory Scale (WMS). The WAIS is the most frequently used general test, and contains six verbal subscales generating a verbal intelligence quotient (VIQ) and five performance subscales generating a performance intelligence quotient (PIQ), and a combined full-scale intelligence quotient (FSIQ). In diffuse, bilateral dementing disease both the verbal and performance score may decrease together, or the performance score may decrease more than the verbal score, resulting in the well-known "verbal/performance split," with the verbal skills "holding" more than performance skills. In dominant hemisphere disease a reverse split is seen with VIQ lower than PIQ. Although physicians should understand that a significant split is roughly 15 to 20 IQ points, such tests must be interpreted in all cases by a competent clinical psychologist in order to be useful to the physician.

The WMS is a sensitive test of memory that generates a memory quotient (MQ) comparable to the IQ of the WAIS, and is capable of detecting subtle defects in both verbal and nonverbal memory. For more sophisticated techniques of neuropsychological localization, there are numerous individual specialized tests and at least two well-known batteries of tests, the Halstead–Reitan Battery and the newer Luria Battery, which the consulting psychologist may employ.[13] In pseudodementia and in organic syndromes with prominent emotional or behavioral features, personality testing is useful, especially the Minnesota Multiphasic Personality Inventory.

Follow-up is the strongest indication for psychometric testing for organicity. After an organic mental diagnosis is already made or suspected, psychometrics can measure the severity of functional deficit and can track the rate of progression serially over time. Because testing is time-consuming and costly, it is most useful in the context of chronic or slowly progressive disorders, rather than acute disorders. Diagnosis is a more variable indication for psychometrics, but is sometimes useful in the diagnosis of equivocal, mild dementias, and this usually requires the addition of the specialized and time-consuming tests described above. When dementia is clinically obvious, psychometrics are merely confirmational, but are useful as a baseline. Psychometric evaluation can sometimes help in the diagnosis of pseudodementia but cannot always be expected to resolve this question. In acute, temporary organic mental syndromes such as delirium, psychological testing is rarely indicated because it is expensive, and the results are questionable due to poor patient cooperation. Specialized psychometric testing of focal brain regions such as frontal, temporal, and parietal regions may be indicated in evaluating and defining complex organic personality syndromes, either occurring alone or as a component of a diffuse lesion. The availability of such testing, however, depends on the training and orientation of the psychologist.

Who should receive psychometric evaluation? In addition to the indications above, young patients who may have a vocational future should probably receive the most extensive testing.

Selective Organic Mental Syndromes

In selective organic mental syndromes a single or specific class of symptom (*e.g.*, personality change, amnesia, delusions, hallucinations, or affect change) predominates without significant overall intellectual disturbance or clouding of consciousness. In the past literature on head injury, epilepsy, and metabolic and toxic conditions, descriptions of such behavioral symptom clusters were frequently described, but they have only recently received formal recognition in the psychiatric nomenclature. DSM-III now recognizes five selective organic mental syndromes: organic personality syndrome, amnestic syndrome, organic hallucinosis, organic delusional syndrome, and organic affective syndrome.

Organic Personality Syndrome[5,9]

It is well known that damage to the prefrontal lobes can result in chronic apathy with superimposed episodes of irritability and impulsiveness. Such permanent personality change often closely imitates functional psychiatric illness, and can easily be misclassified by a naive psychiatrist. Because organic personality syndromes are seen most often in lesions of neurologically silent areas such as the prefrontal or temporal lobes, there are often no clues to organicity such as dementia or an abnormal neurologic exam. In reality such symptoms are not merely nonspecific emotional reactions to brain damage, but are the direct effect of damage to a specific focal portion of the brain and are sometimes called *neurobehavioral syndromes*. Although correlations between behavior and anatomy are only approximate, three patterns of organic personality syndrome have been described: frontal lobe syndrome, interictal temporal lobe personality, and hemisphere syndromes, dominant and nondominant.

Frontal Lobe Syndromes

Frontal lobe syndromes are perhaps the best described of all the organic personality syndromes, because they have been depicted in dramatic accounts of missiles or tumors in the frontal lobes since the early 1800s. Frontal lobe damage may result in states of apathy (abulic syndrome), states of episodic disinhibition and euphoria (disinhibited syndrome), or in some alternating combination of the two. The term *frontal lobe syndrome* actually refers to involvement of the prefrontal cortex, extending from the premotor cortex just in front of the motor strip, around the dorsolateral convexity of the frontal lobes, extending to include the orbitofrontal cortex and undersurface of the frontal lobes. Observations after damage to the frontal lobes are conveniently classified into psychiatric, neurologic, and neuropsychologic; and for accurate diagnosis one should learn to combine all three types.

☐ A 25-year-old, college-educated, white man with a history of a motor vehicle accident four years ago began to show inappropriate sexual approaches; for example, trying to solicit a kiss from someone else's date at a dance, approaching social workers at his rehabilitation center, and even approaching family members (disinhibition). Examination showed euphoria and silliness on a background of apathy (facetiousness). He playfully pretended to refuse to talk, and punned with the names of the examiners (Mr. Daniels—"Jack Daniels"; Dr. Volow—"Vobo, Lobo"). He showed little appreciation of the consequences of his sexual approaches. He said he wanted to be a computer programmer (inability to plan), which seemed to be unrealistic, given his deficits. On mental status he was not clinically depressed but was quite irritable, had a vacuous and hypomimic facial expression (apathy), and moved quite slowly (bradykinesia). His gait was slow and awkward with a spastic left hemiparesis with extreme internal rotation of the left foot. He showed fair preservation of the more elemental intellectual functions (orientation, memory, calculation) but marked disturbances of affect, impulse control, and motor speed; unilateral motor sequence ability was poor. Fluency tests were unaffected. The patient was believed to have a frontal lobe syndrome of the disinhibited variety.

Psychiatrically, patients with frontal lobe syndrome show "irritable euphoric apathy," an emotional state characterized by a tendency to maintain continuous apathy, on which may be superimposed short episodes of irritability or euphoria. Bradykinesia commonly occurs as well, an activity change in which the patient walks and talks slowly, and shows marked paucity and lack of spontaneity in the amount of movement, speech, and even thought. The patient loses interest in previously important relationships and goals and becomes self-centered. His face shows little emotional expression. Other common variations in affect include affect lability, facetiousness, and puerile behavior. In affect lability, discussion of emotional subjects can move the frontal patient to tears with prompt return to apathy moments later. In facetiousness or *witzelsucht,* the patient compulsively employs some form of hostile humor or puns, often at the examiner's expense. In puerile behavior, there is sudden dramatic regression to infantile behavior. Poor judgment and other impulsive phenomena occur frequently in frontal lobe patients, including brief aggressive outbursts and pathologic intoxication. By the time the patient is brought to the psychiatrist, control has returned and the patient is a model of "English valet politeness." There is some suggestion that disinhibition, irritability, and euphoria are more prominent in orbitofrontal damage, and that apathy and indifference are more prominent in dorsolateral convexity damage.

The traditional neurologic exam is usually negative. Frontal release signs are helpful when present (grasp is more reliable than snout or glabellar), but may not always be present if the premotor region happens to be spared by the lesion. Most frontal lobe syndromes are accompanied by a mild gait disturbance characterized by a broadened base and short, shuffling steps; although the more extreme, "glued-to-the-floor" frontal gait apraxia occurs occasionally. Paratonia or *gegenhalten,* a noncogwheeling, nonspastic resistance to passive movement, is also seen fairly often.

Bedside evaluation of neuropsychological data such as orientation, memory, and calculation are typically roughly normal. Surprisingly, traditional psychometrics such as the WAIS and even batteries such as the Halstead–Reitan, are mostly normal. One way to confirm suspected frontal lobe syndrome is by means of specialized neuropsychological tests. Patients with frontal lobe syndromes show three special characteristics not evaluated in the traditional neurologic or psychiatric exam: (1) reduced verbal fluency, (2) poor motor sequence ability, and (3) difficulty in opposing sequence tasks. Tests for these functions are easily performed at the bedside and can be found in the references by Lesak[13] and by Strub and Black.[14]

Many etiologies give rise to frontal lobe dysfunction, of which trauma is perhaps the most important; others include infarcts or aneurysmal bleeds in the anterior cerebral artery circulation, brain abscesses, chronic granulomatous basilar leptomeningitis, normal pressure hydrocephalus, and frontal components of diffuse dementias such as Alzheimer's or Pick's. Syphilis is no longer a common etiology of frontal lobe syndrome.

Hemisphere Syndromes, Dominant[15]

Although it is well known that dominant hemisphere lesions may produce neurologic symptoms such as aphasia and hemiparesis, it is less well known that such lesions may be associated with severe disturbances of mood and behavior. Most of these have to do with mood and language. Most typical is the catastrophic reaction, an emotional storm usually in reaction to frustration, in which the patient may swear, cry, swoon, or throw something. A depressed mood may be continuously present. Even in the absence of clinical aphasia, these patients may have subtle defects in verbal memory and naming under pressure, as well as problems in auditory comprehension. Patients complain of poor memory, and relatives notice that conversations often do not "sink in." In some patients these symptoms all fuse into an episodic behavior spell characterized by emotional confusion, rage, and relative amnesia, sometimes resembling a hysterical seizure. Because of their lesion, these patients seem to have difficulty integrating language and affect.

Hemisphere Syndromes, Nondominant[15]

In contrast with the catastrophic reactions and depressive tone of dominant hemisphere lesions, nondominant hemisphere lesions may produce the opposite, an "unconcern" or denial attitude, even about any neurologic disability. This may or may not be associated with the neurologic syndrome of hemineglect of the contralateral side of the body. Despite this surface unconcern, if patients become depressed, they tend to show it in peculiar ways. They may say that they feel depressed, but seem unable to show sadness nonverbally, except by abrupt crying (affect lability). The physician may ascribe the affect lability to the brain damage and thus fail to detect the depression.

Interictal Temporal Lobe Personality

In the past, a controversial interictal behavior syndrome consisting of irritability, "adhesive thinking," circumstantiality, and hyperreligiosity was described; developing late in the course of chronic temporal lobe epilepsy. The syndrome will be discussed more in detail in Temporal Lobe Epilepsy.

Diagnosis of Organic Personality Syndrome

All organic personality syndromes are diagnosed by the history, often from relatives, of a definite change in personality or behavior, in the presence of a specific organic etiology. This can be difficult if the change is subtle and if the premorbid personality is unknown. There should be no evidence of other organic mental syndromes such as delirium, dementia, or other selective organic syndromes. The change should not be due to functional disorders, such as adjustment disorder after the onset of the brain condition, depression, schizophrenia, or post-traumatic stress disorder; all of which can change the personality temporarily.

Because of slow movement and restricted affect, the main differential diagnoses of frontal lobe syndrome include depression and parkinsonism. Frontal-lobe patients are vacuous and show little improvement with antidepressants, whereas depressed patients show more affective pain and preoccupation, and may improve with treatment. Frontal patients and Parkinson's patients both show bradykinesia, but frontal patients show much more disinclination to act and show a non-cogwheeling type of increased tone, whereas Parkinson patients show cogwheel rigidity and many show a tremor. Although theoretically distinguishable from "psychiatric" depression, hemisphere syndromes with signs of depression often respond well to maintenance antidepressant treatment.

Amnestic Syndrome

Another selective organic syndrome is the amnestic syndrome.[5] This is mainly an isolated disturbance of memory function occurring in a clear sensorium, without associated disturbances in other cognitive functions.

> ☐ Mr. A was transferred to Psychiatry from Medicine for evaluation of long-standing memory problems, wandering around the hospital, wandering into the operating room during surgery, and disorientation. On examination, he seemed bright, slightly ebullient, garrulous, logical in his ideas, and able to carry on excellent but superficial conversations. On mental status he was alert and without clouded consciousness and could read, do simple math and spelling problems, and could write and draw. He could even repeat six numbers forward. However, he could not remember any of three items even at two minutes; and he could recite the presidents forward from Coolidge to Kennedy, but knew no recent presidents. He did not confabulate consistently.

The main features of amnestic syndrome include two types of memory disturbance: a disturbance of long-term memory (retrograde amnesia), as indicated by Mr. A's inability to remember presidents in the past 20 years; and a striking disturbance in the ability to make new memories (anterograde amnesia), as indicated by Mr. A's excellent immediate recall of six digits, but his failure to remember even one of three items after a 2-minute delay. Note that in contrast with his memory problems, Mr. A's other cognitive abilities were roughly intact.

A third feature, disorientation, is frequently present. A fourth feature, confabulation, is less consistently present than previously believed, being more prevalent in the acute state. Confabulations more often represent past memories placed out of time sequence, rather than total fictions contrived to fill gaps.

Often, following recovery from acute Wernicke's encephalopathy, the amnestic syndrome occurs in thiamine-deficient chronic alcoholics, in which case it is called *Korsakoff's disease*. Correction of the thiamine deficiency results in complete memory improvement in roughly one fourth of cases, no improvement in one fourth of cases, and partial improvement in the remainder. In addition to nutrition, other etiologies such as trauma, carbon monoxide poisoning, and herpes simplex encephalitis can also cause a partial amnestic syndrome (in which case the term *Korsakoff's syndrome* is used).

The most frequent differential diagnostic problem is distinguishing amnestic syndrome from delirium, dementia, and psychogenic amnesia. Amnestic syndrome is a selective cognitive syndrome limited to memory dysfunction; whereas syndromes with multiple areas of cognitive dysfunction, with or without clouding of consciousness, suggest delirium or dementia respectively. It is not always possible, however, to make a clear distinction between these syndromes because many amnestic patients act demented at times because of profound disturbances of judgment. In psychogenic amnesia the memory loss is circumscribed and fluctuating, and limited to certain emotionally laden situations.

Organic Hallucinosis[5]

When the patient has hallucinations, without accompanying psychosis and without delirium or dementia, he is diagnosed as having the syndrome *organic hallucinosis*.

> ☐ A 56-year-old man with severe renal disease required chronic hemodialysis for the last 2 years. He then underwent a successful cadaver renal transplant. He had been on steroids for four weeks as part of an immunosuppressive regimen when he began to hear church music that seemed to come from outside his head, did not frighten him, and was not associated with any agitated nor psychotic behavior. (He had been a minister.) Examination showed him to be otherwise completely lucid and without clouding of consciousness, oriented and alert, with excellent intellectual function and good reality testing. Other CNS studies, were normal, including EEG. The steroids were reduced and the hallucinations disappeared.

The most common varieties of hallucinosis are toxic, including acute and chronic auditory hallucinoses and hallucinogen-induced hallucinosis, hallucinatory side effects of medical drugs such as pentazocaine, steroids, digitalis, scopolamine; hallucinosis due to neurologic diseases, especially epilepsy and temporal lobe masses; and physiologic types of hallucinosis, such as with blindness, deafness, or other sensory isolation states.

In acute alcoholic hallucinosis, startling auditory hallucinations suddenly occur during the alcohol withdrawal period in an unconfused, nondelirious patient. The onset of alcoholic hallucinosis is usually quite soon (24–48 hours) after the patient stops or decreases alcohol use, and prolonged heavy intake and high alcohol tolerance are thought to make patients particularly susceptible. For example, men may experience voices calling them deprecatory names or accusing them of homosexuality; women may experience voices accusing them of infidelity. Most often the hallucinations are described as auditory and frightening, but sometimes they may be visual or may be nonfrightening. Fearful affect may be so strong that patients have been known to call the police or hurt themselves fleeing from the voices. Before the voices begin, some patients describe a phase of tinnitus or machine-like buzzing. The course is somewhat variable, with most cases remitting 5 to 30 days after onset, but in a few cases progressing to a chronic hallucinatory state. Studies of premorbid personality and family history do not support the previously held view that alcoholic hallucinosis represents covert schizophrenia released by alcohol withdrawal. Compared to delirium tremens, the hallucinations of alcoholic hallucinosis occur much earlier in the alcohol withdrawal period (1–2 days vs 3–10 days) and are not accompanied by delirium or clouding of consciousness; however, mixtures of the two syndromes are occasionally observed.

Organic Delusional Syndrome

When an organic etiology causes a delusional state without affecting intellect, the diagnosis should be organic delusional syndrome. Hallucinations, when present, are usually not prominent features of the disorder.

> □ A 44-year-old man had an 18-year history of major motor and complex partial seizures and a 16-year history of psychosis. He had had multiple psychiatric hospitalizations between the ages of 30 and 43, usually beginning with an attack on a relative. His upbringing was chaotic, and he had committed violent acts such as hitting a cousin with a shovel. He was transferred to a university-affiliated VA hospital on the premise that psychosurgery might help his violent behavior. He showed surprising behavioral tranquility for the first 6 months, during which some seizures occurred, and during which his EEG showed bitemporal seizure discharges. In December 1972 he experienced a severe paranoid psychotic episode, preceded by a burst of seizures. He became elated, suspicious, preoccupied with the election, and believed that Robert Kennedy was still alive (he had recently been assassinated). After increased medication, the seizures gradually stopped over a 4-week period, but the patient then began a series of unprovoked attacks on the ward staff, breaking someone's hand, and nearly attacking a neurologist. The patient was not disoriented or delirious, but interestingly, his EEG showed no seizure discharges when he was psychotic. Although psychosurgery was considered, his mental state improved greatly when his medication was changed from chloropromazine to haloperidol.

The causes of organic delusional syndrome are restricted to a small range of etiologies, frequently structural brain disease and epilepsy, as in the above example (see Temporal Lobe Epilepsy).[16] Organic delusional syndrome may sometimes be seen in encephalitis due to herpes virus, and also in degenerative conditions such as early Huntington's disease. The syndrome may also be due to certain specific metabolic and toxic disorders; paranoid organic delusional states due to phencyclidine (angel dust, PCP) toxicity have attracted considerable attention recently. The delusions strongly resemble those of schizophrenia and may be accompanied by other schizophrenic-like symptoms, including mutism and posturing similar to catatonia, stereotypes, and feelings of influence and thought control. Paranoid delusions also occur with other drugs of abuse, most frequently with amphetamines, sometimes with cocaine or with hallucinogenic drugs, and occasionally with medical drugs such as bromides and hydantoin anticonvulsants. Delusions may also be present in some metabolic diseases, such as pernicious anemia, porphyria, and Cushing's disease.

Organic Affective Syndrome

Patients with organic affective syndrome experience a prominent disturbance of mood, either depression or elation (less commonly). The mood change may be mild, or occasionally as severe as in a functional affective disorder, but an organic cause is obviously present or suspected. Other symptoms, such as cognitive deficit, clouding of consciousness, delusions, or hallucinations are either completely absent or only minimally present, and less prominent than the mood symptoms. Organic affective syndromes are caused by only a small range of etiologies, most commonly endocrine disorders, toxic disorders, or structural brain disease. Depressive-like pictures may be seen with hypothyroid states, hyperthyroid states, Addison's disease, Cushing's disease, pituitary adenomas, and hyperparathyroid states. Apathy may be seen in hyperthyroid states in the elderly. Elated mood may sometimes be seen in Cushing's disease or hyperthyroidism. Depressive mood-tone is frequent in destructive lesions of the dominant hemisphere, as discussed in Organic Personality Syndromes; and affect change, either depression or anxiety, is rather common in many types of subcortical/extrapyramidal neurologic conditions (*e.g.*, parkinsonism). Depressive syndromes may be caused by drugs such as reserpine, propanolol, steroids, and alpha methyldopa. Elated states can be caused also by sympathetic-like drugs, including the amphetamines, phencyclidine, and synthetic steroids.

Temporal Lobe Epilepsy

Temporal lobe epilepsy is intriguing for the variety of behavioral conditions which may be associated with it. Many clinicians feel that temporal lobe epilepsy is more likely than other epilepsies to cause psychological and psychiatric problems. While the exact percentage of temporal lobe epileptics showing such disturbances is controversial, it is clear that temporal lobe epilepsy is capable of producing many of the organic mental syndromes described earlier in this chapter.[9,16]

Adjustment Disorder With Depressed Mood. As with all patients who develop a chronic disease, patients with epilepsy must make many painful changes in their lives. Following the onset of seizures, patients must begin medication; they may have to give up driving, change jobs or be retrained, move to distant cities with more transportation and work options, and experience some degree of family stress. In the first two years after onset, almost all epileptics develop low mood at some time, as a reaction to the change in health and the stress of readjustment. This may be manifested as poor compliance in some patients; or it may evolve into clinically treatable depression in others; or it may result in sustained chronic depression in patients with premorbid character problems. Although adjustment disorder is not an organic behavioral condition, it is probably the most common behavioral problem in epilepsy, and it may continue unresolved for months or years, and needs to be distinguished from the rarer organic behavioral conditions described below.

Emotion-Triggered Seizures. Some epileptics complain that stress or severe angry or depressed moods may trigger a seizure.

Temporal Lobe Personality (Organic Personality Syndrome). There has been described in temporal lobe epilepsy a peculiar personality change, characterized by irritability and episodic aggressiveness, overdetailed and "sticky" thought patterns, and religious preoccupation. Other features include excessive writing (hypergraphia), humorlessness and moral rigidity, and lowered sex drive and performance. Occurring late (two or more years) after onset of chronic temporal lobe epilepsy, this syndrome primarily characterizes behavior in between seizures (interictally). Only the hyposexuality seems to improve with improved control of seizures; the other symptoms remain, even after operative removal of the epileptic focus. The severity of this syndrome is said to be variable, with some epileptics showing mere behavioral peculiarities, while others are ill enough to require psychiatric hospitalization. The syndrome remains controversial, and its prevalence and differentiation from more common functional psychiatric personality disorders will have to await future research. Our clinical experience seems to indicate that this is a valid diagnosis in only a few chronic, adult, temporal lobe epileptics; moreover, temporal lobe personality must be clearly distinguished from adjustment disorder or depression, which occur more commonly.

In addition, epileptics may show other types of organic personality change in cases where there is substantial lobar structural damage such as described earlier in Organic Personality Syndromes.

Epileptic Psychosis (Organic Delusional Syndrome). Serious psychopathology occurs often in temporal lobe epilepsy, with some studies suggesting a 20% to 30% rate of psychiatric hospitalization. Depression is probably the most common diagnosis, but there is also a 5% to 15% chance of developing a true psychotic illness. Frequently, the psychosis may arise in the aftermath of a recent cluster of seizures, the psychotic symptoms developing interictally after the seizures have died down. Often there may be paranoid-depressive symptoms such as in the case discussed earlier in Organic Delusional Syndrome; but in other cases symptoms may be superficially schizophrenic-like, but without the bizarreness, autism, or thought disturbance of true schizophrenia. An exception to this is the more authentic paranoid schizophrenic picture associated with dominant temporal lobe epilepsy in female patients. Usually the sequence of epilepsy followed by psychosis with a long latency of 10–14 years is highly typical and is important for making the diagnosis of epilepsy-related psychosis. Sometimes, however, when temporal lobe epilepsy is undetected, diagnosis of both seizures and psychosis is made simultaneously. One such patient had symptoms that met all the Schneiderian criteria for schizophrenia, including thought broadcasting and thought insertion. EEG and video monitoring showed numerous brief complex partial seizures, indicating that the patient was postictal much of the day. All of the psychotic symptoms cleared completely after treatment with carbamazepine, without use of antipsychotics.

Postictal Twilight State. The postictal twilight state is a selective organic mental syndrome with mixed affective, amnestic, and dissociative features. Rarely, after a cluster of psychomotor seizures (or after psychomotor status epilepticus), the patient may develop this type of prolonged mental state abnormality, which is characterized either by dissociative symptoms, mood symptoms, or confusional symptoms, and lasting several days to weeks. These states are described separately because they do not behaviorally resemble a functional psychosis as much as does the organic delusional syndrome above. For example, one of our patients suddenly developed a clinical depression after several seizures. Case reports describe rare cases in which patients undergo dissociative spells or fugue states with symptoms of wandering, amnesia, and purposive behavior lasting several days following a burst of seizures. One of our patients experienced a prolonged confusional state resembling a true delirium after an attack of spike-wave stupor (petit mal status epilepticus), and the next year experienced a similar confusional state after an attack of psychomotor status epilepticus. Seizure activity continuing at a subcortical level, or massive inhibitory processes triggered by seizures, have each been proposed as mechanisms for all these behavioral syndromes that seem time-related to clusters of seizures.

Uncinate Hallucinations (Organic Hallucinosis). Some patients with psychomotor seizures have unusual perceptual experiences at the beginning of their seizures. Olfactory sensations are quite common, such as the smell of blood or indescribable odors. Visual hallucinations are also well known to occur; these hallucinations are the same, time after time, and have the quality of memory. Auditory sensations in the form of grinding noises or clicks may occur with posterior temporal foci.

References

1. Reding GR, Daniels RS: Organic brain syndromes in a general hospital. Am J Psychiatry 120:800, 1964
2. American Psychiatric Association: Diagnostic and Statistical Manual of Mental Disorders, 3rd ed. Washington, DC, American Psychiatric Association, 1980
3. Engel GL: Delirium. In Freedman AM, Kaplan H: Comprehensive Textbook of Psychiatry, pp 711–716. Baltimore, Williams & Wilkins, 1967
4. Tyler HR: Neurologic disorders in renal failure. Am J Med 44:734, 1968
5. Volow MR: Delirium, dementia, and other organic mental syndromes. In Cavenar JO Jr, Brodie HKH (eds): Signs and Symptoms in Psychiatry. Philadelphia, JB Lippincott, 1983
6. Seltzer BS, Frazier SH: Organic mental disorders. In Nicholi AM, Jr (ed): The Harvard Guide to Modern Psychiatry. Cambridge, Belknap, 1978
7. Wells CE: Dementia, 2nd ed. Philadelphia, FA Davis, 1977
8. Wells CE, Duncan GW: Neurology for Psychiatrists. Philadelphia, FA Davis, 1980
9. Benson DF, Blumer D: Psychiatric Aspects of Neurologic Disease. New York, Grune & Stratton, 1975
10. Read SL, Jarvik LF: Cerebrovascular disease in the differential diagnosis of dementia. Psychiatr Ann 14:100, 1984
11. Ron MA, Toone BK, Gavralda ME, et al: Diagnostic accuracy in presenile dementia. Br J Psychiatry 134:161–168, 1979
12. Wells CE, Duncan GW: Danger of overreliance on computerized cranial tomography. Am J Psychiatry 134:811–813, 1977a
13. Lezak MD: Neuropsychological Assessment, pp 266–269. New York, Oxford University Press, 1977

14. Strub RL, Black FW: Organic Brain Syndromes. Philadelphia, FA Davis, 1981
15. Heilman KM, Satz P: Neuropsychology of Human Emotion. New York, Guilford Press, 1983
16. Benson DF, Blumer D: Psychiatric Aspects of Neurologic Disease, Vol II. New York, Grune & Stratton, 1982

Bibliography

Heilman KM, Valenstein E: Clinical Neuropsychology. New York, Oxford University Press, 1979

Marvin Swartz

9 Anxiety Disorders

Anxiety, a ubiquitous, unpleasant feeling of tension, worry, and restlessness, becomes pathologic when it is out of proportion in persistence or severity to a particular stressful situation. Pathologic anxiety involves a combination of psychological and somatic symptoms: The psychological complaints include subjective distress, worry, dread, and mental anguish: the somatic symptoms of anxiety include sweating, shortness of breath, rapid pulse, and tremor. Individual patients vary in their emphasis on psychological and somatic complaints. The course of symptoms, which may be acute, subacute, or chronic, has important implications for the diagnosis and management of anxiety disorders. Pathologic anxiety may be classified as an anxiety disorder, but may also be a feature of many other psychiatric and medical disorders. Biological, psychological, and social theories of anxiety will be discussed in this section, followed by a discussion of the diagnosis and treatment of specific anxiety disorders enumerated in the Diagnostic and Statistical Manual of Mental Disorders, American Psychiatric Association (DSM-III).

Social and Psychological Theories of Anxiety

Modern psychoanalytic theories of anxiety focus on anxiety as a signal of disturbed psychic equilibrium. Anxiety signals the threatened conscious awareness of unacceptable thoughts or impulses. Ego defensiveness maneuvers are summoned to keep unacceptable wishes from conscious awareness, and if successful, the anxiety subsides. Repression, an ego defense, keeps unacceptable wishes from consciousness; otherwise, the ego defenses of displacement conversion, denial, and other defenses permit a disguised and partial expression of the unacceptable impulses. Psychoanalytic theory posits that anxiety arises from childhood fears—the fear of annihilation, the fear of loss of the mothering one (separation anxiety), the fear of bodily injury (castration anxiety), and the fear of self-punishing guilt (superego anxiety). The wishes or impulses arising from the unconscious, if acted on, would result in fearful consequences, such as the loss of love. For example, a young child experiences separation anxiety as a result of fantasized rejection in retaliation from aggressive impulses toward the mother figure. In the adult, castration anxiety or other developmental anxieties arise from situations that are psychologically equivalent to the earlier danger situations.

Learning theorists regard anxiety as a conditional response to a number of paradigms. Classically, anxiety represents a conditioned fear response to a stimulus that was associated in the past with punishment. Another learning paradigm posits tension or anxiety arising from conflict situations such as approach–approach, approach–avoidance, or avoidance–avoidance conflicts. In these paradigms, two situations simultaneously arise that have separate consequences leading to conflict over a choice of behaviors. For example, in avoidance–avoidance conflict, the individual is simultaneously presented with a choice of two situations requiring behavior that will lead to two different negative consequences. Hence, anxiety results from the choice of two aversive consequences. Social learning theorists believe that anxiety can also be modeled after important figures in childhood. For example, the child learns from the modeling of a fearful parent that dogs are especially dangerous animals, and as a result the child becomes anxious in the presence of dogs. Cognitive–behavioral theorists regard anxiety as distress from maladaptive thought patterns, such as unrealistic and self-defeating automatic thought patterns. Existential theorists regard anxiety as a uniquely human condition resulting from threats to an individual's value system. Since values give meaning to one's life, a threat to one's value system is a threat to one's actual existence. The existentialists distinguish anxiety from other affects in that it is a uniquely human response to the threat of dissolution and nonbeing.

Social psychologists view anxiety as a response to environmental stressors. They posit that the anxious person has experienced more than the usual amount of recent stressful events, early stresses, or losses. Retrospective studies have not always supported this view; however, a careful case-by-case examination of particular anxiety disorders might reveal different results. Certainly, stressful life events play a role in anxiety states and disorders.

Biological Theories of Anxiety

Some individuals have a genetically determined predisposition to become pathologically anxious when stressed by a situation that most individuals would respond to with little or manageable anxiety. Animal inbreeding studies demonstrate a strong genetic component to anxious predispositions. Human family history data support a partially genetically determined type of anxiety. Certain anxiety disorders, especially panic disorder, have a strong genetic component.

The somatic expression of anxiety is well conceptualized in "fight or flight" reaction. As a result of perceived threat to the individual, the autonomic nervous system is activated by way of increased sympathetic arousal. Increased sympathetic tone results in the shunting of the blood away from the periphery to vital organs and muscle groups. Blood is shunted away from the gut into voluntary muscles, heart, and brain. Vasoconstriction in the extremities and gut, as well as vasodilitation in the voluntary muscles, produce a variety of symptoms, such as palpitations, changes in gastrointestinal (GI) motility, cold extremities, and other anxiety-like symptoms. Blood pressure, respiratory rate, pulse, and cardiac output all rise. Metabolism shifts in the direction of mobilization of glucose through gluconeogenesis and fat through lipolysis. Thus, a general state of arousal, set for activity in flight or fight, occurs through a complex cascade of neuronal pathways involving the limbic system, hypothalamus, pituitary, thyroid and adrenal glands, and general autonomic nervous system. Pathologic anxiety results from a chronic state of central and peripheral arousal activated by a fearful cognitive appraisal of the environment.

Models for the neuroanatomy of anxiety historically have evolved from psychosurgical procedure for incapacitating anxiety. Obviously, these techniques and the models derived from them are often nonspecific. Papez and MacLean introduced the concept of the limbic area of the brain being its seat of emotion. The limbic system comprises the hippocampus and proximal gyri, cingulate gyrus, amygdala, mammillary bodies, and dorsomedial nuclei of the thalamus and hypothalamus. The ventral and medical portions of the frontal cortex and their connections also appear to be part of the limbic system or "emotional brain." Various lesions in these sites from psychosurgical intervention and natural pathologic processes lead to profound alterations in emotional arousal and have obvious implications for the understanding of anxiety as well as other affects.

Redmond proposed a neurophysiological model of anxiety concentrating on the locus ceruleus, a brain stem nucleus, and norepinephrine pathways arising from it.[1] The locus ceruleus is stimulated by afferent sensory or cortical pathways, as well as limbic forebrain pathways potentially aroused by the perception of dander. Efferents from the locus ceruleus mediate higher processes, such as learning, memory, and motivation; but by way of the hypothalamus they also mediate physiological and psychological aspects of anxiety. Redmond postulated that β-adrenergic receptors in the brain mediate the action of anxiolytic (anxiety-reducing) drugs.

Pharmacologic models of anxiety, derived from the anxiolytic class of benzodiazepines, have given rise to other theories of anxiety implicating brain mechanisms subsumed by neurotransmitter systems. The neurotransmitter γ-aminobutyric acid (GABA) seems to be a widespread inhibitory neurotransmitter in the brain. The recent discovery of benzodiazepine receptors in the CNS leads to the recognition that GABA-minergic mechanisms and benzodiazepine receptors are closely related, and that benzodiazepines appear to facilitate the electrophysiologic actions of GABA. Research involving benzodiazepine receptor antagonists have implicated the GABA system and β-adrenergic systems in the mediation of anxiety states. One of the fascinating questions that follows the discovery of benzodiazepine receptors is, What naturally occurring or endogenous substances stimulate benzodiazepine receptors? Is there a naturally occurring endogenous anxiolytic, and what state or behaviors affect or are affected by its activity? The recognition that β-adrenergic antagonists such as propranolol block the peripheral but not the psychological manifestations of anxiety adds complexity to any pharmacologic model of anxiety.

Clinical Features

The anxiety disorders consist of panic, phobic, generalized anxiety, obsessive–compulsive, and post-traumatic stress disorders, in which anxiety is the predominant affect underlying a symptomatic presentation. In panic disorder and generalized anxiety disorder, anxiety itself is the presenting symptoms, whereas in phobic or obsessive–compulsive disorders, anxiety arises only if the patient attempts to confront the feared stimulus or resist the compulsion. In post-traumatic stress disorder (PTSD), anxiety results from disturbing experiences. These disorders will be discussed in this section.

Panic Disorder

Anxiety attacks, which are sudden and overwhelming spells of anxiety, are commonplace. Many people experience occasional anxiety attacks, which can usually be traced to feared situations. DSM-III distinguishes common anxiety attacks from a newly designated disorder called *panic disorder*. Panic attacks are recurrent, severe bouts of anxiety that begin without warning. The unpredictability and severity of panic attacks usually set them apart from common attacks, which can ordinarily be anticipated by the patient. Panic attacks are states of arousal not attributable to life-threatening crises or physical exertion.

Panic attacks are typically described as sudden attacks of overwhelming terror or impending doom. Often the patients report a distinctive unpleasant feeling of being "scared to death." They specifically report a cluster of physical symptoms attributable to hyperventilation and autonomic arousal. Patients may complain of pounding of the chest or palpitations, chest discomfort, and occasionally chest pains. Other patients report severe shortness of breath, air hunger, and a sense of smothering, choking, or pressure in the chest. Others are overcome with dizziness or "wooziness," and "rubbery legs." Numbness, paresthesias, and hot and cold flashes are all common complaints. A sense of unreality or detachment during the attack is common. Some patients are so terrified by their symptoms that they fear they are going crazy or fear a complete loss of control. Most patients report that their attacks last a few minutes, although they may last longer.

The diagnosis of panic disorder requires a constellation of at least four of these symptoms with an average frequency of one attack per week. Often, patients with panic disorder present a diagnostic dilemma because, in part, they present with a monosymptomatic complaint. For example, a patient who presents to his internist with shortness of breath, chest discomfort, and apprehension will usually arouse suspicion of cardiac disease. Sheehan, who refers to panic disorder as the "great imposter," reports that 70% of patients with panic disorder consulted more than 10 physicians for their symptoms before being correctly diagnosed.[2]

A careful history will establish the diagnosis. According to DSM-III, the diagnosis of panic disorder can be made when the following criteria have been met:

1. Three panic attacks occur within a three-week period.
2. These attacks are not secondary to a phobic stimulus.
3. At least four of the following symptoms are present: dyspnea, palpitations, chest discomfort, choking, dizziness, feelings of unreality, paresthesias, sweating, hot and cold flashes, shaking, and fear of dying or being out of control.

Considerable controversy surrounds the concept of panic disorder. Some researchers view it in psychological terms as a reaction to life stresses, maladaptive learning, or unconscious conflicts. These observers place panic attacks on a continuum with other anxiety spectrum disorders. Other researchers have pursued a medical illness model. They argue that panic disorder is a metabolic or biochemical abnormality with distinct genetic vulnerability. They cite evidence that patients with panic disorder, in contrast to normals, experience panic with infusion of sodium lactate. Other evidence includes a higher rate of panic disorder in relatives of affected persons and the greater concordance of panic disorder in monozygotic vs dizygotic twins.

Both theories account for the finding that panic disorder is more common in adults who suffered separation anxiety disorder in childhood. Some argue that separation anxiety, as a predisposition to panic disorder, is evidence for an acquired biochemical disorder in which a psychological phenomenon by an unknown mechanism leads to a later biochemical vulnerability. The following case represents unconscious conflict over separation anxiety:

☐ A 40-year-old woman was referred for psychiatric consultation for evaluation of dizziness after a complete history, physical, neurological evaluation, and laboratory studies including complete blood chemistries, complete blood count, thyroid battery, electrocardiogram, exercise stress test, and chest x-ray had revealed no organic etiology for her symptoms. The patient related a long history of "spells" to the psychiatrist. Her mother had similar attacks, and she recalled similar "spells" in her earlier school years, causing her to miss many days of school. The attacks had disappeared until her early 20s and had waxed and waned since. The attacks recently worsened soon after the departure of her younger child to college. The attacks were especially distressing because they appeared without warning; they varied in intensity but often were so severe that the patient feared she would die of fright. The dizziness followed the fright, and her husband told her that she hyperventilated throughout the attack. She often felt tingling around the mouth and arms and pressure in her chest. The patient doubted that the "spells" were psychological because they were presently unassociated with stressful events. A careful psychiatric evaluation, however, demonstrated a clear relationship between the patient's childhood separation fears and her adult separation fears that were made more acute when her daughter left for college. The patient's symptoms remitted with a combination of alprazolam and supportive psychotherapy.

Panic disorder is more likely a heterogeneous group of anxiety states awaiting further differentiation. Within this heterogeneity, some cases of panic disorder may well represent unconscious conflict, while other cases represent an endogenous anxiety state. Finally, mixed etiologies are also likely.

The prevalence of panic disorder is estimated to be 2% to 5%, affecting women in 80% of the cases. Onset is usually in the early 20s with a chronic fluctuating course. Panic disorder is often complicated by various forms of phobic avoidance conditioned by association with panic attacks. Most commonly, panic disorder is complicated by agoraphobia. Other complications include depression and alcohol, substance and anxiolytic abuse and dependence. The most common complication is costly and unwarranted medical workups.

Differential Diagnosis

In any anxiety disorder, the differential diagnosis must include a number of physical disorders. Metabolic or endocrine disorders or substance abuse disorders should be given high consideration in the differential diagnosis of panic disorder. A careful and thorough history and physical examination, with judicious use of laboratory tests and studies, should be performed. Consideration should also be given to other psychiatric disorders of which panic attacks may be a feature (Table 9-1). These include schizophrenia, major depression, and somatization disorder, and probably the severe personality disorders (borderline, narcissistic, or mixed personality disorders). Generalized anxiety disorders should be distinguished from the anticipatory anxiety that lingers between frequent panic attacks. In social or simple phobias patients may develop panic-like symptoms upon exposure to the feared stimulus, but in panic disorder there is no specific stimulus.

Table 9-1
Disorders Presenting With Panic Symptoms

Disorder	Key Features
Medical disorders (*e.g.*, arrhythmias)	Abnormal physical and laboratory findings
Substance abuse or withdrawal	Physical signs or stigmata of abuse (*e.g.*, needle marks)
Schizophrenia	Delusions, bizarre thought content, odd or flattened affect
Depression	Sad appearance, sleep and appetite disturbance
Somatization	Multiple symptoms in unrelated organ systems
Severe personality disorders	Stormy and unstable interpersonal relationships, self-destructive behavior
Generalized anxiety disorder	"Free-floating" anxiety with motor tension, apprehension, vigilance, autonomic hyperactivity
Social and simple phobias	Anxiety elicited by exposure to feared stimuli

Generalized Anxiety Disorder

Generalized anxiety disorder, the most common anxiety disorder, consists of persistent anxiety that is so ingrained as to be regarded, by many, as a trait of the individual. Commonly the patient cannot pinpoint when the anxiety began, and sees it as "the way I am." Patients with generalized anxiety disorder (GAD) do not have the specific constellation of symptoms characteristic of other anxiety disorders. Although they may have acute exacerbations of anxiety, they do not suffer the acute, frequent, and unpredictable attacks of severe anxiety characteristic of panic disorder. Similarly, while phobic avoidance may supervene, the "free-floating" anxiety characteristic of GAD is not attributable to specific dreaded situations as in phobias. Obsessive–compulsives may suffer chronic anxiety but demonstrate characteristic obsessions and compulsions not found in GAD.

The specific signs and symptoms of GAD are grouped in four areas: motor tension, autonomic hyperactivity, apprehensive expectation, and vigilance and scanning. The patient with GAD has symptoms in three of these areas for a month or longer. In the presence of a preexisting psychiatric disorder (*e.g.*, depression, schizophrenia) the diagnosis is not made.

Motor tension presents as restlessness, fidgeting, trembling, or jitteriness. The patient may complain of fatigue and muscular pain from chronic tension, and his face may show worry in the form of painful apprehension or a furrowed brow.

Autonomic hyperactivity may be observable in diffuse sweating, a cold and clammy handshake, flushing, or pallor. The patient frequently complains of palpitations or an uncomfortable awareness of the heartbeat. The complaints are frequently gastrointestinal with discomfort throughout the GI tract: a lump in the throat, queasiness of the stomach, bloating, or diarrhea. Urinary frequency or other genitourinary complaints are common. Paresthesias in the hands and feet or numbing around the mouth is also frequent. A sense of air hunger may cause respiration to be uncomfortable. Vertigo, "rubber legs," or general lightheadedness or a "band around the head" are also common.

Apprehensive expectation is the cognitive manifestation of the physiologic complaints of anxiety. The patient worries and ruminates unrealistically with a frequent preoccupation with catastrophe or doom. In distinction from panic disorders, the sense of doom or dread is chronic and of a relatively lower grade than in panic attack.

Vigilance and scanning is manifested by painful apprehension. The patient is often irritable from constant vigilance against unknown fear. The apprehension may so interfere with daily activities as to cause insomnia, fatigue, appetite loss, or concentration difficulties.

In DSM-III, GAD replaces the older term *anxiety neurosis,* which was believed to have lost its specificity as a concept. According to psychodynamic theory, neurotics have the psychological conflicts that are primarily related to the oedipal phase of development. Behaviorists argue that neuroses represent various types of conflicts, such as approach–avoidance conflicts, perhaps in the context of maladaptive learning in the family of origin. Most patients with GAD have neurotic conflicts combined with a maladaptive personality; these individuals would be classified as character (personality) neurotics, using psychodynamic terminology (see Chapter 11).

Differential Diagnosis

The distinction between GAD and other disorders, particularly depression, is a difficult one (see Chapter 7). Many patients with major depression present with obvious motor tension, vigilance, autonomic hyperactivity, and apprehensive expectations—the so-called agitated depression. The astute clinician will carefully note the temporal development of symptoms, as obtained from patient or family: In the agitated depression, the depression will precede or begin concurrently with the features of anxiety; in patients with a depression secondary to generalized anxiety disorder, the anxiety is chronic and longstanding with a later development of depression. Even with the most careful history, the differential diagnosis of GAD with depression vs agitated depression may be the most difficult distinction to make in psychiatry (see Differentiating Features of Generalized Anxiety), and a trial of antidepressant medication may be beneficial.

Differentiating Features of Generalized Anxiety (Depression vs Agitated Depression)

Generalized Anxiety With Depression	*Agitated Depression*
Prominent chronic anxiety	Prominent dysphoria
Motor tension	Sleep disturbance
Autonomic hyperactivity	Appetite disturbance
Vigilance and scanning	Loss of interest and pleasure in usual activities
Dysphoria, late and gradual in onset	Loss of libido
Sleep and appetite disturbance, late and gradual in onset.	Guilt
Depression appears to be hopeless response to chronic anxiety	Sense of worthlessness
	Suicidal ruminations
	Onset of anxiety with depression
	Agitation appears to be driven by acute inner pain

□ A 63-year-old man was referred to the outpatient psychiatric clinic for treatment of "depression." He recently had retired from work as a glasscutter because of his constant concern about his health. Two years prior to the visit to the clinic, he underwent vascular surgery for intermittent claudication. Since then he had been convinced that other blood vessels had been verging on insufficiency. He had always been preoccupied with his health, but had been able to suppress his worries. He now worried constantly about his health, finances, and marriage to an extent that was out of proportion to his actual difficulties. He had always had difficulty falling asleep, but slept well once asleep. Despite fatigue, he now always felt "keyed up" and annoyed with his wife. He complained of restlessness, trembling, and jitteriness. He acknowledged that he frequently felt edgy, but denied the biological signs of depression. Because the patient reported no definite symptoms of depression, he was given instructions in relaxation techniques to use at bedtime, and he soon began to sleep better. He was begun on an exercise program and was counseled on reducing caffeine intake, both of which helped reduce his edginess and "keyed-up" feeling. Supportive psychotherapy helped motivate the patient to participate in social activities and volunteer work in his church, thus diminishing his preoccupation with his health. The patient's symptoms gradually remitted without antidepressant medication.

In addition to the secondary development of depression, GAD is often complicated by alcohol, substance, or anxiolytic abuse or dependence. The diagnosis of GAD with underlying substance abuse may also be a difficult distinction. In this case, the diagnosis should be made on the basis of history, because rebound states of autonomic arousal may persist for a month following withdrawal from a central nervous system (CNS) depressant. No good data is yet available on the course, onset, or other characteristics of the natural history of GAD.

GAD is distinguished from adjustment disorder with depressed mood by a less chronic course and the present of a psychological stressor in the latter. In panic disorder, chronic anxiety may develop between attacks. Careful attention should be given to the possibility of panic disorder, even in patients presenting with diffuse anxiety.

Any anxiety disorder raises the diagnostic consideration of an underlying physical disorder. The panoply of symptoms characteristic of GAD prompts extensive medical workups. The clinician needs to carefully evaluate for the presence of intercurrent illness with a careful history and physical examination, and judicious use of laboratory and other studies. A physical disorder and GAD are not mutually exclusive.

Obsessive–Compulsive Disorder

Obsessive–compulsive disorder, a relatively rare disorder, affects less than 0.1% of the population.[3] Disabling and persistent obsessions or compulsions are cardinal features of the disorder. Obsessions are persistent, recurrent or unwelcome thoughts that may take the form of urges, impulses, images, or ideas. The thoughts are ego-alien (abhorrent) to the patient. For example, a common obsession is the intrusive, repugnant thought of running over pedestrians while driving a car—these thoughts cause the individual remorse, but he cannot stop them. Some obsessions consist of neutral ideas: The patient may be obsessively preoccupied with philosophical, religious, or abstract, meaningless topics. Another form of obsession is persistent doubt: Countless hours may be spent in wondering whether an action was completed or a matter settled. Obsessive thoughts cannot be consciously controlled: The individual attempts to suppress or ignore the intrusive ruminations, but the suppression fails.

Compulsions are persistent, repetitive behavior sequences that follow a stereotypic pattern. Common examples are ritualistic cleaning and repetitive hand washing. The compulsive act functions to "prevent" a dreaded occurrence. For example, the obsessive–compulsive who constantly stops his car to check for injured pedestrians is probably fending off expression of his own aggressive wishes. The feared event and the acts to prevent it are recognized to be unrealistic. The patient is aware of the senselessness of the act and finds it unpleasurable but is powerless to resist the compulsion. Failure to carry out the compulsive ritual produces overwhelming anxiety and distress. To a certain extent, then, the compulsive act relieves tension and in that sense reduces the displeasure of resisting the compulsion.

> ☐ A 25-year-old man was admitted to the hospital with an overwhelming compulsion to pick up litter. At the time of admission he was not able to concentrate on his work as a machinist because he constantly looked around the machine shop for litter on the floor. For the past several years the concern about litter had waxed and waned but never interfered with his ability to work. The patient was distraught over the compulsion but could not stop it.
>
> Two years prior to admission he had moved out of his parents' home. He described his parents as good religious people whom he deeply loved. His girlfriend had prodded him to move away from home because she felt he was a "mama's boy" and felt they would have more privacy in an apartment of his own. Over the year prior to that admission they spoke of living together, but the patient was concerned that his girlfriend was not orderly enough and would make the apartment a mess. Often when she visited he would feel an overwhelming desire to clean the apartment. His admission to the hospital followed a bitter argument with his girlfriend over his seeming reluctance to make a commitment to marriage. He argued that he could hardly marry her as long as he had the problem of needing to pick up litter. She responded with an ultimatum to get treatment for the compulsion or she would break off the relationship.
>
> The patient's doctor recommended an inpatient treatment program combining psychotherapy and behavior therapy. His behavior therapy involved progressive muscle relaxation while imagining a hierarchy of increasingly messy apartments that he was not to imagine cleaning up. The daily psychotherapy began to explore the meaning of the compulsions. The patient's compulsive acts responded to behavior therapy; psychotherapy helped him deal with the conflicts over marriage.

Although the course of obsessive–compulsive disorder is variable, it tends to be chronic with periodic exacerbations and remissions. At its worst, the patient may become disabled by the complexity and pervasiveness of ritualistic acts. Many patients develop phobic avoidance of situations related to the obsessions. For example, a patient with fear of contamination may avoid public places or social functions. Chronic states of anticipatory anxiety or depression often develop, and the latter may evolve into a major depression. Alcohol, substance, and anxiolytic abuse or dependence is a common complication of the disorder.

Etiology

Learning theorists view obsessive–compulsive disorder as a repetitive response pattern. They posit that the adult obsessive–compulsive was reared in an environment with strict control and punishment for certain behaviors and thoughts. As a result of the parental punishment of the behavior or thoughts related to it, these behaviors or thoughts were assiduously avoided by the child. Later in an environment where the punishment is more remote, the inhibition removed, or the motivation of the behavior intensified, avoidance behavior may begin to break down. For example, avoidance might wane in the face of increased sexual urges in late adolescence. The urges and impulses are unfamiliar because they have been avoided and are experienced as unreal or "ego-alien" and unpleasant due to their previous relation to punishment. This sets in motion learned reparative responses, which during childhood were used as atonement for forbidden acts.

Early in life the child learns to atone for acts that he may not comprehend to be bad. The atonement behavior is learned in order to reduce parental punishment or deprivation; this atonement process becomes an automatic generalized response for transgressions. The reparative response may then become a powerful anxiety reducer, relied upon in many situations to avoid punishment. The adult, therefore, who is made anxious by unacceptable thoughts may attempt to reduce anxiety through relatively automatic, nonspecific, and ritualistic response. Hence, an unacceptable sexual thought may be followed by compulsive handwashing, although the handwashing has no logical relation to the sexual urges.

Psychodynamic theorists offer a related explanation for the psychogenesis of obsessive-compulsive disorder. The early seat of the disorder seems to be in the conflict between the child and the parent over the child's impulses and parental prohibitions of those impulses. Classically, this struggle occurs over toilet training, cleanliness, and orderliness. The parent often levies rigid, harsh rules and regulations. The child chafes at these demands, and learns to curb the aggression related to these restrictions in order to keep the parents' love. The desire to be loved requires disavowal of the unacceptable impulses that become the source of guilt and shame, leading to the need for atonement. In severe cases, a ritualistic or symbolic act of atonement arises in a disguised form through displacement and symbolization.

The overt obsessive thought in obsessive–compulsive disorder is also seen as a substitute for another wish or impulse that serves to conceal the latent impulse. The latent wish is concealed from consciousness by the ego defense mechanisms of isolation, undoing, and reaction formation. For example, in undoing, a particular act or compulsion serves to "undo" the unconscious forbidden impulse. In reaction formation, the individual consciously feels the opposite of the unacceptable impulse. In isolation of the affect a patient may experience the ideational component of an unacceptable impulse but without the feeling that is usually associated with the impulse. For example, a patient who is disturbed by the intrusive thought that a door is left ajar and needs to be checked, may be found to be concerned with a prohibited wish for "getting out." The painful compulsive "checking" of the door is also atonement for the unacceptable unconscious wishes.

Differential Diagnosis

The differential diagnosis between obsessive–compulsive and schizophreniform disorder may be quite difficult. Stereotypic behavior and peculiar rituals are common features of schizophrenia. Careful inquiry will reveal that the schizophrenic does not find the behavior odd, and his compulsions are often related to the delusional system. The schizophrenic makes little effort to resist compulsive rituals. The withdrawn ruminative state of some schizophrenics may be similarly confused with obsession.

Many behaviors are loosely termed "compulsions." References to "compulsive eating" or gambling are common. Strictly speaking, these behaviors are not compulsions because the behavior is pleasurable, while true compulsions are not. Admittedly, some of these pleasurable behaviors may become aversive in their excess, but this is a secondary development. In a similar vein, many ruminative states are loosely termed "obsessive." An obsessive preoccupation with an upcoming critical exam is not a true obsession, because failing the exam may in fact be disastrous for the patient. The preoccupation in this case, although excessive, is not ego-alien or meaningless, because of the importance of the event.

Obsessions and compulsive behaviors are common features of major depressions, although usually the ideational component of the obsession is mood-congruent; that is, the obsessions and compulsions that are secondary to depression represent an intrusive sense of guilt or a need for punishment. Tourette's syndrome, while characterized by repetitive senseless acts, has an onset before age 13, and is usually accompanied by multiple involuntary tics (see Chapter 16). Patients with organic mental disorders may present with obsessive and compulsive symptoms, but they will also have obvious cognitive deficits as well.

Post-Traumatic Stress Disorder

Post-traumatic stress disorder, a syndrome known since ancient times, gained its first official recognition in DSM-III. Both Virgil and Shakespeare described a constellation of symptoms consequent to military combat such as sleep disturbance, autonomic arousal, and reexperience of trauma among soldiers following combat. Other references in lay and medical literature describe persistent disturbing residua of trauma, variously called "shell shock," "battle fatigue," and other names.

In DSM-III the cardinal feature of PTSD, either of the acute or delayed forms, is the development of a characteristic constellation of symptoms following a traumatic or catastrophic event outside the usual range of human experience. Reactions to bereavement or interpersonal difficulties or other experiences arising in nontraumatic circumstances are excluded. Generally, the stressor would cause significant distress in most people experiencing the trauma, and may result from deliberate human design such as rape, torture, or internment; or natural circumstances such as tornadoes or floods. Stressors caused by human design are thought to result in the most disabling and persistent difficulties.

Symptoms of the disorder include reexperiencing the trauma, diminished interest in usual activities, and a number of dysphoric, autonomic, and cognitive symptoms. Reexperience of the trauma may take the form of recurrent nightmares of the event or persistent intrusive recollections sometimes experienced as vivid reliving of the trauma (flashbacks). Many Vietnam veterans describe vivid dissociative-like states in which they believe they are back in combat, sparked by a stimulus associated with Vietnam, such as the sound of a helicopter overhead. Diminished interest in normal activities is often referred to as "emotional numbing" and can be especially stressful to victims who complain that activities around them seem unreal or distant. Victims often describe a dullness to their normal emotions and a painful distance from loved ones.

Victims often develop a sleep disturbance that may be an initial, middle, or terminal insomnia. They describe a state of autonomic arousal with hypervigilance, a tendency to startle at sudden noises or changes, and difficulty concentrating. Nightmares are a most disturbing symptom, in which the trauma is vividly relived, and which may exacerbate other sleep difficulties. Survivor guilt, if the trauma involves others, may be a painful accompaniment to the other symptoms. Irritability and aggressive outbursts may be particularly vexing problems to the victim's family. The course of the disorder is variable, as is its onset. If the disorder's symptoms arise within six months, it is felt to have a somewhat better prognosis than the chronic disorder, which has a more insidious onset.

☐ A 24-year-old woman presented to her family physician with insomnia. Her sleep was interrupted by vivid nightmares of sexual assault. The nightmares were so vivid that she feared going to sleep, and after a nightmare often paced for hours. The woman was a teacher in a rural town to which she had recently moved. She was raped by an assailant whom she never saw but who threatened to kill her if she went to the police. She was unable to recall the hours following the assault but eventually got dressed and went to work. She moved from her apartment and increased her workload at school, suppressing thoughts of rape. A month after the rape she developed a viral illness and subsequent pneumonia, was put on bedrest, and returned to her parents' home in another state. She began to have nightmares of the assault. She discovered she was pregnant as a result of the rape, and had an abortion, which she anguished over. She also began to have vivid recollections of the assault, quite unexpectedly. On one occasion in the supermarket a man spoke to her, and she believed she was being assaulted. She ran out of the market in fright, realizing later that there had been no call for alarm. She had continuous intrusive thoughts about the rape, and castigated herself for not resisting and for going home alone that night. She tried to distract herself by reading, but couldn't concentrate and couldn't get interested in any of her usual hobbies.

The patient was given a benzodiazepine for sleep and encouraged to return to her physician for regular appointments to discuss the assault. She was encouraged to talk about the assault in detail and to ventilate her feelings about it. She became quite anxious, teary, and grief-stricken while reexperiencing the assault, but seemed to benefit from the sessions with her physician. Her dreams gradually became less vivid and less frequent. She referred herself to a local rape crisis center, which she found helpful and supportive. The symptoms gradually abated over a 6-month period.

By definition, PTSD is a reaction to a stressor that would cause symptoms in almost anyone. Why the disorder reaches the intensity experienced in certain victims is not understood. Investigators have wondered if preexisting psychopathology, character structure, or childhood experience may set the stage for vulnerability to particular responses to stress, but no consistent findings have emerged. Some individuals seem to have unusual resilience to stress, but the variability in stressors and their personal meaning to the individual makes this a difficult phenomenon to evaluate. More puzzling is the recognition that some individuals develop chronic disabling symptoms following relatively minor traumas.

Differential Diagnosis

Since other disorders often coexist with PTSD, especially if it is chronic, it is important to consider coexisting pathology. For example, treatment may rest on the diagnosis of a coexisting major depression. Differential diagnostic consideration should be given to an adjustment disorder whose stressor is less traumatic and for which the full symptom picture of PTSD is not present.

Preexisting psychopathology does not rule out PTSD. In addition, chronic PTSD is especially associated with depression, anxiety, and concomitant substance or alcohol abuse and dependence.

Phobic Disorders

Phobic disorders are a group of disorders linked by the cardinal feature of persistent avoidance behavior driven by an irrational fear of a phobic stimulus. The stimulus may be an object, activity, or situation. The fear is ego-alien in that the individual recognizes the irrationality of the phobia. To be regarded as a phobia, the phobic behavior must cause significant dysfunction for the individual. Three types of phobias are specified in DSM-III: Agoraphobia, social phobia, and simple phobia. These will be discussed separately, although in a given individual various types of phobias can coexist.

Phobias can be viewed in a number of theoretical frameworks. In a psychodynamic view, anxiety is seen as a danger signal arising from the threatened conscious awareness or experience of unacceptable unconscious feelings or impulses. Anxiety signals the ego to fortify its defenses against the awareness of unconscious aggressive or sexual impulses. In the phobic patient, impulses can be kept from awareness by a number of ego defenses: displacement, avoidance, symbolization, and condensation. Through these ego defenses the impulse gains disguised and partial expression by being displaced from the original source of conflict to another situation, person, or object that symbolizes the original source of conflict. The symbolic representation of the conflict is further defended against by avoidance.

The core conflict and other ego-defensive maneuvers can be traced in psychotherapy. For example, a man with a bridge phobia was found to associate all bridges with a particular bridge en route to his work, where he harbored angry feelings toward his boss, a man much like the patient's father. The bridge phobia, in the psychodynamic view, arose when the aggressive impulses toward and fear of his father were displaced to his boss, but they remained too threatening and were symbolized and avoided in the fear of passing over the bridge to work, and then generalized to a fear of any bridge. Psychodynamic formulation of the phobia, then, views the phobia as the product of the ego defenses of displacement, avoidance, and symbolization to prevent awareness or expression of forbidden wishes or impulses.

Learning theorists offer different explanations for phobias. In classical learning paradigms, the feared but harmless stimulus is seen by a process of association to be linked to an original frightening stimulus. For example, a rat who is shocked by the painful stimulus of an electric current paired with the harmless stimulus of a bell going off with the shock, will soon startle when the bell alone rings. Conditioning leads to the association of the bell to the shock and the arousal of the fear to the ball.

In operant conditioning, another learning paradigm, naturally emitted behaviors are shaped by reinforcements. Behaviors that are positively reinforced or rewarded increase because of the reinforcement. Behaviors with negative consequences decrease in frequency.[4] Phobic avoidant behavior is shaped by the reinforcement of avoiding the painful affect of fear. For example, the phobic avoidance of the spider is shaped by the reinforcement of avoiding a naturally feared object.

In social learning theory, yet another learning paradigm, modeling and imitation influence learning. For example, a child whose mother models fear and avoidance of heights may soon imitate or learn that fear. These different theoretical views of phobia are not mutually exclusive. Many clinicians treat phobias through multimodal efforts, reflecting a concept of phobias that is influenced by psychodynamic and learning theories.

Agoraphobia

Agoraphobia is usually the most disabling and common phobia among phobic patients seeking treatment. The core feature of agoraphobia is irrational dread of being alone or of being in a public place from which escape may be impossible. Although agoraphobic patients may present with the fear of crowds or closed spaces, usually they are unable to leave home without companionship. Typically, the phobic behavior follows a period of frequent panic attacks, which are sudden unexpected states of terror. A variety of situations become associated with the panic attacks, and the patient develops the fear of having the attacks in the associated situations, and avoids those situations. Particular dread is associated with the helplessness of having an attack in a confined or crowded public space.

For most patients, agoraphobia seems to develop secondarily after the development of panic attacks. In the minority of patients, no history of panic attacks can be elicited. In agoraphobics who do or do not have panic attacks, phobic avoidance of being alone in a public place leads to increasing restriction of the patient's life. Although the disorder tends to wax and wane in severity, at its worst the patient may become homebound. The patient may develop an associated depression, other anxiety states, or ritualistic behaviors to allay anxiety. Anxiety may also lead to alcohol, substance, or anxiolytic abuse or dependence. The prevalence of agoraphobia is not known, but in some estimates 5% of the population, mostly women, will develop agoraphobia at one time or another.[2]

☐ A 26-year-old woman with a history of intermittent panic attacks began to fear leaving her home. Several months after delivery of a healthy baby girl, complicated by marital discord for which she sought psychotherapy, she found the child to be demanding and oppressive. She was irritated at her husband, who contributed little to the child's care. Although she wanted to arrange for the child to stay with her mother, longstanding discord with her mother made this difficult. She was able to find a woman in the neighborhood to care for the child and began to leave home more frequently to do errands and attend church. With no warning she developed a panic attack in a grocery store, during which she suddenly felt terrified, began to breathe quickly, and was unable to catch her breath. She ran out of the store. Her attacks increased, particularly in church, and she felt the devil was trying to shake her faith. She gradually became fearful of going to church, and avoided stores for fear that she could not leave in the event of panic. For a while the companionship of her husband made church attendance tolerable, but her fears mounted and she could no longer tolerate church or shopping. She became nearly housebound. The patient was treated with a combination of imipramine and psychotherapy. She was gently encouraged to confront the feared situations, beginning with the least threatening ones. Psychotherapy helped her deal with the conflicts of motherhood. The panic attacks subsided within several weeks and she gradually resumed her activities. Within several months she could shop and attend church without distress.

Phobic avoidance may be a feature of a number of psychiatric disorders. When phobic avoidance appears to be a result of another preexisting illness, the phobic behavior should be regarded as a feature or complication of the preexisting illness. Phobic avoidance of any sort may be a feature of schizophrenia, major depression, obsessive–compulsive disorder, or paranoid personality disorder or states. Clinicians may treat the avoidance behavior in these cases, but usually as an adjunct to the treatment of the preexisting syndrome. It would be senseless to treat agoraphobic symptoms in a schizophrenic without a vigorous attempt to treat the schizophrenia.

Social Phobia

The core feature of social phobia is the irrational fear of overwhelming desire to avoid public scrutiny. For example, a common social phobia is fear of public speaking or other types of public performance. Other social phobias include fear of using public restrooms, playing a team sport, or merely eating in a restaurant. The patient usually fears that the public display will lead to embarrassment or humiliation. As with other phobias, the patient recognizes that the fear and phobic avoidance is irrational, but still suffers significant distress as a result of the phobia.

Often a social phobia is manifested by the fear that someone will detect the patient's discomfort. For example, a patient with the fear of public speaking may be concerned that others will detect the shaking of his voice or other signs of nervousness while speaking. This dilemma of being anxious about becoming anxious seems to drive and perpetuate the social phobia.

☐ A 23-year-old man sought treatment because of difficulties in his business. He was a building contractor who frequently spoke to small groups of clients in giving estimates. He worried that the clients thought he was foolish-looking and inept. Although he recognized that these fears were irrational, he felt the clients would stare at his forehead and notice his slowly advancing baldness. He worried that they thought his hands were small and his head funny-shaped. He began to avoid giving estimates in person to his clients. He began to avoid giving estimates and lost jobs when he refused to give estimates in person to his clients. He was concerned that he had begun to avoid groups in general, and had also started drinking.

He was a small but good-looking man with no obvious physical impairments. He had had a stormy relationship with his father, who resented the patient's closeness with his mother. When the patient was a teenager, his father had taunted him about his appearance, saying that he was "queer looking" and had a "pointed head." He told the patient that he would never amount to much and prohibited the patient from contact sports. Over his father's objection, the patient played football in high school. Upon graduation, he started the contracting business. Initially he did well in business, but as his business improved his fear of social embarrassment became overwhelming. Outside his business he began to avoid parties because he felt people thought he looked foolish, and he worried about being humiliated.

In psychodynamically oriented psychotherapy, the patient explored the conflicts with his father and his related fear of success. He became more comfortable in his work, but still strongly felt that "people felt he was funny-looking." He began group psychotherapy in which multiple input from group members helped him confront his belief in his odd appearance. He gradually became more comfortable in social situations, including business encounters.

Social phobia is common; many people, for example, are fearful of speaking or performing in public. The development of a true social phobia causing significant impairment is relatively rare. Its course is usually chronic with a fluctuating severity. Among those who develop the disorder, alcohol, substance or anxiolytic abuse and dependence can be a troubling complication. Commonly, the social phobic also suffers from "free-floating" anxiety or anxiety unassociated with a particular stimulus. A generalized anxiety disorder or other phobias may coexist in individuals with social phobia.

Phobic avoidance may be a feature of a number of other psychiatric disorders. The presence of another major or preexisting condition usually excludes the diagnosis. For example, a schizophrenic with significant social impairment may, in a period of remission of psychosis, present with a social phobia. A history of delusions, hallucinations, grossly disorganized behavior, or a presentation of odd or peculiar affect usually makes the diagnosis of schizophrenia obvious. Similarly, more pervasive impairment in social relations is present in other disorders that are potentially confused with social phobia. The paranoid, schizoid, or avoidant personality may well be fearful of public scrutiny, but their social impairment is more profound and pervasive than the social phobic's. Phobic avoidance may also be a feature of depressive disorders or obsessive-compulsive disorder. The agoraphobic's fear of public places is not a fear of humiliating public scrutiny or embarrassment. The agoraphobic fears abandonment and panic in public. Like social phobias, simple phobias are circumscribed, but social situations with the risk of embarrassment are not involved.

Simple Phobia

The patient with a simple phobia has an irrational and compelling fear of an object or situation. As in other phobias, the phobia causes significant distress even though the patient recognizes that the fear and phobic avoidance are irrational. Simple phobias include the fear of animals (zoophobia), especially snakes, dogs, and insects; as well as the fear of situations such as the fear of heights (acrophobia) or crossing a bridge (gephyrophobia). While phobias are ubiquitous, specific phobias causing significant distress are less common because many phobic stimuli can be avoided. For example, a patient may have a morbid fear of rats. Ordinarily, this would not be a source of significant impairment or distress; however, if the patient is involved in research involving rats, the fear and avoidance may well cause the patient significant problems.

Estimates of the true prevalence of simple phobias await carefully conducted epidemiologic studies. The course of the disorder is variable. Animal phobias, usually beginning in childhood, as well as other phobias of childhood, usually remit without treatment. Phobias beginning or persisting into adulthood more frequently require treatment.

> ☐ A 28-year-old woman sought treatment for the fear of flying in an airplane. As long as she could remember, she had been apprehensive about flying. In the past several years she had avoided it altogether. She was recently promoted to a job that required frequent air travel. She had stopped flying after her father died following a protracted illness. She had been very close to him, but at the time of his diagnosis had been feeling ambivalent toward him. During his illness she frequently flew home to see her father, leaving her boyfriend, despite her increasing fear of a suffocating inferno on the airplane. She was aware of fleeting thoughts of wishing her father's suffering would be over, particularly when thinking of the pleasure of being with her boyfriend and the displeasure of having to visit her father frequently. Her father died a few days after a visit that she had shortened because of pressure from her boss to return to work. She was distraught that she had not been at her father's side when he died and was nearly unable, due to anxiety, to get on the airplane to return for his funeral. Soon thereafter she avoided flying altogether, and the thought of getting on an airplane filled her with dread. In individual psychotherapy, despite her presenting complaint, the patient spoke at length about her grief over her father's death, the heightened conflict with her mother since her father's death, and conflict over her career. The therapist had intended to refer the patient for behaviorally oriented treatment, but the fear of flying remitted spontaneously in the course of psychotherapy.

Simple phobias may be a feature of other psychiatric disorders, as in the case of agoraphobia or social phobia. Careful attention should be given to the possibility of other psychopathology. For example, a patient with the fear of dirt (mysophobia) will commonly be found to have an obsessive–compulsive disorder. Phobic avoidance may be a feature of schizophrenia or paranoid, schizoid, or avoidant personality disorder.

Evaluation of Anxiety Disorders

Symptoms of anxiety are ubiquitous and often signify the challenge we all face in coping with our particular environment. Anxiety can be a stimulus to achieving a successful adaptation to a complex social sphere. The challenge to the clinician is to carefully assess the presenting complaints of the anxious patient in the context of a biopsychosocial model. In most cases anxiety represents a response to particular stressors. Anxiety may result from unconscious psychological conflicts, emotional or environmental stress, an unrecognized medical disorder, a reaction to the illness itself, or, particularly in the elderly, fear of declining health. Of course, an anxiety disorder is most often precipitated by a combination of several of these factors. A careful and collaborative evaluation of the patient's present life circumstances and their association to past events aids in understanding the patient's symptoms.

Medical illnesses often present with symptoms of anxiety (see Medical Disorders Presenting With Anxiety).

Medical Disorders Presenting With Anxiety

Substance Intoxication
- Caffeine
- Stimulants
- Sympathomimetics
- Amphetamines
- Hallucinogens

Substance Withdrawal
- Alcohol
- Barbiturates
- Opioids
- Anxiolytics
- Antidepressants
- Nicotine

Central Nervous System Disorders
- Complex partial seizures
- Transient ischemic attacks
- Benign essential tremor
- Alzheimer's disease

Cardiorespiratory Disorders
- Anemias
- Arrhythmias
- Ischemic heart disease
- Cardiomyopathies
- Pulmonary embolus
- Chronic obstructive lung disease
- Asthma and other respiratory diseases

Gastrointestinal Disorders
- Dysphagias
- Peptic ulcer disease
- Irritable bowel disorders
- Inflammatory bowel diseases

Nutritional and Metabolic Disorders
- Hypoglycemia
- Hypokalemia
- Occult vitamin deficiencies (*e.g.*, folate, thyamine)
- Hyperparathyroidism
- Hyperadrenalism
- Hypercortisolism

The clinician must consider endocrine disturbances, respiratory disturbances, metabolic disturbances, cardiovascular disorders, and gastrointestinal disorders, as well as central nervous system disorders and drug intoxication and withdrawal states. Since these illnesses are in themselves ubiquitous, a review of systems approach to these disorders is helpful. Some disorders, such as peptic ulcer disease, lie at the interface of psychic and somatic disturbances.

The severity of the anxiety, its pervasiveness, and its irrationality are important considerations in the evaluation of anxiety disorders. The clinician develops a working hypothesis or formulation of the patient's problem, taking into account the particular psychiatric syndrome, personality traits, general context of the patient's health, and environmental stressors. In addition, the patient's ego defenses and ego strengths are assessed. Particular attention should be paid to the psychological meaning of the patient's symptoms and coping techniques.

Treatment

Treatment of anxiety disorders depends on the patient's symptoms, vulnerability to stress, and coping techniques. Education, reassurance, and support with appropriate treatment of concurrent or underlying medical illnesses are the cornerstones of treatment for the majority of patients with symptoms of anxiety. Occasionally a brief course of anxiolytics, usually a benzodiazepine, may help the patient to mobilize his own resources so that he may start on his problems. For those patients with good ego strength, the capacity to tolerate painful affects, a reasonable measure of self-observing capacity, and clear intrapsychic conflicts, the treatment of choice is insight-oriented or psychodynamic psychotherapy. For other patients, supportive psychotherapy combining clarification, reassurance, support, and education is the treatment of choice. Adjunctive use of behavior therapy is indicated in many anxiety disorders.

Psychodynamically oriented psychotherapy rests on the development of insight into intrapsychic and interpersonal conflict. Symptom reduction may be a relatively slow process requiring a strong commitment on the part of the patient. The patient may have to tolerate periods of intensified anxiety, as well as other painful affects in the course of treatment.

Behavior therapies strive for symptom reduction, usually through a process of desensitization. A number of different treatment paradigms attempt to diminish the anxious response to aversive situations. These paradigms are more effective in the treatment of specific disorders such as simple phobias, acute anxiety responses to situations such as in social phobias, and relatively circumscribed obsessive–compulsive disorders.

Most behavior therapies rely on relaxation training. Anxiety may be reduced by various relaxation techniques such as progressive muscle relaxation, in which the patient is taught to systematically tense and relax ascending muscle groups. The premise of relaxation techniques is that anxiety and relaxation are compatible. Other relaxation techniques include varieties of meditation to elicit what Bensen has termed the *relaxation response*. Another relaxation technique employs electromyographic biofeedback. In this technique, the patient learns to relax selected muscle groups by altering the rate of feedback from an electromyographic probe that monitors muscle tension. All relaxation techniques require commitment in order to achieve good results.

These various relaxation techniques are usually paired with other interventions. In stress management training a relaxation technique is paired with cognitive coping strategies to identify and reduce stress in the patient's environment. Systematic desensitization, as developed by Wolpe, rests on the principle of reciprocal inhibition, in which relaxation is used to inhibit the anxious response to an aversive stimulus. A hierarchy of anxiety-provoking situations, from least to worst, is constructed, and while the patient practices progressive muscle relaxation he imagines threatening stimuli in stages, progressing from the least to the most troublesome. Systematic desensitization is quite effective for specific phobias.

With implosive therapy, the successive approach to the feared stimulus is substituted with a direct imagined exposure to the most anxiety-provoking stimulus. In flooding, real-life exposure to the actual stimulus is attempted at the outset. Bandura's technique of social learning uses actual modeling of approaches to feared stimuli. For example, the therapist might hold a feared snake and encourage the patient to follow suit. Adjunctive behavior therapies include thought stopping, in which the patient tried to stop obsessional thoughts, and assertiveness training, in which a patient is encouraged to confront fearful avoidance of assertive behavior.

Some patients will require pharmacologic intervention. Generally, anxiolytics are prescribed when anxiety significantly interferes with the patient's functioning. Anxiolytics should be seen as a short-term or intermittent adjuvant therapy. Nearly a dozen benzodiazepines are currently marketed in the United States as hypnotics or anxiolytics. While the half-life and speed of onset vary among the benzodiazepines, there is no evidence of clinical superiority of one compound over another. Cost, an important consideration, varies widely, particularly where generics are available. β-blockers, such as propranolol, which are occasionally prescribed to block the peripheral manifestations of anxiety, must be used with caution. There is little justification for use of older anxiolytic agents such as meprobamate. Other specific medications will be discussed below in consideration of specific anxiety disorders.

Panic Disorder and Agoraphobia

The treatment of panic disorder follows a careful diagnostic assessment. Following this assessment, the clinician is beset with two dilemmas: the panic symptoms and the avoidance behavior that usually complicates the disorder. Some clinicians, because of their orientation, treat panic disorder with insight-oriented psychotherapy, usually with a larger view of the patient as having core neurotic conflicts, of which panic attacks are merely a feature. In carefully diagnosed panic disorder, insight-oriented psychotherapy has not been shown to be efficacious, and results in behaviorally oriented therapy have been inconclusive. The behavioral treatments seem to help with phobic avoidance but had little effect on the panic disorder.

In carefully diagnosed panic disorder, pharmacotherapy is probably the most effective treatment when combined with other therapies. The first-choice pharmacotherapy is either alprazolam, an anxiolytic with antipanic properties, a heterocyclic antidepressant, or a monoamine oxidase inhibitor (MAOI). Imipramine or desipramine are the usual choices for heterocyclics. The only heterocyclic antidepressants that appear not to have antipanic properties are amoxapine and bupropion. MAOIs, and phenelzine in particular, are quite effective but require some caution because of bothersome side effects and the need for a diet low in tyramine. A short course of benzodiazepines for anticipatory anxiety that arises between panic symptoms is often needed.

Although some phobic avoidance and agoraphobia itself may remit with treatment of the panic attacks through pharmacotherapy, supportive psychotherapy and behavioral treatment are often necessary. Recent studies have shown that either modality seems to stimulate the patient to confront the feared and avoided stimuli.[5] Pharmacotherapy for panic disorders should continue six months after symptomatic control is attained. Return of panic attacks is common and requires longer treatment.

Social Phobia and Simple Phobias

Exposure to the feared stimulus is the common element in successful treatments of specific phobias. Considerable controversy surrounds the relative efficacy of specific treatment strategies. Whichever therapy leads the patient to real-life exposure to the feared stimulus and keeps him there long enough to reduce his fear will be the most effective treatment. Some patients will do well with simple encouragement from the clinician in a supportive psychotherapeutic relationship. For others a specific behavioral paradigm is most effective.

Phobics may benefit from assertiveness training as an adjunctive treatment, particularly when the avoidance behavior seems to be part of a reticent personality style. Some civic and religious organizations provide practice in public speaking or public performance. Encouraging a patient to join these organizations is a practical suggestion and may combat the general isolation that is common among phobic patients.

Obsessive–Compulsive Disorder

Obsessive–compulsive disorder is extremely difficult to treat. Clomipramine and other tricyclic antidepressants have been found to be effective for some patients. All other interventions have yielded variable results. A combined regimen of psychodynamically oriented psychotherapy and behavior therapy makes sense clinically, but has not been studied systematically. Severe cases have been treated with psychosurgery.

Post-Traumatic Stress Disorder

Acute PTSD has a favorable prognosis. The goal of treatment is ventilation and abreaction. The patient should be encouraged to speak openly and freely in a supportive atmosphere. Most patients respond well in such a supportive atmosphere where a nonjudgmental and empathic clinician, friend, or family member encourages an open expression of feelings. Specific trauma, such as rape, is effectively treated by peer counselors contacted through rape crisis centers. Occasional patients who find it difficult to express affects related to the trauma, or do not have access to their feelings, benefit from specialized techniques to enhance reexperience of the trauma and related feelings. In these cases sodium amytal infusions or hypnosis are often effective.

Chronic PTSD is more difficult to treat. Careful attention should be directed toward coexisting psychiatric disorders such as major depressions, personality disorders, or schizophrenia. Treatment of these disorders may help PTSD symptoms.

Data from case reports and pilot studies suggest that MAOIs are helpful in the patient with prominent panic-like symptoms. Various behavior therapies such as implosive therapy have helped some patients. For most patients the goal of treatment will be the management of symptoms and assistance in adapting to their disability. Supportive group and individual psychotherapy for the patients and their families is an important ingredient in their care.

Generalized Anxiety Disorder

Persistent anxiety that is unrelated to a particular stressful life event may require anxiolytic therapy. Benzodiazepines are the treatment of choice unless the patient presents with prominent dysphoric features. Some will be best treated with tricyclic antidepressants on an empirical basis. Other patients with anxious depression are best regarded as atypical, and they should be given trials of MAOIs or alprazolam. All patients with GAD should be treated at least adjunctively with a form of psychotherapy. Patients with good ego strength, self-observing capacity, good object relations, and some tolerance for their symptoms should be given a trial of insight-oriented psychotherapy. Stress management training and general relaxation training may also be helpful, but they require a well-motivated patient.

Summary

Anxiety is an ubiquitous symptom requiring careful evaluation by a skillful clinician. Pathologic anxiety may indicate an underlying medical illness, a reaction to illness, some other biopsychosocial stressor, or a wide range of psychiatric disorders. Anxiety disorders are, in this sense, diagnoses of exclusion. They are a heterogeneous group of disorders that require a broad understanding of the multifactorial etiology of psychiatric disorders. Treatment of carefully diagnosed anxiety disorders rests on psychotherapeutic management and communication, combined with the judicious use of pharmacologic agents.

References

1. Lader M: Behavior and anxiety: Physiologic mechanisms. J Clin Psychiatry 44(11, Sec II):5–10, 1983
2. Sheehan DV: Current concepts in psychiatry: Panic attacks and phobias. N Engl J Med 307:3156–3158, 1982
3. Nemiah JC: Obsessive–compulsive disorders. In Kaplan HI, Freedman AM, Sadock BJ (eds): Comprehensive Textbook of Psychiatry, 3rd ed. Baltimore, Williams & Wilkins, 1980
4. Nemiah JC: Phobic disorders. In Kaplan HI, Freedman AM, Sadock BJ (eds): Comprehensive Textbook of Psychiatry, 3rd ed. Baltimore, Williams & Wilkins, 1980
5. Matuzas W, Glass RM: Treatment of agoraphobia and panic attacks. Arch Gen Psychiatry 40:220–222, 1983

Bibliography

American Psychiatric Association: Diagnostic and Statistical Manual of Mental Disorders, 3rd ed. American Psychiatric Association, 1980

Maher BA: Principles of Psychopathology. New York, McGraw-Hill, 1966

Nemiah JC: Anxiety states. In Kaplan HI, Freedman AM, Sadock BJ (eds): Comprehensive Textbook of Psychiatry, 3rd ed. Baltimore, Williams & Wilkins, 1980

Shader RI, Greenblatt DJ: Some current treatment options for symptoms of anxiety. J Clin Psychiatry 44 (11, sec II):21–29, 1983

Skolnick P, Paul SM: New concepts in the neurobiology of anxiety. J Clin Psychiatry 44 (11, sec II):12–19, 1983

James T. McCracken

10 Somatoform Disorders

The somatoform disorders consist of a group of illnesses in which physical complaints exist in the absence of identifiable organic pathology. The symptoms are not produced or maintained voluntarily, and are best understood in terms of psychological processes. Patients with somatoform disorders respond poorly to conventional medical treatment, yet steadfastly refuse psychiatric consultation. The helplessness and confusion engendered in physicians by these patients lead to antipathy, as implied by their nicknames—"squirrels," "crocks," "turkeys," or "gomers." Their excessive demands and great expectations for cure leads to broken physician–patient relationships, doctor-shopping, and failure to obtain appropriate treatment. The five somatoform disorders discussed in this chapter include somatization disorder (Briquet's syndrome), conversion disorder (hysterical neurosis, conversion type), psychogenic pain disorder, hypochondriasis, and atypical somatoform disorder. This group includes patients who were formerly diagnosed as hysterical personality, hysterical, hysterical conversion, hysterical neurosis, Briquet's syndrome, chronic pain syndrome, anxiety neurosis, and other personality diagnoses. Understanding the dynamics of somatoform disorders will allow the physician to better manage these patients.

Somatization Disorder (Briquet's Syndrome)

Somatization disorder, first described by Paul Briquet in 1859, is a chronic disorder predominantly found in women, characterized by multiple somatic complaints involving several organ systems. The symptoms are not due to a diagnosable physical condition, and must be of sufficient intensity to cause the patients to seek medical attention, take medications, or significantly alter their lifestyle. Onset of symptoms usually occurs in adolescence or young adulthood, with a lifelong pattern consisting of frequent clinic visits, doctor-shopping, multiple surgeries, chronic dissatisfaction with medical care, and considerable suffering.

Making the formal diagnosis as defined by the Diagnostic and Statistical Manual of Mental Disorders, American Psychiatric Association (DSM-III), requires an onset prior to 30 years of age, a history of several years' duration of at least 14 symptoms (12 for men) from seven areas:

1. General health felt to be poor
2. Conversion or pseudoneurologic symptoms
3. Gastrointestinal symptoms
4. Female reproductive symptoms
5. Psychosexual symptoms
6. Pain symptoms
7. Cardiopulmonary symptoms

Briquet, in his exhaustive compilation of symptoms from over 400 patients, profiled common symptoms such as epigastric pain, thoracic pain, conversion symptoms, anxiety, and depression. Sexual dysfunction, headaches, abdominal pain, dysmenorrhea, bowel complaints, and musculoskeletal pain are frequent.

The personality characteristics of these patients bear mentioning. Earlier diagnostic classifications included some of these patients as "hysterical personalities;" even by using the more exact diagnostic criteria of DSM-III there may be some overlapping of somatization disorder with histrionic personality disorder. Shared features between somatization disorder and histrionic personality disorder include heightened emotionality, vague impressionistic thought, seductiveness, strong dependency needs, and a preoccupation with symptoms and oneself. Patients with somatization disorder and those with histrionic personality disorder describe symptoms vaguely, along with digressions to past treatment, minor fluctuations of symptoms, and personal frustrations. Their histories are richly colored with feelings of desperateness, despair, and rage. Covertly or even overtly they may be coquettish or seductive with the examiner. Usually, underlying their behavior is a strong wish to be taken care of, admired, or treated specially; and they frequently jump from one physician to the next, enraged when these enormous needs are not met.

The course of somatization disorder typically begins in adolescence or young adulthood, followed by a lifetime of continued symptoms that wax and wane, although recovery from the disorder may occur in a few patients. Suicide attempts, marital discord, and occupational problems are common in the histories of these patients. The following case illustrates the typical features of somatization disorder:

☐ Ms. W was a 36-year-old, white, twice-divorced woman hospitalized on Orthopedics, who was referred for psychiatric consultation as a part of an evaluation of her chronic back pain.

She had had lumbar back pain for many years with two prior laminectomies, but with only transient relief. Her surgical history was replete with other operations for vague pain complaints: cholecystectomy, hysterectomy, and exploratory laporotomy. Her medical history began soon after her first marriage with complaints of fatigue and abdominal pain. In the review of systems she had seemed to accumulate symptoms over the intervening years with the onset of urinary burning and incontinence, frigidity, atypical chest pain, joint pain, mild depression, periodic "blacking out," alternating constipation and diarrhea, dysmenorrhea, frequent vomiting, heartburn, episodic edema, blurred vision, and ataxia.

In the interview she described having married at 16 to escape her turbulent home. The brunt of the patient's rearing had been left to her mother after her father's departure, which occurred when the patient was nine years old. The mother had relied heavily on the patient to keep house and care for the younger children. Even prior to the father's leaving, the patient had served as the mother's confidante, frequently ministering to her mother in bed, where the mother would retreat to on her depressed days, weeping and complaining of headaches and other symptoms.

The patient first married a man who beat her and neglected her, then finally deserted the home. She married again, but sought a divorce within a year. Her later relationships with men had also been stormy and fragile.

The consultant noted her to be dramatic, dressed in a revealing gown, alternately weeping and enraged. Her request for surgery was insistent. She was exquisitely sensitive to the slightest psychological probing, which suggested to her that the examiner believed that the pain was "all in my head." There was no evidence of major depression or psychosis. The diagnosis given was somatization disorder.

The consultant agreed with the surgeon's decision to reject her request for surgery, based on her history of poor pain relief after prior surgeries, history of conversion symptoms, and her current marital strain. The consultant offered a transfer to the psychiatry service for further assessment, which the patient initially accepted; on the following day, however, she angrily left the hospital to return to her local physician.

Prevalence

Large-scale prospective surveys are lacking with respect to somatization disorder, but retrospective analyses of hospital and psychiatric clinic records suggest that the prevalence is approximately 1% to 2% among women. The actual rate among the general population is probably higher. Men who meet the criteria without a covert organic illness or unexpressed major psychiatric illness are quite rare.

Etiology

No comprehensive etiologic theories for somatization disorder have been advanced; however, studies of the family histories of these patients have shown a ten- to twentyfold increase in the incidence of the disorder in female first-degree relatives, along with an increased rate of sociopathy among all first-degree relatives, implying a possible inheritable predisposition. Further investigation of a genetic role by way of twin and adoption studies is lacking at the present time.

Psychodynamic theory emphasizes an early disturbed mother–child relationship in the etiology of somatization disorder. The mother, because of her own conflicts regarding sexuality and dependency, alternately clings to and rejects the child. The child fails to develop an adequate self-soothing capacity. This lack of self-soothing ability is defended against by learning to gain affection and care through illness.

There is little information available concerning the role of the family environment in the genesis of the disorder. Great cultural differences exist between Western and non-Western groups in the expression and perception of emotions; particular cultural attitudes may tend to sanction the channeling of emotional discomfort into somatic symptoms. This theory, however, has not been studied using cross-cultural investigations.

Differential Diagnosis

Somatization disorder overlaps with many diagnoses. Certain physical illnesses such as collagen vascular diseases, systemic lupus erythematosus (SLE), thyroid disease, occult malignancies, Addison's disease, and multiple sclerosis, all have multiple symptoms that defy precise diagnosis, particularly in the early stages of disease, and hence may mimic somatization disorder. Patients with conversion disorders may present with a variety of symptoms but would fail to demonstrate the complete clinical picture of somatization disorder.

Anxiety is an associated symptom of somatization disorder, but patients with panic disorder or phobias would present without the complex physical symptoms characteristic of somatization disorder. Mild depressive symptoms are found in conjunction with somatic complaints that typify somatization disorder; if depressive symptoms are of significant duration and intensity, a full major depressive syndrome should be diagnosed. A diagnosis of major depression can be made in conjunction with somatization disorder. The somatic delusions of patients with schizophrenia would be associated with bizarre delusions, hallucinations, flat affect, illogical thought, and a chronic deteriorating course.

The differential diagnosis highlights the need for a thorough psychiatric and medical history that contains a longitudinal appraisal of the course of symptoms, prior response to treatment, family history, and a complete medical screening.

Treatment

The primary goal of treatment should be to prevent inappropriate medication consumption, drug addiction, unnecessary surgery, or invasive diagnostic procedures.

A solid alliance between patient and physician is crucial. The alliance should be grounded on the understanding that these patients are suffering, and that they tend to express their fears and anxieties through their symptoms. The physician must be able to put aside his frustration over the patient's demandingness and continued complaints in order to provide some constancy and support for problems of living. Over time, these patients may learn to verbalize their thoughts and feelings, allowing them to understand the relationship between somatic complaints and life events.

The majority of these patients will continue to experience symptoms, and physicians will do best to prevent the consequences of unnecessary surgery, drug addiction, and doctor-shopping. Straightforward discussions with the patient's family and members of their support network, detailing the chronicity of the disorder, may also be a powerful intervention toward limiting the morbidity of the disorder. New symptoms or changes in symptom patterns must be evaluated as closely as possible for indications of physical illness, but a conservative approach is indicated for working up new problems. Panic or phobic disorders will respond to standard therapeutic regimens, and secondary major depression should be treated with antidepressants. Traditional uncovering psychotherapy is of no proven value for somatization disorder, and is usually contraindicated.

Conversion Disorder (Hysterical Neurosis, Conversion Type)

Conversion disorder, defined by DSM-III as a sudden alteration of physiologic function that is not due to physical illness, is characterized by the following:

1. The symptom is clearly associated with a psychological stress.
2. The symptom allows the individual to escape from a conflict.
3. The symptom allows the patient to receive a benefit or avoid a noxious activity.
4. The symptom is not under voluntary control.

Additionally, the symptoms must not be limited to pain or psychosexual dysfunction, or be due to another mental disorder such as somatization disorder or schizophrenia.

Conversion disorder receives its name from the "conversion" of anxiety into a physical symptom. The conversion symptom protects the individual from experiencing painful feelings associated with a psychological conflict by keeping the conflict unconscious (primary gain), and simultaneously transforms the conflict into a somatic symptom that allows the individual to receive a benefit or avoid a particular activity (secondary gain). For example, after becoming angered with his boss, a paralyzed hand prevents a man from hitting his employer (primary gain) and allows him to receive a much easier work assignment (secondary gain). Usually there is more than one set of unacceptable wishes or forces that together give rise to the symptom. Forbidden sexual or aggressive wishes, escape from unpleasant duties, or glossing over personal shortcomings may be relieved by the presence of the conversion symptom.

Conversion symptoms can be divided broadly into two categories, sensory and motor symptoms. Sensory symptoms involve disturbances of both skin sensation and of the special senses. Skin sensation alone can be altered in a variety of ways: anesthesia, hypoesthesia, dysesthesia, or hyperesthesia. These alterations can occur over any anatomic distribution, but more commonly present as hemianesthesia, or loss of sensation in an entire limb in a "glove" or "stocking" pattern. All of the special senses may be involved in other conversion symptoms. Visual symptoms range from complete blindness to blurring, scotoma, and monocular diplopia. Conversion deafness is common. A variety of symptoms involving taste have also been described. Paralysis of an extremity, hemiparesis, or hemiplegia are frequent. Generalized weakness (pseudomyasthenia gravis), gait disturbances, dysphonia, tics, and pseudoseizures are among other motor conversion symptoms.

Differentiating the conversion symptoms from symptoms that are due to physical illness varies in difficulty from one patient to the next. With some patients a conversion symptom is easy to diagnose, as in the patient complaining of deafness who is startled by a loud, unexpected noise, for example. Other patients may endure painful examinations without showing evidence that their complaints are functional, as in the patient with glove anesthesia who is stuck with pins until his arm bleeds, yet shows no reaction. At times, even the most highly trained examiner will be unable to differentiate conversion disorder from a neurological disorder based on the physical examination alone.

Presentation

In the past, clinicians placed heavy emphasis on the lack of emotional concern on the part of patients toward their symptoms (la belle indifference) as nearly pathognomonic of conversion reaction. More recent observations refute the importance of la belle indifference. In fact, patients with long-standing symptoms are usually quite distressed about their symptoms in keeping with their more fully established "sick" role. However, if the symptom effectively defends against the underlying conflict as described, anxiety may be minimal.

Conversion symptoms generally arise suddenly, and detailed questioning will reveal external or perceived stress occurring at the time of symptom onset. Less commonly, the disorder appears insidiously.

Acute and chronic conversion symptoms differ in several ways. In the acute situation, a precipitating stress is usually evident for the symptom, and the defensive role of the symptom and underlying conflict are clear-cut. The symptom is usually not associated with other conversion symptoms or major psychopathology, and the prognosis for symptom removal is fair to good.

☐ Mr. P, a 20-year-old recently married man, was brought to the emergency room by his wife after he suddenly lost the use of his right hand and arm.

The psychiatrist obtained a history from both the wife and patient. The couple had been married for 3 months after a courtship of 7 months. Both agreed there had been no obvious problems at first; however, with some encouragement, the patient began to express his feeling that since the marriage, his wife had been pressuring him to devote more time to their relationship, to the exclusion of some important friendships.

On the day of his presentation, Mr. and Mrs. P had made two attempts to discuss the above problem. During the second disagreement, Mr. P noted his right hand and arm suddenly became paralyzed and his fist clenched. Sensation was normal.

The patient's overall health had been good, with no such prior episodes and no discernable prodromal symptoms. Mr. P had grown up in a very religious Southern family that clearly had prohibited the expression of anger. Additionally, a paternal grandfather who lived nearby was hemiparetic and emotionally labile due to a past stroke.

The examiner noted Mr. P's initial indifference to his arm and his reluctance to discuss his marital situation. He seemed a timid, passive man who spoke in a very controlled, precise fashion. During the lengthy interview, as he spoke more freely by himself, it was evident he felt trapped and enraged by his wife's demands. Later, he was able to agree with the examiner's comment that he did harbor significant resentment towards his wife for her stubbornness. At the end of the interview, he noted some relaxation of his fist and arm, and some improved mobility. The examiner's diagnosis was conversion disorder. He was sent home with instructions for follow-up in the outpatient clinic. He declined to pursue psychotherapy, but later reported full resolution of the symptom within two days.

For the patient with a chronic conversion symptom it is much more difficult to trace the genesis of the symptom back to a specific event and unconscious conflict. The patient presents the symptom prominently, and secondary gain in the form of compensation, solicitous behavior from others, or escape from unpleasant activities is paramount. Coexisting psychopathology including somatization disorder, depression, or severe personality disorder is common. Because the illness satisfies powerful wishes to be nurtured and cared for, prognosis is poor.

☐ Ms. N, a 29-year-old single woman, hospitalized on Neurology, was referred to psychiatric consultation of her increased pseudoseizures.

She had had a documented history of major motor seizures since the age of 14, controlled by anticonvulsants, and pseudoseizures documented in the chart since age 18. She was also noted to be mildly mentally retarded.

The psychiatric consultant obtained the history that her pseudoseizures had been less frequent until about 1 month prior, when the patient's parents had begun discussing with the patient plans for her to move to a group home and start vocational rehabilitation. The consultant also noted several past episodes of wrist-slashing when the patient was denied something or when she was frustrated. There was no current evidence of psychosis or major depression.

The consultant recommended that the patient's separation from home be attempted gradually and he encouraged the patient's caseworker to hold family discussions focusing on the patient's fears about moving away.

Relationship to Physical Disorders

Considerable evidence exists that compels the physician to be very cautious in making the diagnosis of conversion disorder only on the basis of the lack of objective examination and laboratory findings. The danger of underdiagnosing subclinical organic disease is clear. An average of 20% to 25% of patients diagnosed as having conversion disorder are later discovered to have physical illnesses that explain their original symptoms. An additional number of patients can be found to have conversion symptoms that exaggerate or muddle the presenting symptoms of an undiagnosed physical illness. For example, most neurologists have at least one patient in their practice who has a documented seizure disorder as well as pseudoseizures. Certain types of physical illness may be highly correlated with conversion disorder. Organic brain disease commonly occurs in association with conversion symptoms; its precise relationship with conversion symptoms has not been elucidated.

Personality Disorders

Studying the personality diagnoses of patients with conversion symptoms dispels the notion that this disorder is limited to a single personality type. These conversion symptoms can be observed in combination with any personality organization, including passive aggressive, histrionic, schizoid, paranoid, and other personality disorders. Similarly, conversion symptoms are not limited to any one developmental level; they may be expressions of conflicts regarding sexuality, dependency, self-esteem, or aggression.

Freud's early clinical experiences had led to his theory of hysterical phenomena arising due to the inadequate resolution of oedipal conflicts. In his postulation, the adult retains the childhood wish for (and fear of) an incestuous relationship with the parent figure, which is repressed from consciousness. The hysterical symptom arises as a result of the blocked drive's being unsuccessfully defended against; the symptom itself symbolizes the underlying wish and a simultaneous fear of punishment for such a wish. For example, the sexual gyrations characteristic of one patient's pseudoseizures revealed the repressed wish for sexual relationships and provided a limited gratification of these wishes, but the frequency of his "spells" prevented him from dating women and contributed to a very restricted life (the punishment for the wish).

Pre-oedipal conflicts can also product conversion symptoms. Conflicts over dependency needs are frequently found in patients with conversion symptoms. Perhaps due to early deprivation or loss, these patients manifest powerful but previously unacceptable wishes to be cared for, which often were defended against by a stoic, hyperindependent lifestyle. If the individual is faced with overwhelming stress or physical illness, these former defensive adaptations can be rendered ineffective, and a conversion symptom may emerge that allows the fearful dependency needs to be gratified in a manner that is less psychologically damaging. Secondary gain in the form of compensation and care from others may further entrench the symptom and make return to the counterdependent lifestyle unlikely.

Conversion symptoms may also be linked to threat to one's self-esteem; according to this view, conversion symptoms become a last-ditch measure to protect the individual from narcissistic injuries to the self. The symptom may mend the profound disappointments incurred from being unable to live up to one's highest expectations, or ego-ideal.

Conflicts over the expression of anger and aggression form the nidus of conversion symptoms in other patients. As described in the case of Mr. P, the symptom of a paralyzed arm with clenched fist occurring at a time of continued marital strain in a submissive, obsequious man represents a safe avenue of expression of his rage. It temporarily halts the fighting, enlists the wife's sympathy, and mitigates the man's fear of killing the wife or driving her away; while symbolically punishing him with new limitations.

Affective Illness

Depression has long been observed to coexist with conversion symptoms. Depression may be covert and only uncovered by symptom removal; however, even excluding patients with "hidden" depressions, moderate to severe depression has been observed in 12% to 30% of patients diagnosed as having conversion disorder. The conversion symptom may serve as a defense against underlying depression. Several follow-up studies have documented a significant incidence of suicide, recurrent depression, and the emergence of hypomania or mania among patients with conversion disorders. These observations underscore the necessity for carefully considering the possibility of an affective disorder in patients with conversion symptoms.

Diagnosis

In making the diagnosis of conversion disorder, the clinician should remember the following:

The presence of a conversion symptom does not exclude the presence of an underlying physical illness.

The diagnosis of conversion disorder should not be made solely on the basis of a negative organic work-up.

In certain patients there may be an additional nonpsychological factor of organic brain disease that contributes to the etiology of the conversion symptom.

Accurate diagnosis rests on a careful, combined physical and psychiatric examination of the patient. All suggestions of physical illness should be fully explored. When taking a psychiatric history, the clinician must avoid, directly or indirectly, implying that the physical symptom may be a product of emotional conflicts. The patient's emotional conflicts are unconscious; suggesting a psychological association with the physical symptoms will only anger the patient. Instead, the examiner should subtly explore the quality of the patient's life, including interpersonal relationships, work history, sexual history, recent losses, medical history, past unexplained physical symptoms, and a history of similar symptoms expressed in a family member, especially during the patient's formative years (symptom model). In addition, an impression of the level of psychological maturity and previous adaptation should be constructed from: characteristic defense mechanisms; the ability to experience and tolerate affects; the capacity to form a trusting, positive relationship with the examiner; and the degree of psychological-mindedness (*i.e.,* can the patient make a connection between physical symptoms and emotional conflicts—most patients with conversion disorder cannot).

While there are no pathognomonic signs of conversion disorder, a variety of criteria have been proposed that assist in gathering evidence for making the diagnosis of conversion disorder. In decreasing order of importance, they are:

1. Past history of conversion disorder
2. Presence of significant emotional stress prior to onset of symptoms
3. The symptom solves a conflict brought on by the current stress.
4. Coexisting major psychopathology (*e.g.,* depression, somatization disorder, schizophrenia, severe personality disorders)

5. Presence of sexual dysfunction
6. The history of a symptom model

Obtaining one or more of the above features does not unequivocally support a conversion diagnosis, but would increase the index of suspicion, and combined with an appropriate clinical context would argue for the diagnosis.

Differential Diagnosis

Organic Illness

The high incidence (25%) of false positive diagnoses of conversion disorder in patients later discovered to have physical illness underscores the physician's need to consider and eliminate the possible physical causes of the patient's complaint. Many systemic illnesses may present early in their course with confusing, attenuated symptoms: Rheumatoid arthritis, systemic lupus erythematosus, perineoplastic syndromes, porphyria, and endocrine disorders are a few examples. Careful neurologic evaluation is crucial in order to rule out causes of cerebral dysfunction such as multiple sclerosis, seizure disorders, brain tumor, or infectious processes.

Schizophrenia

Patients with schizophrenic illness may develop conversion symptoms along with the other manifestations of their disorder. Usually the differential is not difficult because the conversion symptom is present along with the disturbances of behavior, thought, and affect that typify schizophrenia. For the patient who presents with the isolated complaint of hallucinations, primary and secondary gain issues should be evident.

Somatization Disorder

Patients with somatization disorders often have several conversion symptoms in addition to a prodigious list of other associated somatic symptoms and a lifelong pattern of doctor-shopping, disappointment with treatment by physicians, frequent hospitalizations, and possibly unnecessary surgeries and procedures. Onset of somatization disorder is usually in adolescence with a chronic course of continued symptoms that wax and wane in intensity.

Malingering

Malingering patients can confound the best clinician's ability to distinguish this condition from conversion disorder. Determining that a symptom is consciously controlled usually is inferred from evidence that the individual is actively pursuing compensation, attempting to avoid prosecution by authorities or any other situation where secondary gain is paramount. There are also some differences in the type of symptoms chosen by malingerers. They are less likely to complain of pseudoneurologic symptoms and more commonly present with pain or generalized complaints.

Treatment

Treatment of conversion disorders must be determined by the specific clinical situation because, as described, the disorder is commonly associated with other conditions, may be acute or chronic, or may represent a defense against psychosis or depression.

Symptom removal was originally recommended for all patients with hysterical symptoms. Methods still currently employed include hypnosis, narcoanalysis, and persuasion. Hypnosis and narcoanalysis (amytal interview) consist of placing the patient in a relaxed state with diminished anxiety, and by questioning and suggestion, to allow him to reexperience the precipitating stress, abreact fully the repressed affect, and by doing so, free the patient of the psychological need for the symptom. These techniques are highly successful in ameliorating conversion symptoms that are acute, have clearly identifiable stressors, and are not associated with major psychopathology. Chronic conversion symptoms remit less frequently and relapse at a higher rate. Therefore, symptom removal is indicated primarily for acute conversion symptoms.

More ambitious is the second goal of treatment, which consists of furthering the individual's psychological adaptability so that reliance on primitive and inflexible mechanisms of defense is lessened. In this way, the individual is less likely to resort to disabling symptoms with associated morbidity. Psychotherapy, either supportive or insight-oriented, is the treatment of choice. The choice of the particular psychotherapeutic method is based on the attributes that also determine prognosis. Individuals who can tolerate anxiety and depression without developing incapacitating symptoms, who are able to make observations on their feelings and behavior, have developed the capacity for stable, mature interpersonal relationships with satisfying sexual relationships; who verbalize thoughts, feelings, and wishes, and can delay immediate gratification of their impulses, can endure the frustration and regression inherent to insight-oriented therapy and can maximize possible gains from psychotherapy. These patients have the best prognosis. Others, because of their more primitive personality organizations, lack of motivation, resources, time, or similar extenuating circumstances, are more appropriately treated with supportive psychotherapeutic techniques. These patients often carry additional personality diagnoses such as borderline, narcissistic, or passive–dependent. In supportive treatments, the therapy may be individual, but family, group and marital therapies are also used. Here the attempt is made to maximize the patient's adaptation by encouraging appropriate job changes, altering disturbed family interactions or improving specific relationships. Finally, treatment of associated disorders such as major depression should be vigorously pursued.

Psychogenic Pain Disorder

The diagnosis of psychogenic pain disorder should be made when psychological factors contribute to the patient's complaint of pain. The pain must exist in the absence of documentable physical illness, the symptom cannot be under voluntary control, the onset of pain must have a temporal correlation with a stressful environmental event, and the symptom pattern can have no discernable pathophysiologic mechanism. While these patients may have past histories of using somatization as a defense, including past conversion reactions, their current presentation should be limited to the pain complaint with only minor associated symptoms such as sensory changes.

Several psychodynamic formulations have been given as an explanation for psychogenic pain. The unconscious wish to suffer and other masochistic features of chronic pain complainers have been highlighted. The wish to suffer is seen to arise from guilt over hostile and envious feelings that were first experienced in childhood. Often, patients with psychogenic pain present histories that include fantasies of hurting siblings who were specially cared for during illness.

In some families, nurturance and emotional engagement are learned to be solicited by the child's somatic distress, which carries over into adulthood, with health-care personnel serving as surrogate parents. A different conceptualization argues that many of these patients have a fundamental deficit in personality functioning that limits their capacity to consciously experience or verbally express basic affects. These patients have difficulty putting feelings into words (alexithymia); instead, feelings are expressed as somatic symptoms, as in the following case:

> ☐ Mrs. K, a 64-year-old married woman from a rural area, was transferred to the chronic pain unit after an evaluation on Gynecology failed to discover an etiology for her chronic pelvic pain.
>
> The gradual onset of her pain had occurred about 10 years previously, and she had undergone numerous hospitalizations and negative evaluations including a pelvic computed tomography (CT) scan, laparoscopy, and pelvic exams. She complained of a burning, "tearing" vaginal and rectal pain that was relatively constant. She had found little relief from narcotics, antidepressants, or physical therapy. There was no overt depression present by history or examination.
>
> Upon questioning, the patient revealed that she had cared for her mother during the mother's last years with metastatic uterine carcinoma, until her death 14 years previously. During the last 1 to 2 years of the illness, her mother was bedridden, irritable, demanding, incontinent of urine and stool, and suffered from pain.
>
> The diagnosis upon transfer was psychogenic pain disorder. The attending psychiatrist saw the primary dynamic to be unresolved grief over the mother's death due to the extent of unacknowledged anger at the mother for the burden of her last years. The symptom served to maintain an unconscious bond with the mother through the identification with the mother's pain, and at the same time the pain served as a punishment for her unconscious hostile feelings toward her mother. Over a 3-week hospitalization, Mrs. K was reluctant to pursue any psychological issues in psychotherapy, passively refused to comply with suggested behavioral interventions, and insisted on an organic cause for her pain. She was discharged with only slight improvement.

Treatment

There is no treatment of choice for psychogenic pain disorder. However, most pain clinics and pain units offer a multidisciplinary approach after ruling out an obvious separately treatable component such as an organic illness, affective disorder, or neurotic component. The alternatives include:

Behavior modification
Medications
Electrical stimulation

Biofeedback
Nerve blocks
Group therapy

Behavior modification can hold a central role in the management of pain patients. Typically, a behavioral program is developed in-hospital; however, outpatient treatment can also be accomplished. Most behavioral programs have similar goals of enhancing the patient's sense of control over the pain, increasing his physical activity, and decreasing his reliance on habituating medication. In this framework, pain is viewed as a learned behavior, subject to environmental responses that can increase or decrease the behavior. To untangle the complex existing system of reinforcers of pain behavior, the patient's social system, be it the hospital unit or family unit, is set up to take away any positive reinforcers of pain behavior, such as sympathy and contact contingent to pain, and most importantly, instilling praise and positive consequences for a lack of pain and/or adaptive behaviors.

The goal of increasing activity runs parallel to the above. Most pain patients are "overdoers," that is, they tend to set their limits for activity based on pain, not on a programmatic schedule to increase stamina gradually without worsening pain. Treatment is accomplished by developing an activity program of work–rest beginning at a level below the patient's pain threshold and setting specific goals, being careful not to proceed if pain worsens. Here again, the patient experiences his progress as an indication of greater control over pain by use of a systematized method.

An additional important goal is to decrease analgesic medications. This is done by first determining the minimum amount of regularly administered analgesic needed to fully relieve pain, and then followed by a gradual tapering over a 3- to 6-week period until pain returns or until the analgesic is stopped entirely. The taper can be best performed by using the liquid form of the active medicine. This method breaks the pain-reinforcing cycle of having the medication be contingent on pain behavior, and is very successful with the majority of patients.

Other nonanalgesic medications have proven effective in treating patients with significant psychogenic pain. The serotonin-enhancing antidepressants (amitriptyline, doxepin, trazodone, and imipramine) have been shown to partially or fully relieve psychogenic pain, by their antidepressant effect or by other mechanisms. Usual antidepressant doses are recommended. Neuroleptics can be combined with antidepressants; however, the risk of tardive dyskinesia must be fully weighed against clinical benefit. Haloperidol and fluphenazine are used most commonly.

Electrical stimulation can be an important adjunctive treatment. Its effect is thought to be due to inhibition of competing pain signals as explained by the "gate theory." Transcutaneous nerve stimulation (TENS unit), consisting of pulse stimulation from a battery-powered generator through skin electrodes, often affords good short-term relief. Another technique for more intractable pain that is based on the same principle involves the implantation of electrodes into the dorsal column. This is recommended more for patients with documentable organic pathology, and for whom relief with other methods has been poor.

Biofeedback is useful for pain control in patients in whom considerable muscle tension is evident. With continued practice, the relaxation training can be used by the patient without the need for the electromyographic (EMG) feedback.

Nerve blocks can be used for both diagnostic and treatment purposes. Blockage of the appropriate sympathetic nerves by either steroids or neurotoxic agents can effect good pain relief. Typically, pain with a discernable organic component will respond best.

Group therapy may be helpful because it provides a setting where patients can share their experience of illness, learn to verbalize thoughts and feelings, and be confronted by group members and leaders when they reject responsibility for maladaptive behaviors.

Hypochondriasis (Hypochondriacal Neurosis)

Hypochondriasis is characterized by the patient's misinterpretation of physiologic sensations as being pathologic, with the resultant fixed belief that he is suffering from disease. The belief is not shaken by reassurance from the physician or the absence of abnormal laboratory examinations, and significantly shapes the individual's lifestyle. The preoccupation with illness must not be due to another somatoform disorder, major depression, or schizophrenia.

Hypochondriacal patients present with complaints that vary from specific complaints to vague, generalized ones. Solitary symptoms of pain or weakness are common. Organ systems typically involved are the gastrointestinal, musculoskeletal, and central nervous systems. The "complaint" given often represents an amplification of a normal physiologic function such as bowel sounds, that is then attributed with illness or dysfunction. The intensity of the complaint is overridden by the individual's concern and fear of illness, and he tenaciously maintains his preoccupation in spite of any evidence to the contrary. Stressful events lead to an increase in illness behavior. Furthermore, in spite of their dissatisfaction with past medical care, hypochondriacal patients relentlessly pursue contact with the medical system by doctor-shopping, accumulating medications, and visiting emergency rooms. These patients rarely comply with referrals to mental health professionals. They also may accrue iatrogenic morbidity from ill-prescribed medications, procedures, or hospitalizations.

The incidence of hypochondriasis in samples of psychiatric patients is approximately 1%; however, the disorder is extremely common among general medical patients, where patients with "functional" complaints (symptoms without corroborating physical findings) may number between 30% to 80% of the general clinic population. While hypochondriasis represents a fraction of these patients, the importance of the disorder is magnified by the fact that these patients overutilize medical care with repeated presentations of similar complaints that lead to more frequent laboratory examinations, procedures, and consultations. In short, the management of the disorder represents a major concern of general medicine, and its overall impact on the health care system is substantial.

Traditionally, hypochondriacal symptoms have been explained by psychodynamic theory. More recently, however, biological and sociological influences have been advanced that contribute to a broader understanding of the disorder.

Using psychodynamic explanations, hypochondriasis can be thought of as a neurotic illness resulting from one of three conflicts: 1) displaced sexual or aggressive drives, 2) defense against threats to the self, or 3) defense against unpleasant affects.

Freud constructed a mode of hypochondriasis based on his notions of psychic energy. In his view, aggressive impulses are withdrawn from outside objects and redirected to the body, leading to hypochondriasis. Unacceptable aggressive and hostile impulses are transformed into somatic complaints, resulting in a "neurotic compromise." Repeated failures of others to relieve symptoms enable the patient to feel legitimately angry, yet the continued presence of the symptoms serves as punishment. Furthermore, because the cause of the exaggerated hostility springs from past frustrations and trauma, the behavioral cycle also serves as an attempt to undo the past hurts.

A second psychodynamic formulation emphasizes the function of the hypochondriacal symptom in protecting self-esteem. Here, intolerable feelings of low self-regard are channeled into somatic symptoms that are more comfortably distanced from the self. Childhood observation of illness among family members, or childhood illness in which sick behavior elicited parental care and solicitation, may provide a template for hypochondriacal behavior.

Social reinforcement and learning also contribute to the development of hypochondriasis. The hypochondriacal patient unconsciously uses illness behavior as a way of relating to others. Illness provides care and concern from others, escape from life's demands and possible compensation, and a security-providing relationship with the medical care system. Social reinforcements can cumulatively outweigh the individual's genuine desires to regain health behaviors and can interfere with the physician's attempts to encourage the patient to give up the sick role.

Finally, a biological examination of hypochondriasis may at times reveal a coexisting affective disorder. Depression is commonly associated with hypochondriasis, which carries important treatment implications. The hypochondriacal symptom occurring alone may represent an attentuated depressive illness, or the full depressive syndrome may be uncovered along with the presence of the somatic symptom.

☐ Mrs. H, a 53-year-old married woman, was admitted for a psychiatric evaluation. Her past history was significant for her longstanding belief that she was suffering from an undiagnosed abdominal ailment. Over the past 15 years, she had persistently complained of abdominal sensations and her fear of possible malignancy. Her family physician had angrily dispatched her to a colleague after he had been exhausted by her demands for repeated tests and medications. The few medications that he did prescribe led to irritable complaints of side effects or worsening symptoms. Refusing to accept any of the physicians' attempts to persuade her against her belief, she felt "irritated and let down."

Her childhood history was notable for her growing up in a family of three siblings with elderly parents who had been distant from the children. Those early relationships were described as lacking nurturance and support.

A thorough evaluation revealed that, in addition to hypochondriasis, the patient also had a major depression. Depressive symptoms remitted with supportive psychotherapy and antidepressant treatment; however, telephone follow-up with her local physician months later revealed that her hypochondriacal complaints were unchanged.

Differential Diagnosis

The primary differential diagnosis of hypochondriasis consists of covert physical illness, depression, other somatoform disorders, psychophysiologic disorders, and schizophrenia. Somatization disorder has an earlier onset, chronic course, and multiple symptoms, which all separate it from hypochondriasis. Psychophysiologic disorders such as irritable bowel, peptic ulcer disease, and others have demonstrable tissue pathology or pathophysiology, in a setting where psychological factors are evident.

Treatment

Traditionally, hypochondriasis was said to respond poorly to various treatments, and chronicity was said to be the rule rather than the exception. However, given the heterogeneity of the condition and its associated features, response to treatment varies. Depression should be ameliorated by appropriate pharmacotherapy, and some patients will improve with psychotherapeutic interventions. The largest determinant of treatment response may be length of illness. After an extended period of dysfunction, the patient's social milieu may be altered sufficiently to continue to support and maintain the illness in spite of any intervention. With chronic hypochondriasis, a supportive and accepting relationship with a physician who tolerates the patient's behavior without judgment, and who is available during periods of distress and increased symptoms, can help to minimize incapacitating anxiety, doctor-shopping, and further regression. Frequent but brief clinic visits or even regular telephone contacts can serve an important role in stabilizing such patients and preventing morbidity.

Atypical Somatoform Disorder

Atypical somatoform disorder is reserved for somatizing patients who fall short of the formal criteria for other somatoform diagnoses, and yet for whom psychological factors clearly play a role in the etiology of the somatic complaint.

Summary

The somatoform disorders consist of a group of five illnesses in which physical complaints exist in the absence of identifiable pathology. They are best understood in terms of psychological processes, and these disorders range from acute disturbances with good prognoses to chronic, intractable conditions that without appropriate management will accrue significant morbidity. They are common, and it behooves all physicians to be aware of their clinical presentations and guidelines for treatment.

Table 10-1
Frequency of Symptoms in Somatization Disorder

Symptom	Percentage	Symptom	Percentage
Nervous	92	Chest pain	72
Back pain	88	Abdominal bloating	68
Dizziness	84	Anxiety attacks	64
Fatigue	84	Always sickly	40
Weakness	84	Depressed feelings	64
Joint pain	84	Cries a lot	60
Extremity pain	84	Has thought of dying	48
Headache	80	Has thought of suicide	28
Nausea	80	Has attempted suicide	12
Abdominal pain	80	Anorexia	60
Dyspnea	72		

(Adapted from Perley MJ, Guze SB: Hysteria—The stability and usefulness of clinical criteria. N Engl J Med 266:421–426, 1962. By permission.)

Bibliography

American Psychiatric Association: Diagnostic and Statistical Manual of Mental Disorders, 3rd ed. American Psychiatric Association, Washington, DC, 1980

Barsky AJ, Klerman GL: Overview: Hypochondriasis, bodily complaints, and somatic styles. Am J Psychiatry 140:273–283, 1983

Briquet P: Traite clinique et therapeutique de l'hysterie. Paris, Bailliere et Fils, 1859

Engle G: Psychogenic pain and the pain-prone patient. Am J Med 26:899–918, 1959

Gatfield PD, Guze SB: Prognosis and differential diagnosis of conversion reactions. Dis Nerv Syst *23,* 623–631, 1962

Hafeiz HB: Hysterical conversion: A prognostic study. Br J Psychiatry 136:548–551, 1980

Maltbie AA: Conversion disorder. In Cavenar JO, Brodie HKH (eds): Signs and Symptoms in Psychiatry, pp 93–94. Philadelphia, JB Lippincott, 1983

Perley MJ, Guze SB: Hysteria-The stability and usefulness of clinical criteria. N Engl J Med 226:421–426, 1962

Slater E: Hysteria 311. J Ment Sci 107:359, 1961

Woodruff RA, Jr, Clayton PJ, Guze SB: Hysteria: Studies of diagnosis, outcome, and prevalence. JAMA 215:425–428, 1971

Steven Mahorney

11 Personality Disorders

Personality—the distinguishing habits, attitudes, and character traits of an individual, can be considered disordered when the characteristic behavior patterns interfere with the individual's ability to love, work, and enjoy recreation. Typically, an individual with a personality disorder bothers others more than he is bothered by his own behavior: His behavior is ego-syntonic, which means he thinks the fault lies in others rather than in himself. This chapter will discuss the characteristics of patients with personality disorders. Practical methods that physicians can use to manage these difficult patients will be considered in detail.

General Characteristics

Personality disorders and maladaptive personality traits are the most common yet the most rarely recognized conditions in medical practice. The incessant demands, complaints, and manipulations of patients with personality disorders make them a difficult management problem. Nonrecognition and mismanagement leads to countless hours of worry and massive numbers of futile and unnecessary diagnostic tests.

The chief complaint of patients with personality disorders often begins as "nerves," "I can't sleep," "I need help," or chest, back, head, or abdominal pain.

The complaint is usually urgent. A complete physical examination and laboratory evaluation are usually within normal limits. Exotic consultations from microspecialties in medicine rarely produce results. These patients are remarkable for the absence of history and examination findings that are consistent with clear diagnoses of schizophrenia, depression, mania, or organic brain syndrome. They are not psychotic.

Although physical complaints should always be taken seriously and investigated as appropriate, these patients often present with long-standing problems that have failed to respond to treatment. If the problem is "nerves" or pain, previous treatment attempts often "didn't help" or "only helped a little." The patient may even tell of previous diagnostic procedures or treatments that made him worse, the most common of these possibly being spinal tap in patients with low back pain.

Despite repetitive maladaptive behavior, the patient fails to see his behavior as the cause of unpleasant and frustrating situations in life. Consequently, the history obtained by the physician often portrays a helpless individual victimized by pestilent circumstances, without power to influence the events of his life. The patient who left a series of jobs was forced to do so by "headaches," "the boss just had it in for me," and "I couldn't get to work on time" because of traffic, car trouble, his wife, and so forth. The patient who committed crimes did so because "I fell in with the wrong crowd," "I had to get him before he got me," or "I ran into a sheriff who had it in for me."

Maladaptive behavior means failure to adjust to variations in life circumstances, resulting in action taken by the patient that interferes with the accomplishment of basic life goals. Such goals include long-term family relationships, career development, and satisfying recreation. One patient may decide to leave her husband because he doesn't make enough money. Another may overreact or be too sensitive to his supervisor's criticism, leading to resignation from his job.

Each patient feels that he had no alternative and that the control of events was in the hands of others—a process known as externalization. Externalization creates the partial illusion that the patient is helpless and that his problems are being created by others. The problem, by the patient's actions and perceptive apparatus, is being "externalized" onto others. One function of this process is to protect the patient's often fragile sense of self-esteem when things are going painfully bad.

At this point, the essential features of personality disorders have been described. Specific personality disorders are simply named by the behavior styles: compulsive, dependent, histrionic, narcissistic, and so forth. It is much more important to recognize that a personality disorder is present than to be able to identify and name the specific type. Clues for recognizing an individual with a personality disorder include:

Maladaptive behavior as a lifestyle
Rigid and inflexible way of handling situations
Chronic and lifelong pattern of personal problems
Multiple social, personal, and physical problems
Externalization of problems (blaming others and situations)
Free of psychosis

General Management Strategies

It is more appropriate to speak of management of personality disorders rather than treatment. Treatment implies that these patients will be "cured"; that is, their lifestyle pattern of behavior will be completely changed. This task takes many years of psychotherapy with a patient who is motivated to change. The best one can hope in most cases is to manage the problem, which means the physician learns to deal with the patient's personality style so that he can provide that patient with the best general medical care possible. Principles of management include:

- Recognize the patient's personality disorder early.
- "First do no harm" (*primum non nocere*).
- Set limits on maladaptive behavior that interferes with good medical care.
- Delay impulsive action.
- Provide feedback to the patient—let the patient know what is being done and the reasons for the action.

Management of personality disorders is analogous to management of many chronic medical problems such as diabetes mellitus, atherosclerosis, or rheumatoid arthritis. One rarely speaks of cures with these disorders; rather the focus is more commonly on remission, that is relieving discomfort and helping the patient cope with the disorder. Indeed, having unrealistic fantasies of cure may impede the coping process for both the physician and patient. Unrealistic expectations may also lead to transgression of the physician's dictum, "first do no harm."

Often the physician's refusal to "do something" is the most beneficial management technique. When patients present with physical and emotional symptoms in response to the stresses and strains of everyday life that seem unbearably frightening, then *not* to intervene with radical treatment approaches may be the best choice. A thorough examination, reassurance, and encouragement to ventilate concerns often represents the treatment of choice.

After taking a careful history and performing an appropriate physical and mental status examination, the treatment plan can be based on the dictum, "first do no harm" and may range from refusal to prescribe an unwarranted treatment or diagnostic procedure to taking steps to prevent the patient from harming himself or others. These general principles will be supplemented by examples of management techniques for specific personality disorders.

Antisocial Personality

By the strictest diagnostic criteria, an individual with an antisocial personality disorder must have been engaged in antisocial behavior for 5 consecutive years. These individuals break the law and violate the rights of others. These patients often have some explanation for their behavior—an explanation that occasionally involves a physical symptom or disease. Childhood history often includes episodes of fighting, truancy, and delinquency. The adult work history involves frequent job changes, dismissals, and conflicts with co-workers or supervisors that may reach violent proportions. They exhibit a general tendency not to pursue a long-term career over a period of years. These patients tend to have unsuccessful family and marital relations as well. To make the diagnosis of antisocial behavior, the patient's maladaptive behavior must not be due to mental retardation, functional psychosis, or organic brain syndrome. The following case represents a typical presentation of antisocial personality:

> ☐ A 25-year-old white man presented to the emergency room complaining of a headache. Description of the pain was vague. At one point he said the pain had been present for several days; at another point he said it had been with him for years. The patient reported that the pain often caused him to become explosively violent. The patient volunteered a graphic description of an incident in which he brutally assaulted a nurse when he was in the army. The patient reported a history of serving several jail terms for assault, drug trafficking, and burglary. Mental status, neurological, and physical examinations were generally negative with the exception of some mild appearance of agitation. The patient insisted that only narcotics would relieve his headache pain. The patient resisted the idea of further diagnostic tests and of making an appointment at a later date for a more extensive workup of his problem. The patient stated that he must have treatment immediately or "I don't know what will happen!"

Management

Rather than prescribing narcotics to a demanding patient, an option that would contribute to the patient's self-destructive behavior while increasing the likelihood that the patient will repeat the request for further prescriptions, the physician would do best to offer an alternative solution that would offer more lasting benefits. If the physician feels threatened by the patient's demands it may be necessary to summon help from either the police or a security officer in the hospital and have them stand by while negotiations are made with the patient. Force will rarely be required. Once limits are set on acting-out and impulsive behavior, the physician may be able to provide more helpful advice and avoid perpetuating the pattern. In the example given above, the physician may advise the patient that narcotics cause tolerance when used on a long-term basis and are not a solution to the problem that he has. In addition, the physician may suggest to the patient that a drug problem might best be addressed with a more complete work-up and long-term treatment in a drug rehabilitation facility. A more detailed psychiatric evaluation may be done at later date, which could include an evaluation of concurrent conditions, social setting, and current and past family situations.

Histrionic Personality

Histrionic patients are overly dramatic and theatrical. They are vain, self-centered, and demanding. They tend to present themselves to physicians as if they have been overwhelmed by circumstance and accompanying feelings. The physician often feels great pressure to rescue the patient from the situation, but often has difficulty defining the problem in medical terms and coming to a rational form of treatment.

The following case represents a medical presentation of a patient with histrionic personality:

☐ A 24-year-old white woman was seen in the emergency room with a chief complaint of headache. When asked for details about the duration and nature of the problem, the patient stated, "I don't know," and began to cry. After calming down, the patient stated that she had had a great deal of difficulty with her boyfriend. The patient reported that over her mother's objections, she had run away to the coast with her boyfriend, who soon abandoned her. The patient then returned to live with her mother and had been experiencing headaches ever since that time. Further inquiry revealed that the patient recently took an overdose of antidepressant medication in an attempt to kill herself after becoming upset about her mother's demands that she get a job. The patient refused to give any more history and demanded that the doctor "do something" about her headache immediately. When a further workup was suggested, the patient fainted and fell to the floor. On examination the patient was unresponsive to voice but reacted to pain. When the patient's hand was held above her face and released, the hand fell to her side rather than striking her face.

Management

It is important for the physician to understand the distressing affects presented by the patient and to evaluate the reality of the situation. The patient cited above may cause the physician to believe that he should admit her for an extensive workup of headaches and fainting. While this approach might be indicated (depending on other physical findings), it may be more effective to talk calmly and briefly with the patient about her life situation. This reassuring talk may set the stage for a period of observation designed primarily to demonstrate to the patient that someone who is expert in these matters is not as frightened by her situation as she is. Often the demonstration that nothing dramatic needs to be done in response to the patient's feelings has a calming effect. Occasionally, the patient's distress will be so great that if some immediate rescue is not attempted, the patient may become very angry, leading to destructive action toward herself and others. If that becomes the case, either psychiatric or police consultation may be necessary in order to limit the extent of the reactive destructiveness.

When the patient has calmed down, it may be helpful for her to ventilate her fears and concerns. The physician's attitude should be one of calm concern. It may be helpful if the patient feels that the physician appreciates her courage and supports her sense of self-esteem in the face of what seems like overpowering circumstances. After 20 or 30 minutes of ventilation, it may be suggested to the patient that further discussion of her problem may be more helpful than anything else that can be offered. Histrionic patients will often become amenable to psychiatric referral at this point.

Paranoid Personality Disorder

Patients with a paranoid personality disorder often appear distant and suspicious. It is important to rule out schizophrenia, paranoid disorder, psychotic depression, organic brain syndrome, and other disorders that may present in a similar way. Patients with paranoid personality do not have a formal thought disorder or concrete paranoid delusional system, but tend to expect other people to be tricky or harmful toward them. As in all personality disorders, this suspicious attitude becomes a lifelong pattern. The patient has inadequate and maladaptive patterns of behavior but ascribes each instance of failure to the actions or conspiracies of other persons. These patients tend to appear somewhat hypervigilant and anxious and may find it difficult to relax.

As with many personality disorders, patients with paranoid personality disorder may be difficult to recognize. The patient may initially appear to be the victim of a series of unfortunate circumstances. The diagnostic tip-off, however, is the way the patient tenaciously clings to an idea despite evidence to the contrary, as exemplified in the following case:

☐ A 36-year-old black man was seen in the emergency room with a chief complaint of "I have syphilis." The patient stated that he had been preoccupied with the concern that syphilis was harming his nervous system after a recent medical workup revealed that he had a weakly positive VDRL, although follow-up FTA turned out to be negative. Despite assurances from the patient's physician that he did not have syphilis, the patient continued to be very fearful and felt the doctor was not telling the truth. When asked if the patient thought that the doctor might mean to harm him, the patient answered, "I don't know, there was just something about that doctor."

The patient's relatives related that the patient had had several arrests for fighting. He was described as restless and hypervigilant. He tended to blame others for his problems and felt as if people were against him. For example, the relative said that if another driver was slow to respond to a change in a traffic light, the patient would assume that the driver was intentionally trying to frustrate him from getting to his destination. The patient might subsequently become argumentative and even physically assaultive. His three marriages had ended in divorce, and in each case, he ascribed the failure of the marriage to his wife's infidelity. The patient blamed his failure at numerous jobs on the treacherousness of supervisors or conspiracies among his co-workers. Although the patient had left high school in the tenth grade believing that the teachers and principal of the school had developed an unjustifiably negative attitude toward him and made it impossible for him to succeed on assignments and examinations, he had no history of drug or alcohol abuse, psychiatric treatment, hospitalization, or behavioral episodes previously recognized as a psychiatric disturbance.

On mental status examination, the patient was alert and oriented but somewhat suspicious, withdrawn, and anxious. The mood was slightly low without vegetative signs. There was no evidence of formal thought disorder, and no hallucinations or fixed delusions.

Management

Paranoid patients require a warm, nonchalant, and not oversolicitious approach. Because these patients may be frightened of a physician, they should not be rushed, challenged or threatened. Any solicitousness on the part of the physician will be viewed with suspicion. When the patient expresses paranoid ideas, he should be reassured that there appears to be no serious cause for alarm, while being allowed to ventilate his anger, frustration, and fears. If the patient requests medication for his anxiety, low doses of the sedating antipsychotics (*e.g.*, thioridazine 25 mg by mouth q6h, prn) may be helpful for short periods of time. The patient responds best to a longstanding relationship with a nonchallenging but attentive physician.

Schizotypal Personality

Patients with schizotypal personality disorder often display the affective blunting, the autistic appearance, and generally "odd" interpersonal behavior characteristic of patients with schizophrenia. They often exhibit magical thinking, ideas of reference, and paranoid beliefs. These patients appear schizophrenic without meeting formal criteria for schizophrenia (*e.g.*, 6 months' duration of symptoms, deterioration from previous level of care, and so forth).

☐ A 28-year-old black man was seen at the insistence of his mother, who complained that he was afraid to leave the house. The patient reported that there was nothing wrong with him, but that a friend had cast a spell on him. The patient was unable to be more specific about his concern. According to his mother, the patient had always been fearful and excitable: He tended to believe in magic and voodoo, and was always interested in the idea that people can cast spells on other people. He had always been socially isolated, had few friends, and was considered "odd" by his peers. The patient had no previous history of depressive episodes, organic brain syndrome, or other psychiatric disturbance or treatment.

On mental status examination, the patient had a constricted affect and appeared frightened, with a far-away look in his eyes. The patient had no formal delusions other than the belief of having a "spell" cast on him. The patient reported no hallucinations; his speech was vague and digressive, but he was oriented with an intact memory.

Management

The management of these patients is essentially the same as with most forms of schizophrenia. When the patient's behavior becomes extremely bizarre, hospitalization may be required. Generally, support and reassurance combined with low doses of nonsedating antipsychotics (*e.g.*, haloperidol, fluphenazine) are effective in managing symptoms.

Schizoid Personality Disorder

Patients with schizoid personality are characterized by emotional isolation and lack of intimate interpersonal relationships. They tend to lack warmth and a sense of involvement with other people, and usually have few friends or close relationships. Although some clinicians think this condition may deteriorate into schizophrenia, patients with schizoid personality do not have delusions, hallucinations, thought process disorder, or other symptoms of psychosis.

☐ A 30-year-old white man came to the physician's office for examination because he had an earache. The patient had no psychological complaints. The patient lives in his mother's house; he has no close friends nor social contacts. He was always known as a "loner" in school. The patient tended not to be involved in dress and behavior fads typical of other students. The patient graduated from high school with a "C" grade average and has since been employed as a parking lot attendant at night. The patient does not date, and his hobbies consist of watching television and going to the movies.

The mental status reveals an individual with constricted, if not flat, affect. The patient failed to develop rapport easily with the interviewer. He had no sense of humor and failed to respond to attempts by the interviewer to make contact through humor. The patient was oriented in all spheres without evidence of psychosis. Mood was normal and intelligence seemed to be average.

Management

These patients rarely seek psychiatric or medical attention and management is rarely a problem. While they can be taught some social skills, motivation is low and the propensity for isolation and lack of interpersonal involvement tends to be intractable.

Compulsive Personality Disorder

Compulsive personality disorder is quite common. These patients tend to be vocationally successful but less successful in the recreational and interpersonal areas of their lives. They often appear anxious and concerned with time, cleanliness, and often with money. They tend to view life as if it contained not enough time or money and too much dirt. Their preoccupation with triviality often causes them to be inefficient workers. These patients often called "Type A personalities" in the behavioral literature. They are thought to be more prone to cardiovascular disorders than other personality types. They often develop superimposed depression during times of stress.

☐ A 32-year-old white man was admitted to the hospital with a myocardial infarction; he had no previous psychiatric history or psychological complaint. During the patient's period of recovery, he became mildly depressed, with low mood, although lacking neurovegetative features. Subsequent conversations with the patient revealed that he was a heavy equipment salesman considered by his family and friends to be a "workaholic." The patient had been moderately successful in his business, although customers and supervisors had reported that he tended to take longer than necessary doing tasks, even though he always appeared to be very busy. The patient seemed to have no spare time and was practically always working. His only hobby was golf; but he always seemed to return from the golf course angry, frustrated, and with a sense of dissatisfaction with his performance. The patient's wife stated that while she knew that he loved her, he never seemed to express affectionate feelings toward her or other members of the family.

On mental status examination, the patient appeared to be anxious and his mood was low. There were no vegetative signs of depression and the anxiety was easily controlled with low doses of a benzodiazepine. There were no delusions, hallucinations, or other signs of psychotic disturbance. The patient seemed orderly and likeable and seemed particularly ready to accept an explanation of his illness that implied that the illness was a punishment for letting his life get out of control.

Management

Patients with compulsive personality disorder are often concerned with the sensation that things may be getting out of control. When managing them medically, it is important to give concise and accurate descriptions of their condition and appropriate treatment procedures. The patient should be made to feel as if he is a partner in his own treatment. When depression ensues, it should be treated as an affective disorder. Patients with compulsive personality disorder rarely request treatment for the personality disorder itself. When they do, psychological or psychiatric referral is indicated.

Passive–Aggressive Personality Disorder

Passive–aggressive patients often disguise a smoldering hostility with a bubbly and effusive surface. In medical situations, they are often compliant and cooperative on the surface, while sabotaging diagnostic and treatment efforts. These rebellious acts are usually seen by the patient as being "forgetfulness," accidents, or other uncontrollable circumstances. When frustrated or abandoned, these patients can develop depression or rage attacks.

☐ A 36-year-old white woman was undergoing medical workup in a general hospital for vague complaints of abdominal pain. While appearing compliant and cooperative, the patient was often out of her room when diagnostic tests were scheduled, and she failed to comply with her prescribed diabetic diet. The patient's history was poor. She had been released from several jobs due to chronic tardiness and forgetfulness. The patient had two teenage children and had been divorced for ten years. The patient's relatives describe her in glowing terms and find it difficult to understand why she has had so much difficulty with jobs and with her marriage.

The patient's mental status was largely unremarkable. She smiled during most interactions with her doctor and appeared compliant and cooperative. There was no evidence of psychosis, organic brain disease, or depression.

Management

In managing passive–aggressive patients, it is best to be supportive rather than confrontational. For example, the patient may be informed that although the tests that she has missed due to her "forgetfulness" can be rescheduled, there may be a limit to how long the insurance company will pay for her hospital stay. The same is true of office appointments that these patients tend to forget, or arrive late for. It is best for the physician not to go out of his way or inconvenience other patients to accommodate the patient with passive–aggressive personality disorder. Rather, the patient's appointment should be rescheduled at another date and the patient should be sympathetically afforded another opportunity to make her appointment. The condition is fairly intractable to treatment per se, but may be well managed if it is recognized. When these patients develop depression, they may be treated with standard antidepressants.

Avoidant Personality Disorder

Patients with avoidant personality disorder are very sensitive to rejection and criticism and tend to have a chronically low and vulnerable self-esteem. They tend to be socially isolated, displaying a long-term propensity for noninvolvement with others that makes career and recreational pursuits difficult and marriage next to impossible.

□ A 30-year-old white woman was brought to the physician's office for routine examination by her mother. The patient herself had no complaints but the mother was concerned that the patient "just stays around the house" and was neither married nor employed. The patient was described as being shy and having had only one date in school. The patient had no close friends. Her feelings were easily hurt and she cried easily when criticized by her mother. She rejected all attempts by men to date her, according to her mother, because she had felt rejected when the boy with whom she had the date in school did not call back.

On examination the patient was noted to be poorly kempt and slightly obese. The patient had poor eye contact, staring at the floor when answering questions. The patient's answers were brief and unelaborative. The affect was constricted, the mood unremarkable. She showed no evidence of psychosis, and her intelligence appeared to be normal. The patient appeared very shy and self-conscious.

Management

Patients with avoidant personality disorder require a gentle and supportive approach. During examinations the patient may benefit from being repeatedly assured that he or she is "doing fine." Medical procedures and findings should be explained fully to the patient, with consideration for how findings will impact on the patient's self-image. These patients tend to be hungry for affection and often may benefit from developing a relationship outside the family. In the context of a relationship with a minister, counselor, or physician, these patients can occasionally be encouraged to develop some social skills and contacts.

Dependent Personality Disorder

The call of the patient with dependent personality disorder is "You're the doctor!" Whenever an attempt is made to enlist the patient as a partner in defining the problem or in taking responsibility for its management, these patients see themselves as helpless and without influence over their own lives. They see their lives as being in the hands of powerful and omnipotent people such as physicians, spouses, and parents. During periods of stress, these patients may also develop anxiety and depression, and they may resort to suicidal gestures and drug abuse if they feel abandoned.

☐ A 45-year-old white man presented to the emergency room complaining of "nerves." The patient stated that because his wife of 25 years had been recently admitted to the hospital for the first time, he felt anxious and depressed, and had experienced episodes of panic. The patient demanded that the physician provide "help."

The patient had no previous history of psychiatric disturbance. He had held a number of jobs, but tended to either leave the jobs or be discharged due to the development of physical symptoms. The patient had no recreational pursuits and watched television most of his free time.

On examination the patient was healthy. The patient presented in a whining, demanding manner that caused the physician to feel burdened and somewhat overpowered by the demands. The physician felt compelled to admit and to take care of the patient, even though the symptoms did not justify such actions. The patient was mildly anxious and had a lowered mood but had no biological signs of depression. There was no evidence of psychosis.

Management

In the example given, the patient was given reassurance and a follow-up appointment. Dependent personality disorder patients do best when they have regularly established appointment times. They generally need support and reassurance that they will be taken care of. During periods of abandonment by caretaking figures they may require hospitalization for mixed symptoms of anxiety or depression, or to prevent self-destructive or antisocial acts.

Borderline Personality Disorder

Borderline personality disorder is a large and heterogenous diagnostic category. The key to identifying patients with borderline personality is "action." These patients tend to respond to stress with some sort of destructive action that is often designed to elicit a response from others. They tend to be impulsive and are often involved in self-destructive acts such as gambling, antisocial activity, or perverse behavior involving food or sex. They tend to have extremely unstable histories of work, recreation, and interpersonal relationships. A variety of unstable affects are often displayed. Intense and inappropriate anger toward even casual acquaintances is common. They often experience difficulty with their sense of self and identity. These patients are often quite manipulative, as well: in addition to externalizing affects and sense of responsibility onto people around them, they often induce impulsive action in others. For example, the patient with borderline personality often leaves a trail of doctors quarreling over issues associated with the patient.

☐ A 28-year-old white woman presented to the emergency room after having cut her wrists. This was the sixth such cutting, which the patient attributed to her "nerves." The patient stated that after a recent breakup with a boyfriend, she became so depressed and nervous that she cut her wrists. The patient was employed at a local fast-food restaurant. She had no children. Each of the patient's previous hospitalizations had been preceded by an abandonment by her boyfriend, followed by feelings of depression, followed by cutting herself in what she described as a "suicide attempt." The self-slashing episodes were often preceded by several weeks of binge eating and vomiting. The patient also had a history of intermittent cocaine, marihuana, and alcohol abuse.

Upon examination, the patient was disheveled. She cried and appeared quite agitated. The patient gave brief and unelaborative answers to questions. She tended to present herself in a helpless manner but became extremely angry when confronted with her maladaptive behavior. The patient displayed no overt psychosis, but manifested some identity confusion by stating "I just don't know who I am."

Management

The key to managing patients with borderline personality disorder, like those with antisocial personality, is to control the impulsive action. This may involve hospitalization, suicide precautions, or intervention by police. The next step is for physicians and nurses to resist taking on the patient's tendency toward impulsive action. For example, if an impulsive-action-oriented patient with borderline personality also has depressive features, the physician may start the patient on an antidepressant. Antidepressants characteristically take one to three weeks to show efficacious results. Patients with borderline personality often become impatient and feel that their medication should be changed or that they should be discharged from the hospital before therapeutic results can be obtained. Physicians and nurses must be consistent and supportive. Pharmacologically, when these patients present with depression, they may respond to a course of antidepressants. This is best done as an inpatient, as these patients are prone to suicidal gestures, and antidepressants can be toxic. When depression is not a major part of the clinical syndrome, there is some evidence that low doses of neuroleptics may be helpful (*e.g.*, Stelazine 2–10 mg tid).

Narcissistic Personality Disorder

These patients tend to be self-centered and impatient with others who fail to see their "specialness." They tend to be manipulative and often intoxicate others with their grandiosity for purposes of exploitation. They are often exhibitionistic and preoccupied with looks, power, and money, and these preoccupations have a special quality. For example, the compulsive personality may be preoccupied with money as if he fears he is going to lose it. The narcissistic personality is preoccupied with money as it represents a quality of the self; that is to say, persons with money may be seen by him as being magical and grand, and those without money as empty and worthless.

Narcissistic patients' relationships tend to be characterized by brevity and superficiality. They tend to perceive themselves and others as being either grand, magical, and magnificent; or as having no value at all. These patients often have little conception of or concern about the feelings of others.

There is a tendency to confuse narcissistic and histrionic personalities, particularly in women. Both disorders are characterized by exhibitionism and self-centeredness. The narcissistic personality, however, may lack the self-dramatization, labile affectivity, and helplessness often seen in histrionic personalities.

☐ A 30-year-old white woman was seen in a physician's office complaining of headaches. The patient stated that she often developed the headaches at her job, where she felt a great deal of pressure. The patient had been a hairdresser for six months. She stated that she was very excited about the job initially because she had done so well in hairdressing school that she knew she would be an asset to her place of employment. The patient even felt that she was the best hair stylist in the shop and that the business would certainly fail if it were not for her efforts.

The patient left college after her sophomore year because it was "boring." She has had a variety of jobs over the last ten years, few of which lasted for more than one year. The patient left each job either because she found it boring, or because she felt that her employer and co-workers did not appreciate the high quality of her work. Although she was attractive, the patient rarely dated and she had never been married. The patient stated that few men excite her, and that most of the men who have asked her out are not, in her estimation, good-looking enough for her.

On examination, the patient was noted to be well groomed and heavily made up. She wore a low-cut blouse and acted flirtatious. The patient was angry that she had had to wait to see the doctor. Although the patient became flirtatious as her anger passed, there was very little sense of warmth. The mood was unremarkable, and the affect was generally appropriate to content. There was no evidence of psychotic thinking. The patient stated that a number of doctors had unsuccessfully attempted to treat her headaches, but she felt encouraged by the present physician's excellent reputation. The physician initially felt flattered and potent, if not omnipotent, and tended to feel he must do whatever necessary in order to maintain the grandiose sense of importance that the patient had bestowed upon him.

Management

These patients do best when treated with support and respect for their fragile sense of self-esteem. On the other hand, it is wise not to become involved in the projected sense of grandiosity. In the case cited, for example, tests ordered and treatments offered should only be those dictated by the history and physical findings. The patient may occasionally need to be reminded that in spite of the physician's reputation, there is a limit to how helpful his intervention may be. This does not mean that such intervention is worthless, and the patient may occasionally have to be reminded of this, also.

Mixed Personality Disorder

Individual types of personality disorders are named by their characteristics; that is to say, they are named by the groups of personality traits that interfere with the accomplishment of life goals. These traits are so varied that more than one personality disorder may be present in the same patient. Personality disturbances with features of several types may be termed *atypical* or *mixed* personality disorders. What is important is to recognize the presence of a personality disorder; it is an added bonus, from the standpoint of optimal management, to recognize the specific type.

Conclusion

A personality trait becomes a personality disorder when it interferes with the patient's ability to achieve long-term goals in life such as a career, meaningful relationships, and recreational pursuits. Patients with personality disorders are common and the index of suspicion should be high. Recognizing the presence of personality disorder enables the physician to devise a management strategy.

Bibliography

American Psychiatric Association: Diagnostic and Statistical Manual of Mental Disorders, 3rd ed. American Psychiatric Association, 1980

Chodoff P, Lyons H: Hysteria, the hysterical personality, and "hysterical" conversion. Am J Psychiatry 114:734–740, 1958

Vaillant G: Sociopathy of the human process. Arch Gen Psychiatry 32:178–183, 1975

Cavenar J, Walker J: Obsessive compulsive personality and neurosis. In Cavenar J, Brodie H (eds): Signs and Symptoms in Psychiatry. Philadelphia, JB Lippincott Company, 1983

Kernberg O: Borderline Conditions and Pathological Narcissism. New York, Jason Aronson, 1975

Brinkley J, Beitman B, Friedel R: Low dose neuroleptic regimens in the treatment of borderline patients. Arch Gen Psychiatry 36:319–326, 1979

Kohut H: The psychoanalytic treatment of narcissistic personality disorders. Psychoanal Study Child 23:86–113, 1968

Goldberg A: Psychotherapy of narcissistic injuries. Arch Gen Psychiatry 28:722–726, 1973

Mark D. Miller

12 Drug Abuse

In the past two decades, this nation has seen an epidemic increase in the abuse of mind-altering drugs. Drug abuse and its social ramifications are no longer limited to any one sector of society, but are now seen in all populations. The increase, over the past decade, in the number of emergency patients seen for drug addiction may well be a major factor in the disproportionate use of psychiatric emergency services over general medical and surgical emergency services.[1]

In the emergency room, the psychiatrist must be skilled in recognizing the physical signs and symptoms of intoxication by a particular agent, as well as be knowledgeable of the differential diagnosis of the particular alteration in mental status. Two or more drugs may be taken in combination, sometimes without the user's knowledge. Due to the illicit procurement of most drugs of abuse, there is an inherent unreliability as to whether or not the drug a patient says he bought and used is actually that drug, or a cheaper "cut" mixture. To further complicate the diagnostic process, there is a high percentage of drug abuse seen in patients with other psychiatric disorders, where the effects of the drug may compound or confuse the signs and symptoms of the underlying illness. It is therefore implicit that the psychiatrist have a detailed knowledge of even the more subtle physiologic and psychological effects of the drugs of abuse. A familiarity with the common drugs of abuse in the area and their street names, access to a friend or family member who might know the drug habits of the patient, and old records are of particular value in diagnosis. Most emergency rooms have 24-hour availability of blood and urine toxic screening tests as part of their laboratory services. Particular attention should be paid to the "review of systems" in the interview because individuals addicted to drugs are prone to potentially serious medical conditions such as hepatitis, autoimmune deficiency syndrome (AIDS), tuberculosis, and bacterial endocarditis. In instances where such illnesses are suspected, a thorough physical examination and consultation, if necessary, are essential.

Once the correct diagnosis has been made, and the acute toxic state treated, the larger problem of treating the patient's addiction remains. Drug addiction is perhaps the one disorder that most clearly indicates the need for a biopsychosocial model for psychiatric treatment. The physiologic addiction seen in many drugs of abuse, particularly opiates and barbiturates, often requires specific strategies for managing the withdrawal process. An understanding of the psychodynamics of addiction and an ability to communicate in a theoretical framework comprehensible to the patient are necessary tools for psychotherapeutic treatment of the addicted patient. The psychiatrist must use his knowledge of the patient's family and social history, his available social supports, and the community's resources in tailoring a disposition. The limitation inherent in the medical treatment of complex medical–social problems is the lack of stress on the need for social rehabilitation. Programs such as methadone maintenance treatment make possible a first step toward social rehabilitation by stabilizing the pharmacologic conditions of addicts who have been living as criminals on the fringe of society. However, present-day programs often fall short of enabling their patients to feel pride and hope, and to accept social responsibility. The mutual cynicism that ensues often makes such overcrowded facilities seem more like public nuisances than effective treatment centers.[2]

In order to assist the reader in understanding the complexities of diagnosis and management in drug abuse treatment, each drug will first be described as to its nature, pharmacologic properties, and prevalence of abuse. The specific physiologic and psychological toxic effects will then be outlined, as well as the differential diagnosis of these effects. The treatment of acute toxic delirium will then be described, followed, if applicable, by a description of the withdrawal effects of the drug, and the long-term treatment of the addiction.

Sedative–Hypnotics

Among sedative–hypnotics, a widely abused class of non-narcotic drugs, the most common are barbiturates, methaqualone, meprobamate, and benzodiazepines. The barbiturates will be considered separately from the nonbarbiturate sedative hypnotics.

Barbiturates

Since the first therapeutic use of phenobarbital in 1912, over 2500 barbiturates have been synthesized, approximately 50 have been marketed for clinical use, and a dozen or so are still widely used today. Most therapeutic needs would be met by five or six of these.[3] Because of the wide availability of legally manufactured barbiturates, little is manufactured by "black-market" laboratories. The majority of illegal barbiturates are obtained by diverting shipments from manufacturers to foreign addresses and then smuggling them back to this country. Others obtain the drugs by theft. Importantly, a significant number of patients who present with barbiturate intoxication or withdrawal are legitimately prescribed the drug, often for sleep or anxiety problems. This patient may be well off and have little difficulty obtaining refills or prescriptions from several physicians. Often, this pattern of abuse goes undetected until the patient develops withdrawal during a period when he cannot obtain the drug.[4]

Of the barbiturates currently marketed, it is most often the short-acting agents, such as amobarbital, pentobarbital, and secobarbital, that are abused.

Another large percentage of barbiturate abusers are teenagers or young adults who use the drugs to experience euphoria, an effect that often differs from sedation only in the social context of the drug's use. On occasion the same population will use the barbiturates to counter the agitation from an excessive dose of amphetamines on the mistaken assumption that the barbiturate can "take them down."[4]

Other barbiturate abusers use the drug by intravenous injection. This kind of patient is invariably an experienced drug abuser, often concomitantly addicted to opiates, but using barbiturates as a less expensive substitute.[4]

Amobarbital is available as Amytal (Lilly) and combined with secobarbital as Tuinal (Lilly). Tuinal is known illegally as "tooies," "double trouble," or "rainbows." Secobarbital is marketed as Seconal (Lilly) and known on the street as "reds," "downers," or "red devils." Pentobarbital is manufactured as Nembutal (Abbott) and carries the street names "yellows," "yellow jackets," and "nembies." The purity of the street preparations is often highly questionable.

Like alcohol intoxication, the first symptom of barbiturate intoxication is disinhibition, often of sexual and aggressive impulses. The initial euphoria can often change to irritability and combativeness as the patient's mood becomes labile. The dreamlike state can be accompanied by excessive speech and feelings of depersonalization and derealization.

Signs of barbiturate intoxication include ataxia, nystagmus, hyporeflexia, slurred speech, incoordination, dysmetria, dysattention, global memory impairment, poor judgment, and impairment in goal-directed behavior.[1]

The differential diagnosis includes alcohol intoxication, other sedative hypnotic intoxication, or opiate intoxication. Serum toxicology screen tests are extremely helpful and often essential to the diagnosis. Differentiation from opiate intoxication can be made by administration of naloxone, because opiate antagonists will not affect toxic effects that are due to other classes of drugs.[1]

When the diagnosis of barbiturate intoxication has been confirmed, the amount of barbiturate taken daily and the degree of tolerance to the drug must be ascertained. Rapid withdrawal from barbiturates is potentially lethal; the most severe complications are grand mal seizures, delirium, and cardiorespiratory failure. The method of withdrawal is similar to that used in treatment of barbiturate addiction, and the signs and symptoms of acute barbiturate withdrawal in the addicted patient will therefore be described first.

Most striking of the symptoms of even mild withdrawal is marked anxiety and irritability. Mood will be altered ranging from general malaise to depression, and thought disturbance can range from impaired goal-directed thinking and judgment to a full-blown psychosis with visual and tactile hallucinations (formication), confusion, and paranoia. Physical signs of withdrawal include psychomotor agitation tremulousness; blepharospasm; hyperreflexia; muscle weakness; tachycardia; diaphoresis; hypertension; coarse tremor of the tongue, hands, and eyelids; postural hypotension; and in severe cases, convulsions, status epilepticus, and death. Delirium is usually seen approximately 1 week after the drug is stopped and may be clinically indistinguishable from the delirium seen in alcohol withdrawal (Table 12-1).[1]

In treatment of barbiturate intoxication and withdrawal, conservative management is crucial, given the potential lethality of rapid withdrawal. In order to determine the minimal dose of barbiturates needed to cover a patient for withdrawal, a barbiturate tolerance test can be performed on an inpatient basis. The morning after admission an oral test dose of 200 mg of pentobarbital is administered, and the patient is examined for signs of clinical toxicity. If the patient is not tolerant, he will usually be somnolent but arousable. If he is tolerant, but to a dose of less than 500 mg daily, gross neurologic impairment is seen, with ataxia, nystagmus, ptosis hyporeflexia, and a Romberg sign. Tolerance to doses of 500 mg to 600 mg daily produces mild ataxia and nystagmus, and dysarthria. A patient tolerant to 700 mg to 800 mg demonstrates only nystagmus, and tolerance to 900 mg or greater produces no signs of clinical toxicity 1 hour after the test dose. In this last instance, the test is repeated with 200-mg and later 300-mg test doses of pentobarbital. The test must be performed only when a patient is free of signs of intoxication or withdrawal in order to be valid.[1]

In 1971, Smith and Wesson described a clinical technique for withdrawal of patients who are dependent on barbiturates.[5] Phenobarbital is substituted for the addicting agent and the patient is subsequently withdrawn from phenobarbital. The long-acting agent provides a more constant barbiturate blood level than the usual addicting agents, and progressively smaller amounts in the daily dosage are more easily tolerated by the patient. In addition, phenobarbital has a wider margin between the dose in which toxic signs are seen and the serious overdose. Approximately 30 mg of phenobarbital are substituted for every 100 mg of the shorter-acting barbiturates. Once withdrawal is complete, supportive psychotherapy, family, and community resources must be used.[5]

Table 12-1
Seconal or Pentobarbital Withdrawal Syndrome

Dose	Withdrawal Symptoms
200 mg	No physical dependence
400 mg for 90 days or more	Insomnia, tension
600 mg for 6 weeks or more	Nausea, anorexia, vomiting, postural hypotension, autonomic hyperactivity
800 mg for 6 weeks or more	Seizures, delirium

Walker JI: Psychiatric Emergencies: Intervention and Resolution, p. 49. Philadelphia, JB Lippincott, 1983

Methaqualone

The only marketed hypnotic of its class (2,3 disubstituted quinazolinones), methaqualone is now abused more widely than it is clinically prescribed for its sedative hypnotic properties. The drug is marketed as Quaalude by Lemmon, Sopor by Arnar Stone, and Mandrax (with diphenhydramine) in Great Britain.[3] The street names of methaqualone are accordingly "ludes," "soaps" or "soapers," and "mandrakes." The drug is popular among young people, who obtain the drug from prescriptions or illegal sources. It is a popular party drug, often taken in groups.[4]

Symptoms of intoxication include euphoria, increased pain threshold, feelings of indestructability, depersonalization, and derealization. Undesirable effects include dryness of the mouth, dizziness, headache, chills, "hangover," and occasionally anxiety and panic. Physical signs include paresthesia of the fingers, lips, and tongue; diarrhea; epistaxis, and occasionally bruising from falls.[4] Although originally touted clinically for its lack of rapid eye movement (REM) suppression, it has been recently determined that like the barbiturates, dream sleep is suppressed with REM rebound on withdrawal.[4]

Methaqualone is both psychologically and physically addictive. There is a cross tolerance to the barbiturates, and a withdrawal syndrome is seen in patients whose daily doses range from 600 mg to 3000 mg. The withdrawal syndrome consists of anxiety, irritability, anorexia, headache, abdominal cramping, and, rarely, nightmares and hallucinations. The syndrome occurs within 24 hours after the drug is stopped, and the basis for treatment is administration of methaqualone with gradual taper.[4]

Methaqualone overdose can lead to delirium, convulsions, and death. It differs from a barbiturate overdose in that cardiorespiratory suppression is not seen. Most of the fatalities seen have involved the combined use of methaqualone and alcohol.

Meprobamate

Marketed today by Wyeth as Equanil, meprobamate is an anti-anxiety agent that, despite its well-documented physical and psychological dependence, continues to be prescribed extensively. Although not a common drug of intentional abuse for any euphoric effect, excessive use for chronic anxiety often leads to physical dependence.[4]

Toxic effects from overdose include central nervous system (CNS) suppression with somnolence, ataxia, hypotension, and cardiorespiratory collapse.

Rapid withdrawal in the dependent patient leads to headache, insomnia, tremor, gastrointestinal disturbance, and, rarely, convulsions. A syndrome similar to delirium tremens has been described that includes hallucinations, agitation, tremors, and convulsions.[4] Although phenytoin is used to control the seizure activity, the full withdrawal treatment consists of reinstitution of meprobamate or a short-acting barbiturate (to which patients are cross tolerant). A gradual taper of either drug is then instituted, usually in an inpatient setting.

Benzodiazepines

Prescribed as hypnotic or antianxiety agents, this large class of drugs is perhaps the most frequently prescribed class of psychoactive agents. Like meprobamate, their abuse is frequently "unintentional"; these drugs are most often obtained through legitimate prescription. Intended for brief symptomatic control of anxiety during periods of inordinate stress, physicians frequently prescribe the "minor tranquilizers" to patients whose character structure makes them poorly tolerant of even usual levels of daily stress. Although far less euphoria is produced with these drugs than with other agents, the dynamics of the setting in which they are prescribed can lead to a psychological dependence. There appears to be a physiologic dependence with an associated withdrawal syndrome. Withdrawal symptoms can include insomnia, anorexia, agitation, diaphoresis, and occasionally muscle twitching and convulsions. The onset of withdrawal symptoms is variable due to the wide range of half-lives of this class of drugs. Treatment is standard, with a reinstitution of the particular drug and gradual withdrawal. This can often be done on an outpatient basis because this class of drugs has a large margin of safety.[4]

The abuse potential of benzodiazepines lies largely in their availability. Often misrepresented by physicians, patients come to rely on the drugs for relief of even minor stresses of daily living. These patients rapidly develop tolerance which can turn into abuse.

Central Nervous System Stimulant Abuse

CNS stimulants include cocaine, amphetamine, dextroamphetamine, and, to a lesser extent, other sympathomimetic amines, such as phenylpropanolamine, methylphenidate, phentermine, and diethylproprion. In general, they act on both peripheral and central α- and β-receptors for catecholamines. Although the mechanisms are unclear, their stimulant effect appears to depend on local norepinephrine release in the brain. Activation of the reticular arousal system by locally applied amphetamine mimics the effect of norepinephrine. Other CNS effects of the stimulants may involve direct action on catecholamine receptors, but little about this is known at present.

CNS stimulant abuse occurs in individuals seeking a wide range of effects. These include euphoria, decreased hunger, relief from fatigue, feelings of confidence and power, and increased performance. With most of the drugs in this class, tolerance is rapid, yet the narrow margin for the desired effect is narrow. The previous pleasurable effects give rise to intense anxiety, paranoia, or overt psychosis. Often there is repetitive motor behavior and agitation, and occasionally physical violence can ensue.[6] The section on CNS stimulants will be separated into a general discussion of amphetamine and dextroamphetamine. A separate discussion on cocaine will follow because of its increased prevalence of abuse.

Amphetamines

Amphetamine sulfate (Benzedrine) is a white soluble powder, available in 5-mg and 10-mg tablets and 15-mg slow-release capsules. The d-isomer dextroamphetamine is available in phosphate and sulfate (Dexedrine) forms. Methamphetamine is closely related to amphetamine but differs in its ratio between central and peripheral actions. Smaller doses have more prominent central effects without peripheral actions. Methamphetamine hydrochloride (Desoxyn) is available in 2.5-mg or 5-

mg tablets, and in sustained-release tablets containing 5 mg, 10 mg, or 15 mg. An injectable 20 mg/ml solution is available. Combinations exist commercially. There are many street varieties of this class of drug, including "bennies," "black beauties," "crystal," "dexies," "pep pills," "uppers," and "poppers." "Speed," while usually referring to injectable metamphetamine, can also be applied as a general classification.[3]

The drastic reduction in commercial manufacture of these drugs over the past decade has led to a similar reduction in street availability; however, there has been some increase in illegal "basement laboratory" productions. Amphetamine abuse patterns have provided an interesting test case on the effect of drug legislation. The severe restriction of legal medical use through legislation led to a decline in pharmaceutical manufacture of amphetamines. This was followed by an increase in police action against illicit production and traffic of the drug and an overall massive decline in street availability.[6]

The prevalence of amphetamine abuse is higher in populations in which alertness and performance are highly valued, such as students, athletes, and truck drivers. The availability of these drugs in medical settings is also a cause for a high rate of abuse in physicians, nurses, and medical personnel.[6]

Amphetamines are abused most commonly by an oral route, but intravenous injection is often the preferred method for the chronic, high-dose abuser. Occasional users may use a therapeutic dosage (up to 60 mg/d), but dependent heavy users may use dosages in the 250-mg to 300-mg daily range. Rarely, 1000-mg to 1500-mg daily doses are recorded.[6]

In short-term use, subjective CNS effects include restlessness, overstimulation, dizziness, euphoria, mild confusion, dysphoria, panic, reduction of appetite, hyperalertness, reduction of fatigue, and tremor. Peripheral effects are palpitations, tachycardia, arrhythmia, hyperventilation, diarrhea, increased urine output, and either an increase or decrease in libido.[6]

In higher doses, short-term use can lead to intense exhilaration and euphoria, feelings of increased physical strength, agitation, depression, paranoia, or hallucinations. A "rush" similar to the sensation of physical orgasm can occur. In severe overdoses, anginal pain, cardiovascular collapse, high fever, convulsions, cerebral hemorrhage, and death may occur.[6]

Particular patterns of psychosis can occur in sympathomimetic intoxication. A thought disorder with ideas of reference, paranoid ideation (with clear sensorium), and grandiosity can occur. Auditory hallucinations with voices making critical, derogatory remarks can occur as can visual hallucinations with distortions in body image of self and others. The similarity between this psychosis and that of acute paranoid schizophrenia is striking. Qualitative differences are the severity of the thought disorder and the clinical course. An amphetamine-induced delirium can be precipitated by fluctuating levels of consciousness, dysattention, fragmented thinking, and tactile hallucinations.[1]

The differential diagnosis of the toxic state would therefore include cocaine or other sympathomimetic intoxication, paranoid schizophrenia, hypomania, acute excited schizophrenia (catatonia), alcoholic delirium, or acute manic psychosis (Table 12-2).[1]

Table 12-2
Differential Diagnosis Between Paranoid Schizophrenia and Amphetamine Psychosis

Amphetamine Psychosis	Paranoid Schizophrenia
Mental associations accelerated but grossly logical	Loose associations
High level of abstraction	Concrete thinking
Nonbizarre delusions	Bizarre delusions
Orientation intact	Orientation intact
Illusions and visual hallucinations common	Auditory hallucinations
Amphetamines in urine	No amphetamines in urine
Psychosis usually remits within 1 week	Persistent psychotic episodes lead to gradual personality deterioration

Walker JI: Psychiatric Emergencies: Intervention and Resolution, p 59. Philadelphia, JB Lippincott, 1983

Management of amphetamine intoxication will depend on the time of presentation. The symptoms of acute intoxication, including psychosis, usually subside 48 to 72 hours after the drug is stopped. While the hallucinations of an amphetamine psychosis may clear in 48 hours, delusions may persist for a week to 10 days. A long period of sleep usually occurs within a day of the final dose, lasting for 18 to 72 hours, often with vivid dreaming. A psychological depression, "crashing," may ensue and last for several weeks; it differs from major affective illness in its greater degree of apathy and flattening of affect.[1]

Acute management must take into account the intoxicated patient's potential for violence to others or self. Reduction of stimulation with a quiet room or seclusion may be useful. In the first 24 hours, haloperidol in low doses can be of value. In severe overdoses, life support measures may be required.[1]

Long-term use of amphetamines can produce chronic sleep disturbances, anxiety states, arrhythmia, and hypertension. Nutritional deficiencies can occur from chronic appetite suppression.[6]

Withdrawal from amphetamines is peculiar in its predominance of psychological symptoms over physiologic symptoms. Fatigue and deep, dreaming sleep are typical. Of highest clinical concern is the suicide potential in the often profound depression that ensues.

Clinical management of amphetamine withdrawal would include low-dose neuroleptic management in the toxic phase and immediate discontinuation of the sympathomimetic drug. If depression is present, tricyclic antidepressants are helpful, and in severe cases electroconvulsive therapy (ECT) may be indicated. Brief supportive psychotherapy and group therapy are often helpful in initiating treatment of the underlying factors that led to abuse, especially as part of an ongoing treatment program.[1]

Cocaine

Cocaine is a powerful, short-acting sympathomimetic stimulant prepared from the leaf of the coca plant, which is found in South America. Chemically, cocaine is benzoylmethylecgonine, an ester of benzoic acid and a nitrogen-containing base. Its primary clinical action is its ability to block nerve conduction following local application.[3] The drug is abused, however, for its powerful CNS stimulatory effects.

Cocaine hydrochloride is an odorless, white, crystalline powder with a bitter and numbing taste, which is soluble in water and alcohol.[6] Cocaine is rapidly absorbed despite its local vasoconstricting action. This rate rapidly exceeds that of detoxification, hence the highly toxic nature of the drug. Absorption can occur from all application sites, including mucous membranes. Orally administered cocaine is largely hydrolyzed in the gastrointestinal tract and rendered ineffective, however. Once absorbed, the drug is detoxified by the liver.[3]

Street preparations are often adulterated because of the high market value of the drug. Related substances, such as lidocaine or procaine, are frequently used as adulterants because they "fool" the buyer with a similar numbing effect. An increasingly common method of removing these impurities is to extract them with appropriate solvents. The highly flammable nature of these solvents makes this process of free-basing hazardous, as the recent near-death of a popular comedian has graphically illustrated.

The most popular route of administration is inhalation, but injection by all routes is also common. Doses range from 20 mg to several hundred milligrams or more, depending on the frequency of abuse. Some users attempt "sprees" of several grams over several hours.[6]

Patterns of abuse vary; the pure "cokehead" was once rare because of the high expense of the drug, whose use was limited to the higher socioeconomic groups. An almost epidemic rise of abuse in people of this income level has occurred over the past several years. The publicity surrounding this phenomenon no doubt adds to the mystique of the drug and its attractiveness to younger, potential abusers. More commonly, the drug is abused, when available, by polydrug abusers. The classic "speedball" is a mixture of cocaine and heroin in an intravenous (IV) injection.[6]

Today, cocaine use is distributed among all social classes with estimated prevalence rates of up to 100,000,000, a hundred-fold increase in the past 10 years.[7]

Symptoms of cocaine intoxication include physical signs such as pupillary dilation, perspiration and chills, tachycardia, elevated blood pressure, skin pallor, tremor, and elevated body temperature. Psychological symptoms are most notably euphoria, a feeling of mental agility, loquaciousness, a sense of confidence, and insomnia. A toxic delusional syndrome is commonly seen with loose associations, paranoid ideation, ideas of reference, vivid auditory and visual hallucinations, tactile hallucinations, and, at times, violent or assaultive behavior. In short, the syndrome is similar to that seen in amphetamine intoxication, which is in the primary differential diagnosis. Other diagnoses that need to be ruled out include anxiety states, mania, schizophrenia, paranoid schizophrenia, and delirium tremens.[1]

Management of the acutely intoxicated patient is similar to that for patients in other sympathomimetic intoxication states. The self-limited nature of cocaine intoxication (the usual recovery period is 24 hours) makes reassurance and psychological support the primary treatment. Low doses of antipsychotic agents are usually sufficient to control psychotic behavior. Occasionally a rapid-withdrawal "crash" is seen within an hour after acute symptoms have dissipated. This is characterized by irritability, a need for sleep, and drug-demanding behaviors.[1]

There appears to be no demonstration of a physical withdrawal syndrome in pure cocaine abuse. A powerful physical dependence on the drug does seem to exist, although whether the symptoms seen in drug abstinence are truly reflective of drug dependence, is unclear. As seen with other sympathomimetics, these symptoms consist of drug craving, hypersomnia with increased REM activity, hunger, anxiety, and depressed mood.[6] Long-term intranasal abuse can lead to intranasal sores or actual breakdown of the nasal septum. The social effects of long-term abuse are far more devastating than the physical effects. In a recent study surveying callers to a cocaine help "hotline," 44% of abusers reported loss of friends, 34% lost all their financial resources, 25% their spouses, and 10% their jobs. Twenty percent of abusers reported stealing from their employer, family, or friends to support their habit and 36% were dealing in cocaine.[7]

The most common management of cocaine dependence is psychotherapeutic, focusing on goals of structuring emotional and social support. Where cocaine use is associated with an underlying psychiatric condition, treatment is targeted toward the primary illness, with appropriate drug education.

Opiates and Opioids: The Narcotic Analgesics

Narcotic analgesics include opium, opium alkaloids, and synthetic narcotic analgesics. They are all characterized by the powerful physical dependence they produce and by the transient but extreme abstinence syndrome that develops when the drug is withdrawn. To this extent, the *Diagnostic and Statistical Manual of Mental Disorders,* 3rd ed (DSM-III), has established a subdivision in opioid-related diagnoses. *Opioid abuse* is characterized by two diagnostic criteria: (1) impairment in social or occupational functioning secondary to the drug use (including absenteeism from work, legal difficulties, loss of job, fights, and loss of friends); and (2) a duration of abuse for at least 1 month.[8] *Opioid dependence* is essentially characterized by the presence of drug tolerance or withdrawal: *Tolerance* is the need for markedly increased amounts of opioid to achieve the desired effect, or markedly diminished effect with regular use of the same amount; *withdrawal* is a syndrome that occurs after reduction in prolonged, heavy use occurs.[8] Separate diagnoses exist for opiate intoxication and opiate withdrawal; their features will be described later.

Some narcotic analgesics occur naturally, and others are semisynthetic or wholly synthetic. Opium is produced naturally as an exudate from the unripe pods of *Papaver somniferum,* the poppy flower. This plant is an annual found in widespread areas of Asia and Asia Minor. The opiates morphine and codeine are refined products of opium, and they constitute the only two products of approximately 20 alkaloids of opium that have psychoactive properties. Morphine composes 10% to 15% of the opium exudate and codeine 1% to 2%. The semisynthetic opiates, which include heroin and hydrocodone, are chemically derived from either morphine or codeine. The wholly synthetic agents, distinguished from opiates as *opioids,* mimic opiate effects; they include methadone and meperidine. The potency of these opiate and opioid compounds varies, but they all share the property of being able to relieve pain. Sedation and sleep are produced in higher doses, hence the name *narcotic*. Several narcotic agents are used clinically for other purposes, such as cough suppression or bowel motility. Some are used entirely to manage physical dependence on other narcotics. All of the opiates and opioids share the property of causing physical dependence, which is an unfortunate complication because no other agents are as effective in palliating moderate to severe levels of pain.[6]

The analgesic effect of narcotics may be twofold in nature when one considers that pain is composed of both a physical sensation and the emotional reaction to that sensation. Recently, specific narcotic receptor sites have been located in the ascending pain pathways of the CNS. The mechanism is poorly understood, but narcotic drugs are believed to bind to these sites and interfere with transmission of pain impulses to the higher cortical centers responsible for the perception of pain. Recent research has again discovered high concentrations of narcotic analgesic receptors in the limbic system structures believed to regulate emotional sensations. Endogenously produced analogues of opiates, called *endorphins,* are believed to play a role in CNS regulation of sensations of pain and well-being, and act at these sites. The euphoric effect of narcotics that is desired by abusers may well be governed by these limbic receptors. The narcotic analgesics may therefore relieve the emotional component of pain as well. Curiously, many initial experiences with narcotic analgesics produce dysphoria, anxiety, and depression. Some degree of tolerance appears to be necessary before the euphoric effect of the drugs is appreciated. Separately, the specific narcotic analgesic agents will be briefly discussed.[6]

Opium

Opium is prepared from the thick exudate of the unripe seed pods of the poppy plant. The exudate is collected from scored pods and allowed to dry in the shade, where the crude exudate darkens into a brown, tar-like resin, which is then shaped into bricks.[6]

Opium users often increase the purity of the substance by dissolving it into solution and filtering the extract, often many times. The resulting paste is dried and smoked.

Today, the majority of opium use is restricted to rural areas of Asia and the Middle East. It has a potential for dependence that is similar to that of morphine. The most notable side effect of acute intoxication is nausea.[6]

Although many synthetic analgesics have replaced opium in clinical use, a highly purified form, Pantopon, is prepared for injection. A tincture of opium with camphor, benzoic acid, and anise oil is available as a paregoric, and is contained in several widely used antidiarrhetics, such as Donnagel PG.

Codeine

Codeine is a naturally occurring opiate that produces mild euphoric and analgesic effects. It is effective in controlling moderate to mild pain and is widely used as an antitussive agent. It is an uncommon drug of abuse because of its only mild euphoric effects and its potential for dangerous side effects, such as seizures.[6]

Codeine phosphate is an odorless, white crystalline powder, fully soluble in water and slightly soluble in alcohol. Isolated from crude opium, it is marketed either as paveral syrup or under its generic name. It is also available in combination products compounded with other analgesics, such as aspirin and acetaminophen. Cough preparations may include codeine in combination with diphenhydramine, phenylpropanolamine, and terpin hydrate, as well as other agents.[6]

CNS effects usually consist of lightheadedness, drowsiness, mild euphoria or anxiety, clouding of cognitive functions, and a slight pupillary constriction. Gastrointestinal effects include nausea, vomiting, and constipation. In higher doses, blood pressure is lowered, and tachycardia and arrhythmia can occur. In severe overdoses, tremors, seizures, delirium, coma, respiratory depression, pulmonary edema, and hypotension can occur. Long-term abuse can lead to constipation, decreased libido, restlessness, anxiety states, and affective lability. Gradual tolerance develops with chronic and frequent use. While physical dependence is rare, a withdrawal syndrome is seen in abrupt terminations of high-dose use. The symptoms include yawning, anxiety, diaphoresis, lacrimation, nasal discharge, and insomnia. These symptoms may progress to anorexia, flushing of skin, chills and "gooseflesh," and muscle twitching.[6]

Although infrequent, deaths from overdose of codeine occur with seizures, coma, delirium, cardiac and respiratory arrest as antecedents. Overdoses may be complicated with salicylate and acetominophen toxicity as well.[6]

Morphine

Morphine is the other naturally occurring opiate and is used clinically for control of moderate to severe levels of pain. Next to heroin, it has the second greatest degree of dependency potential. Morphine is available as a water-soluble salt, most commonly as a sulfate or hydrochloride. Both preparations are fine, crystalline, white powders soluble in water and alcohol.[6]

For clinical use in controlling moderate to severe pain, the usual intramuscular dose is 10 mg per 70 kg of body weight every 4 hours. The oral dose is between 8 mg and 20 mg, but is far less effective because of rapid hepatic metabolism. Intravenous injection delivers immediate effect and is used for emergent or severe postoperative pain.[6]

Patterns of abuse vary, intravenous injection being the most common, but morphine is also abused in oral tablet form, subcutaneously ("skin popping"), or intramuscularly. Because of its availability in hospitals, a significant rate of abuse exists among health-care personnel. Street names for the drug include "M," "morph," "Miss Emma," and "Sister M."[6]

Initial effects include euphoria, analgesia, drowsiness, relaxation, cognitive impairment, psychomotor slowing, pupillary constriction, and blurred vision. Peripheral effects are decreased body temperature, sweating, and decreased respirations. Constipation, anorexia, nausea and vomiting, and lowered gastric motility may occur. Parasthesias and decreased libido are other short-term effects. In higher doses, sleep often occurs; if not, higher levels of cognitive impairment are reached. After immediate injection a "rush" is often the most desired effect with almost orgasmic levels of euphoria. In overdoses, morphine produces a progression from deep sleep to coma, pinpoint pupils, hypotension, arrhythmias, respiratory depression, loss of muscle tone, vascular collapse, and occasionally pulmonary edema. The lethal dose is estimated to be between 120 mg and 250 mg, although tolerant long-term abusers have been known to survive much higher doses.[6]

Marked tolerance develops at a fairly rapid rate with heavy use, although not with occasional abuse. Tolerance develops not only to the euphoric and analgesic effects but also to the respiratory-depressant and nausea-producing effects. Tolerance, however, is not seen with the drug's pupillary-constricting and constipating effects. The pattern seen in chronic, heavy abuse is that of increasing tolerance until a plateau is reached, where no amount of the drug produces the desired effect. The user will then usually inject himself with the sole purpose of avoiding the withdrawal syndrome, which commonly begins within 12 hours of the last dose.[6]

Initial withdrawal symptoms include lacrimation, nasal discharge, yawning, and sweating. An irritable period of sleep follows, and upon awakening the user experiences agitation, depression, dilated pupils, and gross tremor. The withdrawal syndrome peaks between 36 and 72 hours after the last dose, with autonomic symptoms of chills and flushing, "gooseflesh," nausea, vomiting, insomnia, anorexia, abdominal cramping, hypertension, and tachycardia. Aches in muscles and joints can occur with muscle spasms and twitching movements of the legs. The withdrawal commonly runs its course within 7 to 10 days.[6]

Heroin

Heroin is a semisynthetic opioid. A derivative of morphine, it is the most widely abused of the narcotic analgesics. No longer clinically used in this country, it is still used in some areas of the world for control of severe pain. Heroin is a crystalline white powder, although on the black market it is diluted with such a wide variety of substances that its appearance is highly variable. Some dilutants include quinine, dextrose, and lactose. Legal manufacture of heroin is under strict surveillance; small quantities are produced for research, and in Great Britain it is manufactured to treat opium dependence. Most heroin production is illegal. Morphine alkaloid is altered with acetic acid to produce the drug, which has a far greater potential for tolerance and dependence than the parent compound.[6]

The drug is usually taken intravenously, although inexperienced users may inhale the drug nasally or smoke it in combination with tobacco or marihuana. Analgesic effects begin between a 1-mg and 8-mg dosage. Abusers may begin at doses of less than 2 mg, but chronic dependent abusers have reported daily dosages of 200 mg to 300 mg. This range, of course, is unreliable because of the variable estimates of illegal-drug purity.[6]

The population of heroin abusers is heterogeneous, but a significant number are male, of lower socioeconomic background, and from minority groups. A large concentration of abusers reside in urban areas. Heroin abusers begin at a young age and are usually experienced with other drugs of abuse. As with morphine, tolerance develops rapidly, and the daily dose of the chronic, dependent abuser will increase until no euphoric effects can be produced any longer. The drug will then be taken primarily to avoid withdrawal symptoms. The expense and intermittent availability of heroin make it a common component of polydrug abuse.[6]

The short-term effects on the CNS include euphoria and a far greater "rush" than experienced with morphine. Clouding of conciousness, analgesia, and relaxation occur. This may progress to a twilight "sleepy" state or even full sleep. Pupillary constriction, ptosis, and decreased visual acuity occurs. Cardiorespiratory effects are decreased body temperature, sleeplessness, and lowered respiratory rate. Nausea and vomiting, anorexia, and constipation are common gastrointestinal effects. At higher doses, the above effects are increased and deep sleep or coma can occur. At overdose, blood pressure is lowered, bradycardia or arrhythmia occur, and cardiorespiratory failure can ensue. Death, when it occurs, is typically due to respiratory arrest.[6]

The lifestyle and conditions experienced by heroin abusers greatly increase the mortality rate for intravenous drug abuse. Medical complications result from the unsanitary use of needles, and they include subcutaneous infections, endocarditis, pneumonia, tuberculosis, and hepatitis. It has been estimated that up to 40% of deaths of heroin addicts are violent.[6]

Although tolerance develops quickly in regular abuse, with intermittent use, especially by other than intravenous routes, this phenomenon can be avoided. Tolerance is primarily developed to the euphoric, analgesic, and sedative effects, as well as the nauseating and respiratory-depressant effects. It does not appear to occur, however, with the constipating or pupillary-constricting effects.[6]

The severity and duration of withdrawal sickness appear to be related to the regularity of use and the amount of daily dosage. Onset usually occurs 8 to 12 hours after the last dose. Initial symptoms are lacrimation and nasal discharge, yawning, and diaphoresis. An agitated sleep may follow with subsequent depression, agitation, "gooseflesh," pupillary dilatation, and tremor. The withdrawal sickness peaks between 36 and 72 hours. Autonomic dysfunction occurs with alternating chills and flushing, "gooseflesh," intestinal spasms, elevated heart rate and blood pressure, and nausea and vomiting. Muscle spasms and involuntary kicking movements can occur. In most cases, the symptoms wane and are no longer present within 7 to 10 days. Deaths from withdrawal are rare, and are far exceeded by deaths from overdose or other complications of drug use.[6]

Hydromorphone

Hydromorphone, available commercially as Dilaudid, is a semisynthetic narcotic analgesic. A derivative of morphine, it is a fine, white crystalline powder that is soluble in water and alcohol. It is also available in a combination cough syrup. Clinical uses include control of moderately severe and severe levels of pain, as well as severe levels of cough.[6]

Dosage for pain control is 1 mg to 2 mg every 4 to 6 hours orally or by injection in subcutaneous and intramuscular sites. When abused, the drug is taken orally or by injection, including intravenous injection. Doses of up to 100 mg per day have been reported.[6]

The abuse of hydromorphone has increased over the past decade because abusers have gained access to the drug through theft from hospitals and pharmacies, or by forging prescriptions. Because of its wide medical use it is easily available and therefore inexpensive.

Short-term CNS effects are similar to those of morphine and heroin, but without the "rush" reported with these drugs. When injected, local pain and irritation occurs at the injection site. Higher doses produce intensification of effects, and the symptoms of overdose are similar to that of morphine. Long-term effects include sclerosing of the skin at injection sites. Importantly, nontolerant individuals have a significantly lower lethal dosage than with other opiates, which is estimated at 100 mg.[6]

Tolerance develops more gradually than with other opiates, but tolerance to the analgesic, sedative, euphoric, and respiratory-depressant effects is clearly defined.[6]

Withdrawal sickness is similar in character to that of morphine, but usually disappears within a week of the last dose administered.

Meperidine

Meperidine is an entirely synthetic opioid. Although its potency is far less than that of morphine, it has the property of retaining its potency after oral administration. In addition, tolerance develops gradually, making dosage adjustments infrequent. Meperidine's principle clinical use is in control of moderate to severe pain levels. The drug is marketed as Demerol, and it is manufactured exclusively by the pharmaceutical industry. The drug is a white crystalline powder, and is soluble in water and alcohol.[6]

Clinical dosage for moderate pain is 50 mg to 100 mg orally or by subcutaneous or intramuscular injection, at a frequency of up to 3 hours. This dosage can be increased up to 150 mg at the same schedule for severe levels of pain. When abused, single doses of meperidine can reach 200 mg to 300 mg. Daily doses can reach 3 g to 4 g. The drug is taken orally or by injection, with all routes used.[6]

Short-term effects are similar to those of morphine, although the duration is far shorter, lasting only 3 to 4 hours. In contrast to other narcotic analgesics, meperidine can produce pupillary dilatation, and occasionally CNS excitation rather than depression. In overdose, meperidine may cause hallucinations, seizures, and coma, as well as respiratory depression and cardiovascular collapse.[6]

As with hydromorphone, meperidine will sclerose the skin around injection sites. When high-dose chronic use occurs, intractable twitching, tremor, psychomotor agitation, seizures, and toxic psychosis are long-term effects. A lethal dose for nontolerant users is estimated at 1 g.[6]

The tolerance pattern for meperidine is similar to that of hydromorphone where analgesia is concerned. In contrast, however, its euphoric and sedative effects have similar tolerance patterns to the more potent opiates.

Physical dependence varies with chronicity of use. The withdrawal syndrome is qualitatively less severe and of shorter duration than with morphine and heroin. The symptoms are comparable to those of the other opiates but with much less nausea, vomiting, and diarrhea.[6]

Although meperidine is an infrequent drug of abuse on the street, a high incidence is reported among hospital personnel because of the drug's availability in that setting.

Oxycodone

This semisynthetic opiate is a derivative of codeine and is used for control of moderate to severe levels of pain. Like meperidine, its principle advantage is that it retains much of its potency after oral administration. Oxycodone is a white crystalline powder that is soluble in water and alcohol. Oxycodone is available in pure form as Supendol or in combination with other analgesics as Percodan (with aspirin and caffeine), Percocet (with acetaminophen), and Percobarb (with hexobarbitol). Dosage for Percocet and Percodan is 2.25 mg up to four times daily for moderate pain and 4.5 mg for severe pain.

When abused, the drug is usually taken orally in doses of up to 100 mg. Because of its wide use in outpatient populations, oxycodone is regularly available from legal or forged prescriptions. It is also available illegally.[6]

Early effects are similar to those of codeine, and in long-term abuse there appears to be less physical deterioration than with other narcotic analgesics. Tolerance is rapid with regular abuse but does not develop to the drug's effects of pupillary constriction or constipation. The withdrawal sickness syndrome lasts a week after the last dosage and is of similar intensity to the withdrawal seen with morphine.[6]

Pentazocine

Pentazocine is unique among the narcotic analgesics because it is a mild opiate antagonist. It has a high affinity for opiate receptors and has the mixed property of producing both analgesia and withdrawal in narcotic-dependent patients. Pentazocine is a moderately potent analgesic that is stronger than Demerol but weaker than morphine. It is also available in combination with tripelennamine, called "T's and blues" by abusers. The drug is used clinically for relief of moderate to severe pain at a dosage of 50 mg to 100 mg every 4 hours orally or 30 mg every 8 hours by injection. A wholly synthetic opioid, pentazocine is a white crystalline substance that is soluble in water and alcohol. It is marketed as Talwin.[6]

Pentazocine is not abused widely in the pure form because it does not postpone withdrawal in narcotic-dependent users. The "T's and blues" combination is a powerful euphoric, however, and is growing in popularity in certain areas. Tolerant abusers may take over 1 g per day. The drug is taken orally, by rectal suppository, or is crushed and prepared into solution for IV injection.[6]

The effects of pentazocine are similar to Demerol at approximately twice the potency. It differs from other narcotics in its ability to precipitate withdrawal in a narcotic-dependent patient. Long-term use appears to have several unique effects, most notably toxic psychoses, depression, and sleep disturbances. When injection is the method of chronic abuse, intradermal fibrosis and deep ulceration of the skin can occur. There are no reports to date of death from overdose.[6]

Tolerance has been reported but not widely studied. Recent evidence has indicated that dependence can occur in even small doses when use is regular; its withdrawal syndrome is similar to that of meperidine.

Methadone

Methadone is an entirely synthetic narcotic analgesic. Although its effects are comparable to morphine, it retains much of its potency when taken orally, and its effects last longer than those of morphine or heroin. The drug also lacks a euphoric or sedative effect with the usual oral dosage in drug-tolerant users. These properties have earned the drug a major role in the treatment of narcotic addiction because it avoids the dangerous concomitants of unsanitary needle administration. The drug is a white crystalline substance, and in maintenance programs it is dissolved in an orange-flavored drink.[6]

Clinical uses in this country are almost exclusively in drug treatment programs, where an initial dosage is usually 20 mg to 40 mg per day in a divided dose. This is increased to the level where a maintenance dose is achieved in which avoidance of withdrawal symptoms is stable. A maintenance program is then instituted in which patients are stabilized with avoidance of health problems other than the dependence itself.[6]

Although illegal use of methadone was widespread 10 years ago, strict manufacturing guidelines have substantially diminished street use. When abused, the drug is typically injected intravenously, but the manufacture of compounds that make intravenous injection difficult has reduced the rate of abuse.

Short-term effects are similar to morphine and heroin. The drug is potentially of higher lethality, and the minimum lethal dose in nontolerant users is approximately 75 mg.[6]

Of significant importance is the lack of euphoric effect when tolerance is achieved. It is this property that allows methadone maintenance patients to attempt to achieve productivity and stable employment. The potential for dependence is higher than heroin or morphine, but since the drug is excreted slowly, there is a higher degree of CNS adaptation to the withdrawal of the drug. Therefore, the withdrawal state is less severe but more prolonged. The course of abrupt withdrawal is 6 to 7 weeks. Withdrawal programs typically withdraw methadone gradually over several months.[6]

Treatment of Opiate Intoxication

The acute treatment of opiate intoxication is usually limited to conservative management unless life-threatening overdose exists. Observation and support as well as treatment of associated medical or psychiatric conditions suffice.

In several instances, however, the use of opiate antagonists is indicated. Where overdose has occurred, and respiratory depression is severe, these drugs can reverse narcotic analgesic effects. They are also useful in diagnosing narcotic intoxication where history of laboratory diagnosis is insufficient. Naloxone (Narcan) is a pure antagonist; that is, it has a high affinity for opiate receptor sites but no pharmacologic action or effect at that site. It will precipitate withdrawal in drug-dependent individuals, often within minutes. The usual dosage for adults is between 0.1 mg and 0.8 mg by injection.[6]

Naltrexone, also a potent narcotic antagonist, is derived from a naturally occurring opium alkaloid, thelaine. Fifty milligrams on oral administration will block opiate effects. It is longer-acting than naloxone and is currently being used only in experimental programs.[9]

Treatment of Opiate Dependence

The current models of treatment for opiate dependence largely fall into two categories of pharmacologic management: opiate antagonist treatment and methadone maintenance. There are complicating phenomena in each approach, and an optimal drug treatment program has yet to be devised.

In the antagonist model, opiate antagonists such as naloxone or naltrexone are administered on a daily basis. The philosophy of this program is that these drugs will block the withdrawal-alleviating effects of any illegal narcotics the dependent patient might obtain during the treatment course. It is felt that drug-seeking behavior could therefore be deconditioned.[10]

In methadone maintenance programs, methadone is substituted for the opiate on which the patient is dependent. As outlined above, a dosage to which the patient is just tolerant is achieved and no euphoric or sedative effects occur. The patient is maintained at this dose for a period of time until methadone is withdrawn over a protracted course and discomfort minimized.[2]

The pros and cons of each program are manifold. While the antagonist model allows for narcotic-free management of withdrawal, there is little incentive for patients to return. Yet if such a patient were to abort a treatment program, little adverse effect would occur because the antagonists are not addicting substances. In methadone maintenance programs, the drug is addicting, and patients will return daily. It is a more comfortable and hence more humane withdrawal; however, there is little guarantee that drug-seeking patients would not supplement such a program with illegally obtained narcotics, risking poor medical control or even serious overdose. The necessity for frequent visits makes these programs expensive from both manpower and financial considerations.[10]

A recent development in the management of opiate dependence has been experimental detoxification with α-adrenergic agonists such as clonidine and Lofexidine. In these experimental programs, clonidine is given in daily divided doses of 0.1 mg to 1.5 mg. The drug appears to completely block withdrawal symptoms in narcotic-addicted patients. The dose is tapered over a 5-day period, with careful monitoring of the side effects of hypotension and sedation. The narcotic dose must be entirely stopped rather than tapered, because narcotics and clonidine will potentiate each other's sedative effects. Lofexidine seems to lack the sedative and hypotensive properties of clonidine and may be a useful alternative in the future. Optimal use of the α-adrenergic agonists is recommended as a transition to narcotic-antagonist programs employing naloxone or naltrexone.[11]

Recent experimental approaches to treatment of narcotic addiction include acupuncture, levo-alpha-acetyl-methadol (LAAM), and propoxyphene napsylate. Acupuncture appears to partially relieve the symptoms of opiate withdrawal, but the efficacy and mechanism of this procedure is not well understood. LAAM is a long-acting synthetic variant similar to methadone that can be delivered at a frequency of three times weekly at daily doses of 30 mg to 80 mg. The financial and manpower costs of maintenance programs could therefore be reduced; the success of such programs is still under investigation. Propoxyphene-N (Darvon-N) is absorbed slowly from the gastrointestinal tract and may be an alternative to methadone for gradual withdrawal programs; however, its weak potency makes it a poor choice when opiate dependence is severe.[9]

Cannabis

Perhaps the most widely abused illegal drug in the United States, cannabis has a long history of use for its psychoactive effects, dating back to 2737 BC in China.[4] Obtained from the Indian hemp plant, *Cannabis sativa,* the principle psychoactive component is tetrahydrocannabinol (THC). Drug preparations from the plant vary but all are more or less derived from the resinous exudate of the leaves and top clusters of the ripe plant. Three varieties of preparations exist: low-grade *bhang* from tops of uncultivated plants; higher-quality *ganja* from flowers and top leaves of selected plants; and highest-grade *charas,* a purified resin preparation. The name *marihuana* is a Mexican derivative for the lower-grade preparations of stems and leaves. *Hashish* is the dried cannabis resin and flowers, available in compressed cubes of brown or black color. An extract of hashish using organic solvents is hash oil, which is highly concentrated THC and other components of the cannabis plant.[4]

Cannabis is obtained illegally; legal uses are restricted to investigational approaches to epilepsy, antiemetic therapy for cancer, anorexia nervosa, severe pain, and wide-angle glaucoma. The cannabis plants are grown in many parts of the world, and their illegal cultivation is a multibillion dollar enterprise. Colombia, Mexico, Panama, Hawaii, Jamaica and the United States are all large producers of marihuana. Slang names for marihuana usually include geographic origin such as "Acapulco gold," "Panama red," "Hawaiian," and so forth. Other common names are "pot," "grass," "reefer," and "weed." Hashish is generally referred to as "hash," its extract as "hash oil."[6]

The extent and patterns of use vary geographically, but in all areas of the country, cannabis use has grown astronomically. Occasional use has been reported in as much as 90% of the population in some areas. A 1980 study showed a 60% incidence of use of cannabis "at least once," and a "9% daily use" among American high school students.[9] As such patterns approach the rates of alcohol and nicotine use, the definition of "abuse" must necessarily be narrowed and sociocultural norms taken into consideration. DSM-III defines cannabis abuse by a pattern of pathologic use on a daily basis for at least 1 month and by impairment in social and occupational functioning due to cannabis use. Cannabis dependence, on the other hand, is defined by the presence of tolerance to the drug's effects. Two organic mental syndromes are defined: cannabis intoxication and cannabis delusional disorder. Both are diagnosed by maladaptive behavioral effects, and the latter by persecutory delusions following drug use.[8]

A typical marihuana cigarette or "joint" contains 2.5 mg to 5.0 mg of THC. Typically, only small doses are needed to produce the desired effect, but heavy users may smoke up to five joints daily.[6]

Marihuana is usually ingested by inhalation of smoked preparations. The dried leaves are rolled into joints and smoked as cigarettes, with deep inhalation to maximize alveolar absorption of THC. Water-cooled pipes may be used to make the smoke less harsh. Hashish is usually smoked from a pipe, and hash oil applied to joints or cigarettes. On occasion, marihuana and hashish may be baked into food for gastrointestinal absorption. In research uses, THC is available in gelatinized capsules for oral ingestion.[6]

The short-term effects of marihuana use are early disinhibition, relaxation, talkativeness, and drowsiness. Then a progression to a state of euphoria and exhiliration occurs, with increased perceptual acuity in visual, auditory, tactile, and gustatory areas. The user may smile and laugh excessively. Cognitive impairment further occurs to a point where distortions in time (usually time-expansive) and body perception occur. Perceptual–motor integration is impaired to a level at which driving or operating machinery can become dangerous. In rare cases, frank hallucinations and paranoia occur with feelings of panic and intense anxiety, which may be related either to the setting of the drug ingestion or an idiosyncratic reaction and constitutes the cannabis delusional syndrome. Peripheral drug effects include tachycardia, hypotension, and reddening of the conjunctiva. Irritation of the respiratory mucosa occurs, as well as bronchodilatation. Gastrointestinal effects are dryness of the mouth and markedly increased appetite. Libido may increase as well. The effects normally last several hours after marihuana is smoked, longer if ingested.[6]

In high doses, synesthesia, the blending of sensory stimuli, may occur. True hallucinations are rare; they are usually subjectively perceived as "unreal." Depersonalization may also occur, in which the user believes that his experience is not real. Rarely, acute psychosis may be precipitated with paranoia, agitation, and loss of insight.[6]

Tolerance is unusual with cannabis. In short-term daily use, reverse tolerance may occur, in which less of the drug is needed for the desired effect. In long-term daily use, however, true tolerance to cannabis occurs with resultant heavy use. Among the effects prone to tolerance are euphoria, cardiovascular effects, and psychomotor impairment. Cross tolerance to other drugs is not known.[6]

Dependence occurs in several ways. Psychological dependence may occur to the extent that marihuana users cannot cope with normal stresses of life without the drug. Physical dependence appears to exist in mild form in heavy users. Abrupt cessation may lead to withdrawal symptoms of sleep and appetite disturbance, gastrointestinal upset, anxiety and depression, and occasionally chills and tremors. The duration is several days to a week.[6]

Treatment of cannabis intoxication is largely supportive. After assessment of concomitant psychiatric or medical conditions is made, patients can usually be "talked down" when anxiety and panic are present. Low-dose benzodiazepines may help curb anxiety. When delusional symptoms are present, neuroleptics in low dosages are helpful. An important aspect of treatment is diagnosis of intoxication by other agents, which the user may not be aware of ingesting. Phencyclidine is not uncommonly mixed with cannabis to enhance the effects.[1]

Follow-up and supportive psychotherapy may be helpful because chronic use and dependence often mask underlying psychopathology. The chronic abuser of marihuana may require a period of social readjustment after cessation of drug use.

Phencyclidine

Phencyclidine (PCP) is an arylcyclohexamine originally developed as an anaesthetic, but discontinued when patients awakening from anesthesia reported confusion, hallucinations, fear, and disorientation. Its veterinary use continued as an immobilizing agent. In the early 1960s the drug appeared on the illegal market as PCP or "angel dust." The drug was initially unpopular due to its unpleasant side effects. In 1979, further use of the drug by veterinarians was banned when it became known that over seven million people in the United States had tried the drug and its abuse rate was soaring.[9]

Although phencyclidine is often called a hallucinogen, it is rare that hallucinations occur; in fact, the intoxication state can be distinguished from that of lysergic acid diethylamide (LSD) and mescaline by the relative absence of hallucinations. A crystalline white powder, it is soluble in water and alcohol. On the black market the drug is often off-white because of impurities, or incorporated into capsules and pills. It is often misrepresented as THC, mescaline, psilocybin, or LSD because it is much less expensive to manufacture. Needless to say, this can complicate the diagnosis of the toxic state tremendously. It may also be smoked in combination with marihuana to "enhance" the euphoric effects. The drug may also be smoked with joints made from parsley or other neutral substances.[6]

The usual route of administration is oral, as a liquid, capsule, or tablet, but the drug may also be inhaled as described above. Rarely, the drug may be injected intravenously in solution.[6]

The psychological effects of phencyclidine are notably more unpleasant and less dependent on the personality structure of the user. Initial symptoms include distortions in body image, followed by depersonalization and depression lasting for hours. Negativism, hostility, and apathy are prominent features, making the differential diagnosis between PCP intoxication and schizophreniform psychosis difficult.[12] In lower doses, mild euphoria and relaxation are the desired effects, but because of the drug's illegal manufacture, phencyclidine dosage is unreliable. The typical dosage is 5 mg to 10 mg, but abusers may consume up to 100 mg in a dose.[6]

The production of psychosis is a prominent feature of the intoxicated state. Sensory modalities are impaired and additional schizophreniformlike symptoms include blocking, impaired motor function, impairment of abstract symbolic cognition (as in proverb interpretation), and sequential thinking. Violent behavior or suicidal gestures have been reported (Table 12-3).[12]

Physiologic effects include ataxia, slurring of speech, parasthesias, paralysis, and analgesia. Increased blood pressure and heart rate occur, but without respira-

Table 12-3
Clinical Effects of PCP Use

Dose	Serum Level	Clinical Effects*
<5 mg	20–30 mg/ml	Numbness, mild euphoria, mood changes
5–10 mg	30–100 mg/ml	Catatonic-like stupor with eyes open, repetitive motor movements, muscle rigidity, hypertension, nystagmus
20 mg	>100 mg/ml	Prolonged coma, hypertension, convulsions, vomiting, diaphoresis, possible death

* May vary widely from individual to individual
Walker JI: Psychiatric Emergencies: Intervention and Resolution, p 61. Philadelphia, JB Lippincott, 1983

tory depression. In severe overdose coma, convulsions and death from respiratory arrest can occur.[12]

Long-term effects of phencyclidine abuse include memory and thought impairment. "Flashbacks," recurrences of the toxic state, have been reported after drug use is discontinued. Chronic anxiety and depressive states are not uncommon. The probability of violent or self-destructive behavior increases with frequent use.[6]

Tolerance to phencyclidine has not been reported, and while withdrawal has been observed in animal subjects, no such syndrome exists in humans. A psychological dependence may occur, however, with chronic use.[6]

Because of the potent neurologic effects, the acute intoxicated state should be considered as emergent with careful assessment of medical status. In states of mild intoxication the symptoms can clear fairly rapidly, but in some cases (often with no relation to dosage) the psychosis can persist for weeks. Rapid neuroleptic tranquilization may be indicated, with seclusion and restraint for violent patients.[1]

In severe overdoses, gastric lavage and ventilatory support may be indicated, and if severe hypertension occurs, diazoxide or propanalol may be used. Excretion can be enhanced with furosemide and ascorbate. Supportive measures are essential.[12]

Because of the variability of phencyclidine's effects and its widespread use, patient education is essential. It is hoped that once the dangers of phencyclidine become known, its epidemic abuse can be curbed.

Hallucinogens

Hallucinogens represent a broad category of psychoactive drugs, including many chemically unrelated substances. Many are naturally occurring derivatives of plants, but others are wholly synthetic. They all produce varying degrees of sensory disturbances as well as alterations of mood and thinking. More frequently, visual hallucinations and distortions are prominent, but all sensory modalities including hearing, taste, touch, and smell can occur as well. Synesthesia, in which one sensory modality is experienced as another (*e.g.*, colors are tasted or smelled), may be experienced. The quality of sensory, affective, and thought impairment is idiosyncratic. The psychological makeup of the user, his previous experience with the drug, the setting or context in which the drug is taken, and the dosage will all greatly influence the drug's effect.[6]

Documented use of hallucinogens dates to ancient Asian civilizations, where they are known to have played a part in many cultural and religious rites. In the Americas, Mayan and Aztec cultures employed and cultivated hallucinogenic plants, and many North American Indian tribes incorporated drugs into their rituals. In the 1960s, hallucinogens played a major role in "counterculture" societies as well as in personal explorations by many young people in our country. Over the past decade, however, the frequency of hallucinogen abuse declined among drug abusers, in favor of cannabis, cocaine, and amphetamines.[6]

Today, hallucinogens remain as active drugs of abuse but rarely are they used on a regular basis. Tolerance to the drug's effects is generally rapid, and chronic users are rare. More often, users experiment with hallucinogens or supplement their use of other drugs with occasional "weekend trips."[6]

The only legal use of hallucinogens has been restricted to investigational techniques in psychotherapy of various disorders. The Native American Church, composed of various American Indian tribes, has legal permission to incorporate peyote as a sacrament in religious rituals.[6]

The DSM-III defines hallucinogen abuse as a pattern of pathologic use that the user is unable to reduce or stop, with resultant impairment in social and occupational functioning. In addition, three organic mental disorders are defined: hallucinogen delusional disorder, with belief that the disturbances from the drug correspond to reality; hallucinogen hallucinosis, with perceptual changes, physical symptoms, and maladaptive behaviors due to the drug; and hallucinogen affective disorder, with affective disturbances persisting beyond the effects of the hallucinogen.[8]

Due to the variety of hallucinogenic substances, the major individual drugs will be discussed separately. As outlined above, the effects vary enormously, and the descriptions below are intended only as generalities.

LSD

Often considered a prototype for hallucinogenic drug effects, LSD is a powerful synthetic drug capable of producing extreme psychotic symptoms in a minority of individuals, but usually producing changes in visual perception, synesthesia, mood, and thought. Chemically it is lysergic acid diethylamide, a derivative of the ergot fungus. It is available as a crystalline white substance (LSD tartrate) soluble in water and packaged in a variety of ways including capsules, tablets, gelatin, blotting paper, and liquid. Street names include "acid," "orange sunshine," "purple haze," "windowpane," or simply colors such as "brown," "red," and so forth. It is extremely common to find phencyclidine being sold as "acid," or to find LSD altered with PCP or amphetamine. A high percentage of users take the drug once or twice for experimentation only. Rarely, the drug may be administered to unwitting users when slipped into a drink or food at a party because it is entirely odorless, colorless, and tasteless. The usual "street" dosage of an LSD "tab" is 40 mg to 500 mg. The drug is almost always taken orally, although it may in rare cases be injected or inhaled.[6]

The early effects of LSD include numbness and physical relaxation, or in some cases tremulousness and twitching. Pupillary dilatation occurs. Euphoria or anxiety may occur as affective changes begin.[6]

Early sensory distortions occur as "illusions"; that is, the user is aware that the perceptions are not real. Later, spatial perception and body image become disorganized, and time perception is also impaired. An "oceanic" experience, in which the user loses sense of his physical boundaries, can be an exhilirating or terrifying experience. Synesthesias occur and in fact different emotions may blend. Some users become preoccupied with trivial thoughts or objects and perceive them as having deep importance. All sensory modalities may be heightened in acuity.[6]

Not uncommonly, the affective and perceptual changes may change to extreme fearfulness, panic, and fear of losing one's mind. The illusory nature of the perceptual changes can become terrifyingly realistic hallucinations, and an overtly psychotic state can ensue. Behavior may change in conjunction with delusional thinking and progress to overt disorientation. These negative reactions or "bad trips" are highly influenced by the setting and the user's expectations when the drug is taken.[6]

Cardiovascular effects of LSD range from tachycardia and hypertension to a general state of sympathetic activation with increased body temperature and chills. Breathing may become rapid, and nausea and vomiting can occur.[6]

The effects of LSD begin within an hour of administration, reach a climax or peak at 3 to 5 hours, then wane and dissipate within 12 hours. A prolonged sleep may follow.[6]

The long-term effects of LSD include flashbacks, amotivational syndrome, and psychosis. Flashbacks are brief recurrences of perceptual changes usually lasting only several seconds or minutes. They range from intensification of colors and halos around lights to geometric images or, rarely, formed hallucinations. The disturbances are typically visual, but may occur across sensory modalities. They appear to be relieved by some agents such as benzodiazepines, and exacerbated by others, such as phenothiazines or cannabis. In general, flashbacks are rare among users.[6]

Amotivational syndrome, seen also with other drugs such as cannabis and cocaine, consists of increased apathy and withdrawal from social activity. Whether this is a true drug effect or due to underlying psychopathology is not known.[6]

In rare cases, unremitting psychosis has followed a single dose or chronic use of LSD. It is schizophreniform in nature and may mimic true schizophrenia. The etiology is poorly understood; the drug may indeed have unmasked a latent schizophrenic illness.[6]

Reports of chromosomal abnormalities in LSD users generated much debate in the late 1960s and early 1970s. Current understanding remains inconclusive, and the only documented risk appears to be to pregnant women who use LSD and then spontaneously abort. Many such women have been polydrug abusers, further complicating the picture. Clearly, any illicit or unsupervised drug use during pregnancy is unwise.[6]

Tolerance to LSD is extremely rapid and daily use is therefore rare. Cross tolerance to other hallucinogens also occurs. Physical dependence has never been demonstrated and there is no known withdrawal syndrome. Psychological dependence is known to occur, but the pure "acid head" is rare among hallucinogen abusers.[6]

Methylenedioxyamphetamine (MDA)

MDA represents a class of hallucinogen that is intermediate between LSD and amphetamines, sharing properties of both these drugs. It is wholly synthetic and manufactured illegally, its having no clinical uses. It is a hydrochloride salt of white crystalline nature, but may vary in appearance because of impurities. MDA's street name is "love drug." The dosage is typically over 120 mg, usually taken orally.[6]

The effects are similar to those described for LSD, but of much lesser intensity. True hallucinations almost never occur and the drug is typically euphoric rather than anxiety-provoking. Physical effects are sympathetic in nature with decreased appetite, pupillary dilatation, and increased cardiovascular function and perspiration. MDA begins to take effect within half an hour, peaks at 90 minutes, and usually disappears by 12 hours.[6]

The drug is uncommon on street markets, and typically phencyclidine is misrepresented as MDA to naive purchasers.

Mescaline and Peyote

Mescaline is a naturally occurring hallucinogen derived from the peyote cactus *Lophophora williamsii,* grown in the southwestern United States, Mexico, and Central America. It may also be wholly synthetic, made in illegal laboratories. In pure form, mescaline sulfate is a white crystalline powder. The dried "buttons" from the peyote cactus are tufted with white fibers and contain at least 14 other psychoactive substances other than mescaline; the buttons may also be ground to a powder.[6]

The drug is taken orally in capsule, liquid, or tablet form. In the case of peyote, the cactus is chewed, although the taste is unpleasant. With peyote, severe nausea and vomiting typically occur before any psychological effects are noted. A typical dose is 300 mg to 500 mg of mescaline, equivalent to three or four peyote buttons.[6]

Mescaline and peyote effects are essentially the same as those described for LSD, and are of similar intensity and duration. As with LSD, sympathetic nervous system activation occurs.[6]

Tolerance develops rapidly and therefore chronic use is rare. Psychological dependence may occur but physical dependence or withdrawal has not been demonstrated.[6]

Use of these drugs is currently uncommon among drug users, and phencyclidine is often sold under the false label of mescaline. Peyote abuse is also rare due to the unpleasant gastrointestinal effects, but legal use of the cactus occurs in the Native American Church.[6]

Psilocybin

A naturally occurring hallucinogen, psilocybin is found in the mushroom *Psilocybe mexicana*. Due to chemical instability and technical difficulty in synthesis, artificial psilocybin is rarely manufactured. The mushrooms are usually obtained intact in dried form or are ground into powder and placed in capsules; on occasion the powder may be mixed with juice. Administration is by oral route, the usual dosage being between 4 mg and 10 mg.[6]

The effects of psilocybin mimic those of LSD in a low dosage, with sensory distortion, illusions, synesthesias, and loss of a physical sense of boundaries. The physical effects are all of short duration and tend to be sympathetic in nature. The duration of effects is approximately half that of LSD, usually lasting approximately 6 hours. As with LSD and mescaline, tolerance is rapid and only rarely is the drug used chronically. There is no physical or psychological dependence seen with psilocybin.[6]

Like the other hallucinogens, phencyclidine is often misrepresented as psilocybin. Occasionally, ordinary mushrooms are altered with LSD and sold as psilocybin.

Paramethoxyamphetamine (PMA)

PMA is a synthetic hallucinogen derived from amphetamine. It retains its stimulant properties, and is highly toxic because it excessively stimulates the CNS. This action has led to its nickname, "death drug." Produced in illegal laboratories, it is a white or yellow–white crystalline powder, placed in capsules or wrapped in foil packets. The usual dosage is 50 mg to 75 mg and the drug is taken orally, inhaled, or injected. While the effects are similar to mescaline, the minimum dose for the same effect is much less. Adverse effects are frequent, which include CNS effects such as hallucinations, delirium, convulsions, hyperactivity, and rigidity. Tachycardia, hypertension, and fever occur also, accompanied by nausea and vomiting. High doses can lead to coma and death.[6]

Because of its high lethality, PMA is rarely found as a drug of abuse.

Dimethyltryptamine (DMT)

DMT is a synthetic hallucinogen of similar structure to psilocin, one of the alkaloids found in the *Psilocybe mexicana* mushroom.

A white crystalline powder, DMT is more effective when inhaled, curiously, and is often smoked in conjunction with marijuana. The effect is powerful and 50 mg to 60 mg of DMT will approximate the effects of LSD. The duration is extremely brief, however, lasting half an hour to an hour. Anxiety states are frequent.[6]

No physical or psychological dependence is reported for DMT, and tolerance is not well studied. Interestingly, cross tolerance with other hallucinogens does not occur, causing many researchers to speculate that the drug is atypical in its mechanism for hallucinogenic action.[6]

Trimethoxyamphetamine (TMA) and Dimethoxymethylamphetamine (DOM)

TMA and DOM are both synthetic hallucinogens derived from amphetamine, and are both white crystalline substances synthesized illegally. DOM is also called "STP."[6]

In low doses the drugs produce euphoria and CNS stimulation, but in higher doses mescaline-like visual hallucinations and distortions occur.[6] TMA has the peculiar property of producing aggressive behavior in high dosage.[6] Both drugs are infrequently abused but occasionally misrepresented as other hallucinogens.

Treatment of Hallucinogen Intoxication

The emotional state of the drug user, environmental setting of the drug ingestion, and the context of the drug abuse: these influences on hallucinogen effects have already been described. It follows that manipulation of these factors plays a major role in the treatment of dysphoric intoxication states.

Patients should be placed in rooms that are well-lit and quiet, with minimal distracting stimuli. The physician should reassure the patient that his psychological experiences are due to the drug, and he should help orient him to the treatment setting. The presence of a friend or family member may help, and they should be enlisted to assist in this process of "talking down."[1]

Benzodiazepines in low dosage are helpful adjuncts when anxiety is overwhelming. Higher doses of 20 mg to 40 mg can be used when sedation is indicated.

If psychosis is present, phenothiazines may be used in low doses, but unfortunately, they may exacerbate dysphoric hallucinogen effects.[1]

Because of the frequent misrepresentation of street drugs, all available laboratory studies should be secured to properly identify the drug.

Unresponsiveness to the above measures may necessitate hospitalization. Once the toxic state has cleared, underlying psychiatric or medical conditions should be properly identified and treated.

Inhalants

Inhalants represent a category of diverse psychoactive drugs that are characterized by their physical state. On exposure to air at room temperature they change from liquids to vapors. The vapors are then inhaled and rapidly absorbed from the nasal mucosa into the bloodstream.

Intentional inhalation of volatile substances for psychological effect began in the 1800s with the advent of nitrous oxide, ether, and chloroform, prior to the introduction of these drugs as anasthetics. The 20th century introduced gasoline-sniffing and glue-sniffing, but the widespread experimentation with psychoactive substances in the 1960s gave rise to even more inhalants as drugs of abuse.[13]

The typical abuser of inhalants begins in very early adolescence, although a continuous pattern of abuse through adolescence is rare. Inhalants are usually substances intended for various innocuous uses such as airplane glue, gasoline, kerosene, or cleaning fluid. Their availability therefore makes them attractive drugs of abuse among those to whom controlled substances would be unavailable, such as young adolescents or indigents. Hispanic Americans and American Indians are overrepresented in recent studies.[13]

Some inhalants are controlled substances that are only available to the medical community. The anesthetics ether, halothane, and nitrous oxide have recently become popular drugs of abuse. Amyl nitrite and butyl nitrate are popular drugs among the homosexual community for their purported enhancing effects on sexual performance.[9]

The general properties of inhalants include rapid absorption and almost immediate CNS effect. The desired sensations range from euphoria to overt delirium with identifiable neurologic impairment. The toxic effects are usually short-lived, but mild to severe medical complications may result. The predictability of these effects is hindered by the complex chemical nature of many inhalants. Gasoline, for example, contains benzine, tolnene, xylene, and napthalene, all aromatic hydrocarbons; as well as n-hexane and n-heptane, both aliphatic hydrocarbons. The presence of different toxic substances may lead to synergistic toxic actions. It is typically the medical complications of inhalants, rather than the behavioral or psychiatric effects, that bring inhalant abusers to medical attention. These major adverse effects will be briefly discussed.[13]

A sudden death syndrome has been demonstrated in rare cases of inhalant abuse. Although it is not well understood, it appears to be caused by the potentiating action of fluorocarbons on epinephrine effects on the heart, causing heart failure and sudden death.[13]

Neurologic damage, with direct damage to neurons and peripheral neuropathic effects, are produced by tolnene, n-hexane, gasoline, gasoline additives such as lead and triorthocresyl phosphate, and benzenes. Muscular atrophy, cerebellar dysfunction, paresthesias, decreased reflexes, and positive Babinski's signs can occur, as well as CNS depression, with initial disinhibition and euphoria progressing to dizziness, memory impairment, slurred speech, and acute psychosis.[9] Bone marrow depression and leukemia can occur with benzene exposure; carbon tetrachloride is highly toxic to renal and hepatic tissue.[9]

Treatment of solvent abuse should be directed first to identification of medical complications, and appropriate interventions. If a pattern of abuse is present, discontinuation of the drug is insufficient despite the lack of physical dependence or withdrawal syndromes. Underlying psychiatric problems should be identified and treated. Because of the particularly young population that is prone to inhalant abuse, school and community drug education programs may be of great value.

Miscellaneous Drugs of Abuse

This section is devoted to brief descriptions of a variety of drugs that occasionally lend themselves to abuse, but that do not necessarily relate to the major categories of drugs of abuse previously described. Most are naturally occurring substances that might lead to unintentional psychoactive effects following normal patterns of use (*e.g.*, caffeine, nutmeg, bromides). Others are deliberately abused for their psychoactive properties, but because of their inherent toxicity, do not lend themselves to common use.

Amanita Muscaria

This hallucinogenic mushroom is also known as *fly agaric* because of its insecticidal properties. The North American variant has a yellow, orange, or white cap with white, red, or yellow markings. It contains the alkaloid muscarine along with ibotenic acid and muscimol. Early effects of oral ingestion include dizziness and anxiety, rapid respiration, muscle twitches and parasthesias, and gastrointestinal effects of nausea and vomiting. Later effects are euphoria, sensory enhancement, and altered perceptions similar to psilocybin or mescaline. After 3 to 4 hours, depressant effects begin, followed by sleep. Rarely, overt psychosis can occur. Coma, convulsions, and death from cardiac arrest may occur, although they are rare.

Angel's Trumpet—Atropine, Scopalomine, Hyoscyamine

Angel's trumpet, also known as *Datura sauvealeus,* is a flowering plant found in the Southeastern United States. Its flowers are eaten directly, or brewed and then orally ingested. A toxic anticholinergic syndrome is produced with hallucinations, confusion, paranoid delusions, and disorientation. The naturally occurring alkaloids atropine, scopalomine, and hyoscyamine are the psychoactive agents. Other related plants include *Atropa belladonna* ("deadly nightshade") and *Datura stramonium* (jimson weed).[6]

Initial stimulation and then depression of cortical function occurs. Physical effects include widening of pulse pressure, flushing and dryness of the skin, glandular secretions, and arrythmias.

In treating angel's trumpet intoxication, supportive measures are essential because behavior can be violent. Gastric lavage should be performed, and physostigmine 1 mg to 4 mg will counteract the alkaloid's effects. Because of the anticholinergic properties of phenothiazines, they are absolutely contraindicated.[1]

Bromides

Once used in pharmacologic treatment of seizures and as sedative hypnotics, bromides have now been replaced by safer and more effective medications. Occasionally they are still found, largely in the form of their sodium, potassium, or ammonium salts.[6]

Because of their irritating gastrointestinal effects, true abuse is rare, but unintentional overdosing used to lead to a wide variety of psychiatric symptoms. The major factor in overdosage was the relatively slow renal excretion of bromide and the long half-life of 12 days.

Psychiatric symptoms of bromism may include schizophreniform psychosis, mania, depression, or organic mental states of delirium and dementia. Photophobia, headache, vertigo, and blurred vision occur. An idiosyncratic acneiform rash occurs with bromide intoxication, and other physical signs include pupillary dilation, "furring" of the tongue, positive Babinski's sign, cyanosis, tremor, ataxia, papilledema, decreased reflexes, and bradykinesia. Diagnosis is by serum bromide levels of greater than 50 mg/100 ml.[1]

Treatment involves administration of sodium chloride orally or by IV saline at dosages of up to 6 g to 12 g daily. In extreme cases, dialysis may be needed. Paraldehyde at oral doses of 10 ml to 15 ml every 4 to 6 hours or 4 ml intramuscularly every 6 hours can help control psychosis. Low-dose neuroleptics may also be of use, although careful monitoring of blood pressure is essential. Symptoms typically last 2 to 6 weeks after the last intake of bromide.[1]

Caffeine

Undoubtedly the most commonly ingested psychoactive drug, caffeine may cause anxiety, restlessness, insomnia, and early-phase insomnia when high amounts are taken. Physical symptoms include diarrhea, tinnitus, diuresis, nausea and vomiting, with signs of muscle twitching, arrythmias, and tachypnea.[1]

Caffeine is not only present in coffee, tea, chocolate, and soft drinks, but is often a component of over-the-counter analgesics, stimulants, and diet pills.

Tolerance to caffeine has not been clearly demonstrated, but psychological dependence and physical dependence unquestionably exist. The withdrawal syndrome is mild and characterized typically by headache. Other withdrawal symptoms include irritability, lethargy, and psychomotor restlessness. The duration of withdrawal is brief, rarely over 48 hours.[6]

Morning-Glory Seeds

The seeds of the morning-glory plants, *Rivea corymbosa* and *Ipomoea violacea,* contain psychoactive components that are chemically analogous to LSD. These compounds, d-lysergic amide and d-isolysergic acid amide, are hallucinogenic, albeit far less potent than LSD. Their effects include sensory distortions, affective impairment, and pseudohallucinations, but rarely true hallucinations. Physical effects are far more common and mostly gastrointestinal in nature, with nausea, vomiting, and diarrhea.[6]

Although popular in the 1960s, abuse of morning-glory seeds is rare today.

Nutmeg

Nutmeg is a spice derived from the evergreen *Myristiea fragrans*. The seed coat and seed oil appear to contain a hallucinogenic compound, myristicine, which produces euphoria, elation, dissociative states, perceptual distortions, and disorientation. Physical signs of intoxication include headaches, restlessness, paraesthesia, flushing of the skin, and muscle twitching, as well as nausea and vomiting.[6] In extreme dosages, liver damage from fatty degeneration can occur.[1] Hallucinogenic effects can be promoted by as little as 1 teaspoon of ground nutmeg, and the effects may not be experienced for several hours. Recovery is often slow and associated with headache, bone, and muscle aches.[6]

Intentional abuse of nutmeg is rare today; most frequently it constitutes an inexpensive "high" for young or indigent drug abusers.

Polydrug Abuse

In evaluation of the drug-abusing patient, the psychiatrist should be careful to take as complete a drug history as possible. Due to the patient's intoxicated state, he may need to rely on information supplied by friends or family of the patients. It is uncommon today to find a drug-abusing patient who is limited to abuse of one drug alone, with the possible exception of those who use cannabis.

The diagnostic picture is further complicated by the unreliability of the street drug market. As described previously, phencyclidine may be misrepresented as

LSD, mescaline, or THC. Heroin may be adulterated with substances ranging from lactose to strychnine; marihuana may be "enhanced" with phencyclidine. In any of these cases, the user is entirely unaware of which drug has been ingested.

Drug-abusing patients usually refer to drugs by street names. These names can vary widely according to region, and colloquial terms can change within a short time. Some street names can apply equally to completely different classes of drugs; for example, "meth" may refer to methadone or methamphetamine. Acronyms do not always give an accurate clue as to chemical composition; STP, for example, does not indicate any known compound, but may stand for "serenity, tranquility, and peace."[6]

In confusing cases of polydrug abuse, physical diagnosis may be extremely helpful in identifying the toxic state. Sympathetic nervous system activation, such as occurs with sympathomimetics like amphetamines and cocaine, as well as certain hallucinogens, results in pupillary dilatation with reactivity tachycardia, muscular tension, perspiration, elevated blood pressure and body temperature, and nausea and vomiting. By contrast, opiates and opioids cause pupillary constriction, decreased heart rate, psychomotor retardation, flushing, and decreased blood pressure and body temperature, although they also lead to nausea and vomiting. When working in an emergency setting, a psychiatrist must be familiar with the particular signs and symptoms of intoxication by the major classes of drugs.

Laboratory analyses are of great diagnostic assistance when available; unfortunately, the prolonged turnover time for most of these tests limits their usefulness in the acute setting. Most major medical centers have serum toxicology screens for barbiturates and benzodiazepines. Urine and gastric contents toxicology screens offer a wide variety of detectable agents, including methaqualone, phencyclidine, amphetamines, meprobamate, and benzodiazepines. In the case of narcotic abuse, thin-layer chromatography can detect heroin up to 24 hours after use, as well as the presence of quinine, antihistamines, and other fillers of street narcotic preparations. More sensitive tests, such as gas chromatography, hemagglutination inhibition, enzyme-multiplied immunoassay, and radioimmunoassay techniques, can be applied in highly uncertain cases.[9]

In cases where opiate intoxication is suspected, narcotic antagonists, such as naloxone, can be administered to reverse opiate effects, although withdrawal will be rapidly precipitated in addicted patients.

In addition to diagnostic concerns, it is essential for psychiatrists to be aware of the medical concomitants of polydrug abuse. Scarring and hyperpigmentation of the skin over veins and puncture marks, brawny edema, and ulcerations are all symptoms of repetitive needle use. Insterility of drug abusers' equipment should be assumed, and liver function tests as well as hepatitis antigen levels must be obtained. Typically, the total serum protein is elevated, both in albumin and globulin fractions, with globulin slightly higher. Transaminases and immunoglobulins are often elevated, as are bilirubin and alkaline phosphatase.[9] None of these tests are indicative of active hepatitis, and are chronically elevated in many intravenous drug abusers. To detect active disease, liver biopsy or viral titers may be needed. Opiates can cause false positive serology tests for syphilis, so fluorescent-treponemal antibody tests are indicated, because syphilis is frequent in drug-abusing populations.

In addition to the above findings, polydrug abusers may have elevated lymphocyte and polymorphonuclear cell counts, elevated hemoglobin, and high blood urea nitrogen levels.[9] While these are idiosyncratic and poorly understood findings, and often without underlying disease, the general poor physical health of many drug abusers may necessitate their workup. Acutely intoxicated patients may have fallen down and sustained closed skull fractures. If there is any history or physical finding suggestive of this, immediate workup is indicated.

The skills of the psychiatrist define his role beyond the detoxification stage of drug treatment. When more than casual drug use occurs, underlying psychopathology is strongly suggested. Associated psychiatric conditions may range from the "self-medicating" depressed patient to the latently psychotic schizophrenic seeking relief from or responding to delusional thoughts. Adolescent adjustment reactions frequently present initially through drug abuse. Drug abuse is also associated with a wide variety of personality disorders and antisocial character traits. The identification and treatment of latent psychiatric conditions in drug abusers is an essential aspect of drug rehabilitation.

Psychopathology is an important adjunctive tool in treating polydrug abuse. Supportive psychotherapy and manipulation of social factors are universally beneficial in drug rehabilitation. In appropriate cases, more insight-directed psychotherapy or psychoanalysis may give patients opportunities for understanding the unconscious determinants of their drug abuse. An opportunity for global behavioral and personality change may then be provided.

The psychiatrist has a number of perspectives and skills with which to synthesize a comprehensive treatment program for the drug-abusing patient. A thorough knowledge of the specific physical and laboratory findings, appropriate therapeutic interventions, and long-term follow-up treatment for drug abuse syndromes allow for successful drug rehabilitation. As current psychiatric training begins to transmit this knowledge to psychiatric residents, it is hoped that the cynicism and pessimism that characterized drug rehabilitation programs in the past decade can be transformed into successful treatment strategies and optimism.

References

1. Slaby AE, Lieb J, Tancredi LR: Handbook of Psychiatric Emergencies. Garden City, Medical Examination Publishing Company, 1981
2. Dole VP, Nyswander ME: Methadone Maintenance Treatment—A Ten Year Perspective. J Am Med Assoc 235:2117, 1976
3. Goodman LS, Gilman A: The Pharmacologic Basis of Therapeutics, 5th ed. New York, Macmillan, 1975
4. Grinspoon L, Bakalar JB: Drug Dependence: Non-narcotic Agents. In Kaplan HI, Freedman AM, Sadock BJ (eds): Comprehensive Textbook of Psychiatry, 3rd ed. Baltimore, Williams & Wilkins, 1980
5. Smith DE, Wesson DR: Phenobarbital Technique for Treatment of Barbiturate Dependence. Arch Gen Psychiatry 24:56–60, 1971
6. Cox C, Jacobs MR, Leblanc AE, et al: Drugs and Drug Abuse: A Reference Text. Toronto, Alcoholism and Drug Addiction Research Foundation, 1983
7. International Medical News Service, Clinical Psychiatry News 12(6):15, 1984

8. American Psychiatric Association: Diagnostic and Statistical Manual of Mental Disorders, 3rd ed. Washington, DC, American Psychiatric Association, 1980
9. Senay EC: Substance Abuse Disorders in Clinical Practice. Boston, John Wright, PSG Inc, 1983
10. Freedman AM: Opiate Dependence. In Kaplan HI, Freedman AM, Sadock BJ (eds): Comprehensive Textbook of Psychiatry, 3rd ed. Baltimore, Williams & Wilkins, 1980
11. Washton AM, Resnick RB: Outpatient Opiate Detoxification with Clonidine. J Clin Psychiatry, 43:39 (Sec 2), 1982
12. Showalter CV, Thornton WE: Clinical Pharmacology of Phencyclidine Toxicity. Am J Psychiatry, 134:1234, 1977
13. Nicholi AM: The Inhalants: An overview. Psychosomatics 24:914, 1983

Samuel B. Thielman

13 Alcohol Abuse

Alcohol abuse presents a major challenge to the clinician because it is a common disorder, with psychological, medical, and social ramifications. It involves people in almost every age group, and cuts across economic and cultural barriers. In 1975, alcohol abuse cost the United States economy $43 billion. In addition to the cost in health expenditures for alcohol-related problems, which accounted for approximately one fourth of the alcohol burden on the American economy, society was forced to pay for $19.6 billion in lost production of goods and services, $5.1 billion in motor vehicle damages, $2.9 billion in alcohol-related violent crime, $1.9 billion in costs for social agencies dealing with alcoholism, and $430 million in alcohol-related fire losses.

Some 7% of the population 18 years of age and older are problem drinkers, and among youths aged 14 to 17 years, almost one in five is a problem drinker. In 1978, estimates of alcohol-related deaths in this country were as high as 205,000. Assuredly, any physician involved in the clinical care of patients will frequently be faced with alcohol-related medical and behavioral disorders.

Etiology of Alcoholism

The etiology of alcoholism is only partially understood, but recent research on patients with alcohol abuse problems has challenged some earlier thinking about the development of pathologic alcohol use.

Inheritance

The inheritance of alcoholism is still a subject of much debate, and considerable evidence suggests that alcohol-dependent behavior is, at least in part, genetically determined. This notion is supported most convincingly by a number of studies that showed that adopted sons of alcoholic parents were as likely as nonadopted sons to develop alcoholism, and that both groups were more likely to develop the disorder than controls. Twin studies have demonstrated that monozygotic twins show a greater propensity for drinking behavior and alcoholism than fraternal twins.

What exactly one might inherit that would predispose him to alcoholism is not currently understood. Although there is little research evidence to suggest the existence of an inherited defect of alcohol metabolism in alcohol-abusing individuals, some have suggested that a physiologic aversion to alcohol may be inherited. For example, some have suggested that the lack of alcoholism among Orientals is the result of the presence of skin-flushing and unpleasant sensations in most Orientals when they consume alcohol. Such ideas are still speculative, however, and there is no consensus on the nature of the inheritance of a disposition toward alcohol.

Premorbid Personality Characteristics

The role of premorbid personality characteristics in producing alcoholic behavior is a subject of considerable interest. Some have suggested that there are certain personality disorders that are predisposed to the development of alcoholism, but George Vaillant reported that although future alcoholics in his study tended to exhibit antisocial and extroverted personality traits, the development of alcoholism was not significantly associated with premorbid psychological irritability. In fact, prior psychological health seems to have little to do with the development of alcoholism, and alcohol abuse appears to be the cause of psychological problems rather than a symptom of preexisting ones. Nonetheless, the perpetuation of established alcohol-abusing behavior seems to have a great deal to do with the social environment of the individual, and one must not neglect social exacerbations of the alcohol-abusing condition.

Family Environment

The role of family environment in the development of alcoholism has undergone close scrutiny in recent years. Prior to the last decade, there had been considerable attention paid to family environment as a factor in the development of alcoholism in certain individuals. Although the contribution of family environment is difficult to assess, mounting evidence indicates that the family plays a less important role in the genesis of alcoholic behavior than was once thought. Among the most interesting work done on this question is Vaillant's recently published work. Based on his own and previous work, Vaillant has suggested that family instability alone is insufficient to account for the development of alcoholism. Indeed, in one of his cohort groups, individuals from stable families who nonetheless had an alcoholic parent were five times more likely to develop alcoholism than individuals from unstable families with nonalcoholic parents.

Cultural and Ethnic Factors

Cultural and ethnic factors also appear to be related to drinking behavior. Research concerning cultural perspectives on pathologic alcohol use suggests that individuals from cultural groups that view alcohol consumption negatively are at low risk for alcohol abuse if they follow their cultural norms, but at high risk if they drink. On the other hand, individuals from cultural groups that incorporate alcohol use into daily life and cultural functions in a structured and nonpathologic way are at low risk for the development of problem alcohol use. In Vaillant's work and the work of others, alcoholic individuals appear to come from cultural backgrounds that are tolerant of adult drunkenness, but that did not provide an acceptable cultural context in which people could use alcohol nonabusively (such as consumption of low-alcohol-content beverages such as wine during religious ceremonies or with meals). Thus, cultural styles may account for differences in rates of alcoholism among ethnic groups, as may the ethnic differences in physiologic response to alcohol, mentioned above.

Diagnosis of Alcoholism

Though the term *alcoholism* is in widespread clinical use, how to define the term is open to considerable debate. E. M. Jellinek defined alcoholism as "any use of alcoholic beverages that causes any damage to the individual or society or both." That definition, though unwieldy because of its breadth, serves to illustrate the problem of how to define alcoholism as a clinical entity.

Pattison and his co-workers have extensively assessed the current research evidence on the nature of alcoholism and have pointed out that research evidence contradicts many popular conceptions of alcohol abuse. They note that alcohol dependence is a term covering a variety of syndromes rather than one distinct entity and that the pathologic use of alcohol can be viewed as existing on a continuum that stretches from nonuse of alcohol to pronounced abuse. Thus, not all problem drinkers are "born" alcoholics, and the distinction between the nature of the alcoholic individual and that of the nonalcoholic is not as clear as was once thought.

Further, Pattison and his co-workers have indicated that evidence is insufficient to support the idea that there is a particular pattern of progression that is characteristic of alcohol abuse. Indeed, the course of alcohol abuse varies considerably from individual to individual, and in individuals who are long-time abusers, the course of alcohol-associated problems is often related to other life events.

DSM-III, the official manual of nomenclature for the American Psychiatric Association, avoids some of the problems associated with the use of the concept "alcoholism" by minimizing that term and using instead two separate designations for pathologic alcohol use—alcohol abuse and alcohol dependence. Alcohol abuse is a disorder marked by a pattern of pathologic alcohol use, by impairment in social or occupational functioning as a result of alcohol use, and by a duration of the disorder for at least 1 month. Alcohol dependence involves either the pathologic use of alcohol, social or occupational disruption as a result of alcohol use, tolerance to the effects of alcohol, or at least one episode of alcohol withdrawal.

A critical part of the diagnosis of disorders of alcohol use is the determination of pathologic use. Clinically, this determination is made by interviewing the patient, a family member, or close acquaintance. When interviewing a patient or his family about alcohol use, one must attempt to ask questions in a nonjudgmental, nonhostile manner. Not only does a demeaning attitude on the part of the examining physician ensure poor cooperation from the patient, but it suggests that the physician will deliver substandard care to the patient.

Questions that the examiner should be able to answer as a result of interviewing the patient or the family include the following:

Has the patient ever drunk as much as a fifth of liquor in a day?
Does the patient sometimes feel that his drinking is out of control?
Has anyone ever suggested to the patient that he has a problem with alcohol?
Does he ever drink in the morning?
Does he have episodes of drinking to excess for a day or more?
Does he have alcohol-related absences from work?
Has alcohol use ever become an issue in his marriage?
Has the patient received treatment for alcohol abuse in the past?
Has he ever experienced loss of memory after drinking ("blackouts")?
Does he drink in spite of the knowledge that he may be exacerbating a preexisting physical disorder?
Does he feel the need to drink alcohol in order to function normally?
Has he ever drunk nonbeverage alcohol?

Absorption and Metabolism

Alcohol is readily absorbed from the stomach, small intestine, and colon. Absorption of alcohol by the gastric mucosa is initially rapid, but later slows, and complete absorption may take 2 to 6 hours. A number of factors may affect the rate of absorption, including the amount and rate of alcohol ingestion, the presence of food in the stomach, and the type of spirits consumed.

The stomach may in fact serve to delay the absorption of alcohol, because once it crosses the mucosa of the small intestine, alcohol is absorbed very quickly, and the rate of absorption is less contingent upon factors such as the presence of food in the intestinal lumen than is absorption in the stomach. The rate of gastric emptying is therefore an important factor in determining the rate of introduction of alcohol into the bloodstream.

More than 90% of the alcohol that enters the blood is oxidized, the unoxidized fraction being excreted primarily by the kidneys and lungs. Alcohol metabolism takes place primarily in the liver, where it is oxidized to acetaldehyde. There are three mechanisms by which the liver is known to metabolize alcohol to acetaldehyde. The primary one occurs in the cytosol of the hepatocyte, where alcohol dehydrogenase catalyzes the conversion of alcohol to acetaldehyde using nicotinamide-adenine dinucleotide (NAD^+) as a hydrogen ion acceptor. In the second mechanism, alcohol is converted to acetaldehyde in the hepatocyte microsomes by the microsomal ethanol oxidizing system. In the third, the enzyme catalase, located in the hepatocyte peroxisomes, mediates the conversion. Following the conversion of alcohol to acetaldehyde, acetaldehyde is converted to acetate by liver aldehyde dehydrogenase. Acetate is then converted to acetyl CoA, and acetyl CoA is metabolized by way of the citric acid cycle. In the chronic alcohol abuser, alterations occur in the hepatic enzyme systems that metabolize alcohol, and alcohol is consequently metabolized more rapidly.

Alcohol interacts with a large number of drugs to produce undesirable side effects. Knowledge of these side effects can be of considerable importance to the clinician who is frequently confronted with the task of sorting out an array of puzzling symptoms in the alcoholic patient. The effects of mixing alcohol and commonly used drugs are summarized in Table 13-1.

Alcohol Intoxication

Alcohol intoxication is a common phenomenon in Western societies, but the range of effects that alcohol can produce is not widely appreciated. The response of an individual to alcohol depends on a number of factors, including personality, genetic makeup, the degree of previous exposure to alcohol, and to some extent the social setting in which alcohol is used. The mental effects of alcohol intoxication range from disinhibition to coma; the physical effects range from mild incoordination to death.

Mild to Moderate Intoxication

Mild to moderate intoxication produces mild euphoria, a sense of increased energy, loquaciousness, emotional lability, and decreased behavioral inhibition. The individual's ability to judge the social appropriateness of his behavior is impaired, and an individual's usual inhibitions are attenuated. Under such circumstances, individuals with marginally effective ego mechanisms of defense under normal conditions may resort to behavior that is unquestionably maladaptive. A man with poorly controlled anger who normally shouts at his family may resort to physical violence. A depressed individual who has contemplated suicide over a period of time might actually attempt the act. Physiologic effects include lengthened reaction time, decreased control of motor movements, and mild slurring of speech. In individuals who are not heavy drinkers, mild to moderate intoxication occurs when serum blood alcohol is 30 mg/dl to 70 mg/dl.

Severe Intoxication and Coma

With increased intoxication (100 mg/dl to 200 mg/dl), an individual becomes increasingly lethargic. Selective disinhibition of the central nervous system (CNS) becomes more generalized CNS depression. Feelings of detachment may ensue. The individual becomes increasingly disoriented and emotionally labile and may exhibit angry outbursts or withdrawal. Speech becomes slow and slurred, the pulse strong and rapid, breathing heavier, and bladder and bowel control sometimes impaired. One may see an ataxic gait and gross motor incoordination. If the serum alcohol level is above 300 mg/dl, many individuals become stuporous and exhibit respiratory and, to a smaller degree, myocardial dysfunction; a serum alcohol level

Table 13-1
Interactions of Drugs With Alcohol

Interacting Drugs	Adverse Effect	Probable Mechanism
Acetaminophen	Increased hepatotoxicity	Increased production of toxic metabolites
Oral anticoagulants	Decreased anticoagulant effect with chronic alcohol abuse	Increased metabolism
	Increased anticoagulant effect with acute intoxication	Decreased metabolism
Antihistamines	Increased CNS depression with acute intoxication	Additive
Barbiturates	Decreased sedative effect with chronic alcohol abuse	Increased metabolism
	Increased CNS depression with acute intoxication	Additive; decreased metabolism
Benzodiazepines	Increased CNS depression	Additive
Chloral hydrate	Prolonged hypnotic effect	Synergism
Disulfiram	Abdominal cramps, flushing, vomiting, psychotic episodes, confusion	Inhibition of intermediary metabolism of alcohol
Isoniazid	Increased incidence of hepatitis	Not established
	Decreased isoniazid effect in some patients with chronic alcohol abuse	Increased metabolism
Meprobamate	Decreased sedative effect with chronic alcohol abuse	Increased metabolism
	Increased CNS depression with acute Intoxication	Additive; decreased metabolism
Metronidazole	Similar to disulfiram reaction but milder	Not established
Narcotics	Increased CNS depression with acute intoxication	Additive
Phenothiazines	Increased CNS depression	Additive
Phenytoin	Decreased anticonvulsant effect with chronic alcohol abuse	Increased metabolism
	Increased anticonvulsant effect with acute intoxication	Decreased metabolism
Propranolol	Masks tachycardia and tremor of alcoholic hypoglycemia	Beta-receptor blockade
Quinacrine	Similar to disulfiram reaction but milder	Inhibition of intermediary metabolism of alcohol
Salicylates	Gastrointestinal bleeding	Additive
Sulfonylureas	Decreased hypoglycemic effect with chronic alcohol abuse	Increased metabolism
	Increased hypoglycemic effect with ingestion of alcohol, particularly in fasting patients	Suppression of gluconeogenesis
	Reaction similar to disulfiram reaction but milder	Inhibition of intermediary metabolism of alcohol

(Modified from Medical Letter 23:34, 1981)

of 500 mg/dl is fatal in 50% of patients. Interestingly, although individuals who are heavy users of alcohol are able to perform difficult tasks at high blood–alcohol concentrations, the lethal dose of alcohol is similar for alcoholics and nonalcoholics.

Alcohol Idiosyncratic Intoxication

Certain individuals exhibit an atypical response to intoxication that is described in DSM-III as *alcohol idiosyncratic intoxication,* in which an individual exhibits uncharacteristic aggressive behavior after ingesting an amount of alcohol insufficient to produce intoxication in most individuals. The duration of the episode is usually brief, and the individual may not even recall the event. This condition is a relatively uncommon one, and there is some indication that it occurs more commonly in persons with brain damage.

Alcohol Withdrawal Syndromes

Sudden cessation of alcohol intake in an individual whose CNS has undergone prolonged continuous exposure to alcohol may produce symptoms of alcohol withdrawal. Alcohol withdrawal takes a number of forms, including uncomplicated withdrawal, withdrawal hallucinosis, withdrawal seizures, and withdrawal delirium.

Uncomplicated Withdrawal

Uncomplicated withdrawal usually has its onset within several hours after an individual who has been drinking steadily for some time reduces his alcohol intake. Malaise and tremor are experienced initially and are commonly accompanied by nausea and vomiting; the individual also exhibits signs of autonomic hyperactivity, such as diaphoresis, bounding pulse, and hypertension. Such patients are usually fully oriented and frequently exhibit grave concern about their physical condition. Symptoms reach their peak intensity in the first 24 hours following abstinence, but symptoms may persist for 3 or 4 days, and a sense of overalertness and malaise may last 1 or 2 weeks.

Assessment of affective status in the individual undergoing alcohol withdrawal is most difficult. The affect may be transiently anxious, irritable, or depressed, but following resolution of withdrawal symptoms, dramatic improvement is often made in these symptoms.

☐ A 58-year-old white woman was admitted to an inpatient ophthalmology service for cataract extraction. While on the ward her behavior became bizarre and her physicians requested psychiatric consultation. A psychiatric history revealed that the patient had been a long-time alcohol abuser, had had multiple alcohol-related hospital admissions, and had experienced delirium tremens at least once in the past.

On mental status examination the patient was dishevelled, uncooperative, and lying in a fetal position on her bed. Her affect was depressed and she had psychomotor retardation. She was oriented in all three spheres and her speech was distinct, but there was marked response latency. She denied auditory or visual hallucinations, and she rejected suicidal ideation. The psychiatrist diagnosed alcohol withdrawal and advised observation and treatment with benzodiazepines for symptoms of withdrawal. The following day the patient's affect was appropriate, she was spontaneous in her interactions, her psychomotor retardation had resolved, and she was requesting discharge.

The above case illustrates the difficulty in establishing a diagnosis of affective disorder in a person with alcohol withdrawal syndrome.

Alcoholic Hallucinosis

Alcoholic hallucinosis is a disorder involving the onset of vivid hallucinations following cessation of drinking; the sensorium, however, remains clear. Thus, while the individual complains of auditory, visual, or even tactile or olfactory hallucinations, he does not experience disorientation, impairment of memory, confusion, or impairment of consciousness. The patient's affect is appropriate to the content of the hallucinations.

Hallucinosis usually occurs in the first day or so following the cessation of alcohol use, with 85% of cases occurring within 6 days following abstinence. Sometimes a chronic hallucinosis evolves, in which the patient is unable to overcome the hallucinatory experience. The relationship between chronic alcoholic hallucinosis and schizophrenia is controversial, but these disorders appear to be distinct, hallucinosis having a much less clear hereditary contribution and an older age of onset.

Alcohol Withdrawal Seizures

Alcohol withdrawal seizures, sometimes known as "rum fits," are generalized tonic–clonic seizures that usually occur 7 to 48 hours following significant reduction in alcohol intake. Approximately one third of patients with withdrawal seizures develop delirium tremens (DT). The distinction between withdrawal seizures and seizures of another etiology is an important one since withdrawal seizures are not treated with antiseizure medication, as are seizure disorders. Particularly significant causes of seizures in alcohol abusers other than "rum fits" are post-traumatic seizures related to prior head injury and exacerbation of idiopathic epilepsy following the heavy use of alcohol.

Withdrawal Delirium

DT, described in DSM-III as *withdrawal delirium,* is a pathologic mental state associated with alcohol abuse and characterized by disorientation, clouding of sensorium, auditory and sometimes visual hallucinations, suggestibility, and frequently confabulation. It is accompanied by autonomic hyperactivity, including such symptoms as diaphoresis, tachycardia, pupillary dilatation, transient hypertension, and sometimes fever. DT occurs after a relative or absolute decrease in alcohol intake in chronic users of alcohol. Although DT occurs in less than 5% of patients hospitalized for treatment of alcohol withdrawal, it is the most serious of the withdrawal states. In older studies, the syndrome was associated with a mortality rate of 5% to 15%, although the current mortality rate for this disorder is probably lower given the advancements in the ability to diagnose and monitor severely ill individuals. Withdrawal seizures are unusual after the onset of DT, and the development of seizures in a patient with DT should prompt a careful search for a cause other than withdrawal.

☐ A 34-year-old construction worker was admitted to the orthopedic service of a general hospital with a complaint of back pain after a poorly constructed carport had collapsed on him. There was no history of loss of consciousness, paralysis, or paresis.

The physical examination as recorded by the orthopedics resident showed the patient to be alert and oriented, and to have normal blood pressure. Examination of the head, neck, chest, and abdomen was normal. The patient had lower back pain that did not radiate. His reflexes were symmetrical. Radiographs of the lumbar spine revealed fracture of the transverse spinal processes of L_1, L_2, and L_3.

On the third day of hospitalization, the patient had a grand mal seizure lasting 2 minutes and became combative in the postictal state. He was noted by the orthopedics resident to be uncooperative and disoriented to place and time. The patient became diaphoretic and tremulous and was noted to be very suggestible. Hallucinations were also noted. A history of heavy drinking and previous seizures was obtained. The patient was treated with sedatives and anticonvulsant medication and was discharged on the 7th day after admission.

A recent Danish study of DT found that the disorder occurred overwhelmingly in men, with a men-to-women ratio of 8 : 1. The mean age of DT patients was 46 years, the majority of patients falling between the ages of 40 and 59. The onset of symptoms occurred from 0 to 8 days following cessation of drinking, and one third of the patients diagnosed with DT had been previously admitted with the disorder.

Treatment of Withdrawal States

The management of uncomplicated alcohol withdrawal syndrome varies depending on the severity of the symptoms and the medical and social status of the individual involved. Withdrawal symptoms respond to a number of drugs for which cross tolerance with alcohol exists. A common practice is to administer a benzodiazepine to the patient. Benzodiazepines lessen the severity of withdrawal symptoms markedly and provide some prophylaxis against withdrawal seizures as well. Diazepam 10 mg every 6 hours or the dose equivalent of another benzodiazepine may be administered. The total daily dose should be reduced by 25% each day following control of withdrawal symptoms. On occasion, larger doses are necessary, but one must guard against oversedating the withdrawing patient, because oversedation masks mental status changes and is dangerous in certain physically impaired patients, such as those with severe lung disease. Older drugs such as barbiturates, paraldehyde, and chloral hydrate have been used to treat alcohol withdrawal, but these drugs are not as safe in higher doses as the benzodiazepines.

Since alcohol abusers frequently have underlying medical problems, a medi-

Indications for Hospitalization for Alcohol Withdrawal

Severe tremulousness or hallucinosis

Significant dehydration

Fever > 101

Documented seizure in a patient without a history of seizure disorder

Clouding of sensorium

Evidence of Wernike's encephalopathy (disturbance of consciousness and mentation, ataxia, and abnormalities of ocular movements)

Head trauma with a documented episode of unconsciousness

Present of major complicating or associated disease:

- Hepatic decompensation
- Respiratory failure
- Respiratory infection
- Gastrointestinal bleeding
- Pancreatitis
- Severe malnutrition

Known history of previous episodes of withdrawal that progressed to full-blown delirium, psychosis, or seizures if untreated

(Modified from Greenblatt D, Shader RI: Treatment of alcohol withdrawal syndrome. In Shader RI (ed): Manual of Psychiatric Therapeutics. Boston, Little, Brown, 1975)

cal history, physical examination, and indicated laboratory examination should be performed on withdrawing individuals who come to the attention of a physician. Although not always necessary, hospitalization is indicated in many cases of withdrawal (see Indications for Hospitalization for Alcohol Withdrawal). Thiamine (50 mg–100 mg intramuscularly [IM]) and daily multivitamins should be routinely given because their administration is attended by minimal risk, and they may prevent or arrest the development of certain neurologic syndromes described below.

Patients without a history of severe withdrawal and with no complicating medical illnesses have been managed successfully without medications with *social setting detoxification.* Such treatment requires the participation of a staff dedicated to the concept of social setting detoxification. This treatment should be offered only in selected cases.

Alcoholic hallucinosis may be treated by the administration of a high-potency neuroleptic; such as haloperidol 5 mg to 15 mg daily. Lower-potency neuroleptics should be avoided because of the risks of postural hypotension in a population already prone to falls and to compromised cardiovascular function. One should also be alert to the potential for the development of DT in hallucinosis patients.

There is no specific therapy for DT, and treatment is aimed toward managing complications of the syndrome, such as dehydration, infection, malnutrition, and seizures. General management involves providing the patient with enough sedation and physical restraint to ensure that he does not harm himself through injury or physical exhaustion. Diazepam 2.5 to 5 mg should be administered slowly, intravenously, every 5 minutes or so to obtain adequate sedation, with upward administration of the dose if adequate sedation has not been achieved after half an hour. Intravenous (IV) diazepam should be administered only when the patient can be placed under close medical supervision. Too-rapid IV administration of larger doses of this drug may cause respiratory or cardiac arrest.

Medical Implications of Alcohol Abuse

Neurologic Complications

Wernike's Encephalopathy

Wernike's encephalopathy is characterized by a triad of neurologic signs: disturbance of consciousness and mentation, ataxia, and abnormalities of ocular movements, although not all of these symptoms are present in every case. The disorder is caused by thiamine deficiency, and although it appears primarily in alcoholics (in this country) it is not peculiar to alcohol-dependent patients and may appear in anyone who is thiamine-deficient. Resolution of this condition may be followed by the appearance of Korsakoff's psychosis (described below); therefore, the term Wernike–Korsakoff's syndrome is commonly used to designate the combined disorder.

The disturbance of consciousness and mentation in Wernike's encephalopathy is characterized by confusion, apathy, lethargy, and impaired concentration. These features are not invariably present, and some 10% of patients with Wernike's encephalopathy do not have altered mental status.

Patients may exhibit the gait of cerebellar ataxia, characterized by a wide-based stationary position and an unsteady broad-based gait. The ataxia may vary in severity; sometimes it may be so prominent that the patient cannot walk, or it may only become evident on observing impaired tandem walking during the neurologic examination.

Impairment of ocular movements may be present, as sixth-nerve palsies, paralysis of conjugate gaze, and horizontal and sometimes vertical nystagmus. Any or all of these eye movement findings may be present in a particular individual.

The presence of Wernike's encephalopathy in a patient is a serious finding, and therapy with thiamine must be instituted immediately to facilitate the reversal of the disease as early in its course as possible. It is particularly important to initiate thiamine replacement therapy prior to the administration of intravenous glucose in any malnourished alcoholic patient who is to receive intravenous glucose therapy. Administration of glucose without thiamine may precipitate the Wernike's encephalopathy in previously asymptomatic thiamine-deficient patients. In patients with the disease, glucose may worsen the clinical picture. After thiamine replacement, a rapid improvement is generally made in the patient's condition. The mental symptoms generally clear within hours, followed by a more gradual resolution of ataxia and eye movement abnormalities.

Pathologically, this disorder is characterized by multiple sites of degenerative change in the brain. The mammillary nuclei of the hypothalamus are the most common brain regions to be affected in this disorder. Lesions frequently occur as well in the thalamus, other regions of the hypothalamus, the midbrain, the pons, the medulla, and occasionally the fornix.

Alcohol Amnestic Disorder

The term *alcohol amnestic disorder* is used in DSM-III to include the disorder known as *Korsakoff's psychosis*. Korsakoff's psychosis is not a psychosis in the modern sense of that term, but is rather a defect of memory involving impairment of the patient's ability to recall information from his past (retrograde amnesia) and an inability to learn new information (anterograde amnesia). In patients who have this disease, this memory defect is out of proportion to any other defect in mental functioning, and thought processes that do not rely on memory (*e.g.*, alertness, affect, attentiveness) remain relatively intact. Confabulation may or may not be present. The disease usually appears following the resolution of the disturbances of sensorium in Wernike's disease. Only about 20% of those exhibiting signs of the disease fully recover, although with adequate treatment the majority of patients eventually show improvement in memory.

Dementia Associated With Alcoholism

The notion that chronic alcohol use can lead to intellectual deterioration is a relatively old one. The idea that alcohol itself has a toxic effect on the brain, however, is one that has been controversial during the past four decades, because many researchers see the cognitive deficits in alcoholics as being secondary to other factors, such as Korsakoff's psychosis, trauma, or general nutritional deficiency. Nonetheless, in the past 10 years, a new appreciation has emerged of the direct toxic influence of chronic alcohol use on brain function and morphology. Alcoholic dementia, as opposed to Korsakoff's psychosis, is characterized by a general cognitive decline: Although some individuals demonstrate memory and intellectual deficits in the clinical mental status examination, other individuals reveal the neuropsychological characteristics of dementia only after careful psychological testing. A number of studies have demonstrated ventricular enlargement and cortical atrophy in patients with alcoholic dementia. With abstinence, the prognosis of this disorder is hopeful, and although patients seldom regain their full intellectual capacity, up to two thirds of patients improve, the bulk of the improvement occurring during the first 2 months following cessation of alcohol use.

Alcoholic Cerebellar Degeneration

Abnormality of gait and of movement coordination in the lower extremities is a relatively common finding among chronic alcohol abusers. The gait is typically broad-based and unsteady. Other evidence of cerebellar involvement, such as upper extremity tremor or dysarthria, may be seen later in the course of the disease. The condition results from atrophy of the cerebellar cortex in the region of the anterior portion of the vermis and of the anterior lobes of the cerebellum. The disorder may be the result of a nutritional deficiency.

Alcoholic Polyneuropathy

Alcoholic polyneuropathy, a relatively common condition (occurring in 9% of alcoholics studied by Maurice Victor in his Boston City Hospital series), may also be the result of nutritional deficiency. The severity of the condition varies considerably among patients; in some, it may be uncovered only by neurologic examination, but in others it is a recognized source of distress. Symptomatic patients complain of the insidious onset of weakness, tingling, or pain. Lower extremities are affected before upper extremities and distal portions of limbs before proximal. On examination, patients may reveal muscular atrophy in the affected extremities. Frequently, a loss or diminution of ankle and knee reflexes occurs. Sensory deficits of all types are also common. Provision of an adequate diet is the primary mode of treatment.

Alcohol–Tobacco Amblyopias

Alcohol–tobacco amblyopia is a condition in which alcohol-abusing or tobacco-abusing patients complain of blurred vision and have a bilateral decrease in visual acuity. The disorder is thought to be secondary to an optic nerve lesion, and it generally improves with better nutrition.

Marchiafava–Bignami Disease

Marchiafava–Bignami disease is a very rare disorder associated with alcohol abuse, that is characterized by degeneration of the central portion of the corpus callosum. The exact nature of the clinical syndrome associated with this pathologic finding is unclear, since many of the patients who have been diagnosed with the disease were in the terminal phase of alcoholism when they came to medical attention.

Central Pontine Myelinolysis

Central pontine myelinolysis is another uncommon condition seen in alcoholics that involves demyelinations of neurons in the central pons. It cannot generally be recognized as a distinct clinical entity during life.

Alcohol Abuse and the Heart

Alcohol has both acute and chronic effects on the heart. Acutely, alcohol acts as a myocardial depressant and reduces cardiac contractility. Since alcohol also increases heart rate and, in most patients, decreases peripheral vascular resistance, its myocardial depressant effect is frequently masked in younger individuals. In individuals with heart disease, however, even moderate amounts of alcohol present a threat to hemodynamic stability.

Alcoholic Cardiomyopathy

Chronic (more than 10 years) ingestion of large amounts of alcohol may lead to the development of alcoholic cardiomyopathy. This condition, resulting from the toxic effects of alcohol and its metabolites on the cardiac muscle, is characterized clinically by dyspnea on exertion, paroxysmal nocturnal dyspnea, palpitations, and edema. The onset usually occurs in middle age, although the disease may occur in much younger individuals. Improvement is associated with abstinence from alcohol.

Holiday Heart Syndrome

Heavy alcohol consumption may also produce cardiac arrhythmias. Transient arrhythmias may occur after heavy drinking, particularly in abusers. The condition is known as *holiday heart syndrome* because of its occurrence in affected individuals after holiday binges. Most commonly the rhythm disturbance is atrial fibrillation, but sinus tachycardia, paroxysmal atrial tachycardia, and paroxysmal ventricular contractions may also occur.

Alcohol and the Liver

Hepatic Steatosis

Hepatic steatosis or "fatty liver" is the most common alteration of liver morphology and function produced by alcohol abuse. This disease, which is not specific to alcohol but may appear in various conditions that produce liver insult, is characterized pathologically by the appearance of fat-containing vacuoles in hepatocytes. It usually occurs following a period of several weeks of heavy alcohol ingestion. Patients are often asymptomatic and have only hepatomegaly on clinical examination. More severe cases involve symptoms such as right upper quadrant tenderness, nausea, vomiting, and anorexia, and may be characterized by jaundice. Laboratory testing may reveal elevated serum glutamic-oxaloacetic transaminase values (SGOT) and serum glutamic-pyruvic transaminase (SGPT) values and decreased prothrombin time. With supportive care and abstinence from alcohol, these laboratory values return to normal.

Alcoholic Hepatitis

Alcoholic hepatitis, a potentially life-threatening development, occurs following years of heavy alcohol intake. Clinically, the disorder has a range of presentations, from relatively mild symptomatology to coma and death. Patients may develop fatigue, anorexia, right upper quadrant tenderness, hepatomegaly, jaundice, and ascites as well as leukocytosis and intermittent fever. SGOT and SGPT are elevated, as are, in most cases, alkaline phosphatase and bilirubin. Pathologically, one sees polymorphonuclear leukocytic infiltration into the liver parenchyma, ballooning of the hepatocytes, fat accumulation, and often hyaline bodies and focal lymphocytic infiltration.

Alcoholic Cirrhosis

Alcoholic cirrhosis, the fifth leading cause of death among men 25 to 64 years of age, was once thought to be a nutritional deficiency disease. Current evidence, however, indicates that this condition is the result of the toxic effect of alcohol on the liver. Clinically, the disease is manifested by anorexia, weakness, weight loss, jaundice, and hepatomegaly, although hepatomegaly disappears as the liver becomes progressively smaller and more sclerotic in the advanced stages of the disease. Other physical manifestations of liver dysfunction in cirrhosis are ascites, splenomegaly, and prominent venous collaterals (hemorrhoids, esophageal varices, and visible venous collaterals on the abdomen [caput medusa]), all secondary to portal hypertension. Incomplete hepatic degradation of estrogens results in the gynecomastia prominent in so many patients with advanced cirrhosis.

Pathologically, the liver becomes increasingly nodular and hard during the course of the disease. Fibrous tissue distorts the normal hepatic architecture, and total blood flow to the liver decreases. The five-year survival rate is 75% for uncomplicated cirrhosis and 40% for patients with ascites.

Pancreatitis

Pancreatitis is associated with alcoholism and several other medical conditions, particularly cholelithiasis. Patients with acute pancreatitis complain of severe abdominal pain, often radiating to the back, that may diminish when the patient leans forward. Nausea and vomiting are usually present. The patient frequently exhibits diffuse abdominal tenderness, although the tenderness may be localized to the epigastrium. Since other gastrointestinal disorders may present with similar symptoms, an elevated serum amylase determination, although not infallible, is the single most important laboratory test used to differentiate pancreatitis from other diseases with similar clinical presentation. Acute pancreatitis may be attended by hypotension, and severe cases are associated with a high mortality rate. The presence of the disease is cause for immediate hospitalization.

In chronic pancreatitis, attacks of pancreatitis are recurrent; the disease most frequently occurs in alcohol abusers of many years. The condition may result in diabetes and malabsorption as a result of compromised endocrine and exocrine function of the pancreas. Management of the disorder's chronic pain may become a particularly difficult problem to solve. Abstinence from alcohol may lead to clinical improvement.

Treatment of Alcoholism

The number of treatment modalities used to deal with alcohol abuse is very large. The degree to which some of these modalities address common problem areas is summarized in Table 13-2. Although no single psychiatric approach is appropriate for every case, the most effective approaches to alcohol treatment emphasize the role of the alcoholic in recovering from alcohol abuse, as well as the dangers of alcohol abuse, the availability of care givers in time of crisis, and the dignity of the individual alcohol abuser.

Treatment of alcoholism based on a contemporary medical understanding of the disorder generally incorporates a variety of approaches and may include individual supportive psychotherapy, group psychotherapy, family therapy, aversive drug therapy, and encouragement of participation by the patient and his family in lay-run groups, such as Alcoholics Anonymous (AA), Alanon, and Alateen. Only three of the most common elements in the clinical approach to the treatment of alcoholism will be discussed here.

Table 13-2
Degree of Focus of Community Treatment Programs on Particular Problem Areas

Community treatment program	Drinking behavior	Physical health	Work performance	Residential stability	Social deviancy
Pastoral services	+				+
Alcoholics Anonymous	+ +				+
Inpatient alcoholism therapy	+ +	+ +	+	+	+
Outpatient alcoholism therapy	+ +	+	+		+
Missions/shelters	+	+	+	+	
Halfway houses	+ +	+		+ +	
Psychiatric treatment	+	+	+		+
General hospitals		+ +			

(Modified from Shore JH, Kofoed L: The treatment of alcoholism in the community. In Gallanter M, Pattison EM (eds): Advances in the Psychosocial Treatment of Alcoholism. Washington, American Psychiatric Press, 1984).

Group Therapy

Group therapy is one of the most effective means of dealing with alcohol abuse. There are a number of different sorts of groups that can be used for the treatment of alcoholism, but the most commonly used group is Alcoholics Anonymous, a nonmedical organization that uses certain fairly stringent behavioral and quasi-religious principles to help the alcoholic become abstinent. Although a number of the assumptions of AA about the disease nature of alcoholism are no longer shared by the medical community, and although the organization's use of the concept that an individual must depend on a higher being for help in overcoming alcohol dependence is generally foreign to psychiatric treatment, the organization appears to be the most effective group treatment for alcoholism and therefore should not be neglected by the medical practitioner.

Pharmacologic Deterrence Therapy

Pharmacologic deterrence therapy may be a useful adjunct to other treatment modalities, but should only be used when a physician is actively involved in the care of the alcoholic patient. The most common agent used to produce physiologic aversion to alcohol is disulfiram (Antabuse). Disulfiram produces an adverse physiologic reaction to alcohol, thus deterring the patient from drinking. The drug alters the action of aldehyde dehydrogenase, thereby interrupting the second step in alcohol metabolism, that of the conversion of acetaldehyde to acetate. When alcohol is ingested, therefore, the patient experiences the toxic symptoms of acetaldehyde. The ingestion of even small amounts of alcohol may produce symptoms such as vasodilatation, headache, nausea, vomiting, diaphoresis, dyspnea, postural syncope, anxiety, and confusion. Rarely, fatalities have occurred.

Disulfiram is given to those patients who want to abstain from alcohol, but who are given to impulsive drinking. Its administration requires the cooperation of the patient. The usual dose is 500 mg daily for 5 days and then 250 mg daily for maintenance. Higher doses have been used in the past, but were associated with a higher incidence of undesirable effects. Patients should be thoroughly informed of the toxicity of the drug after consumption of alcohol and should sign a contract stating that they understand the potential adverse effects of the drug. They should also be given an Antabuse wallet card to notify emergency personnel that the patient is taking the drug, should a severe alcohol reaction occur. Antabuse, although effective in certain patients, is almost never of long-term value when used alone, and for that reason it should be used only in combination with other means of treatment.

Psychiatric Coordination of Treatment

A common approach of physicians to the treatment of alcoholism is to combine the use of more traditional psychiatric therapeutic modalities with an insistence that the patient presenting for treatment engage in AA as part of the overall plan of treatment. Like any large organization with numerous local branches, AA groups vary in quality from one local group to another. The physician who wishes seriously to undertake treatment for alcoholic patients should become as familiar as possible with the nature of the AA groups in his area.

Two additional factors about the treatment of alcoholism should be kept in mind. First, recovery from alcoholism may occur without intervention from the mental health community. In fact, there is an estimated 2% to 3% annual spontaneous recovery rate among alcoholics. Second, certain nontreatment factors appear to be important in the establishment of sustained abstinence in the alcohol abuser. As described by Vaillant in his 1983 study of alcoholism, some of these factors are:

- The discovery by the alcoholic of a "substitute dependency"
- The presence of external reminders of the deleterious nature of alcohol for the individual (disulfiram or a physical disease related to alcohol abuse)
- The availability of sincere, compassionate social support for the patient
- Involvement in a group offering the patient release from guilt and enhanced self-esteem (*e.g.*, the offering of a sense of personal redemption and group acceptance provided by some types of religious groups)

Thus, although the recovery from alcoholism is a difficult process, the prognosis for this disorder is not entirely dismal. With active concern on the part of the physician and a desire on the part of the affected individual to alter his destructive use of alcohol, there is hope for recovery from pathologic alcohol use.

Bibliography

Cutting J: Alcoholic dementia. In Benson F, Blumer D: Psychiatric Aspects of Neurological Disorder. New York: Grune and Stratton, 1982

Gallanter M, Pattison EM (eds): Advances in the Psychosocial Treatment of Alcoholism. Washington, American Psychiatric Press, 1984

Goodwin DW: Alcoholism and heredity: A review and hypothesis. Arch Gen Psychiatry 36:57–61, 1979
Greenblatt D, Shader RI: Treatment of alcohol withdrawal syndrome. In Shader RI (ed): Manual of Psychiatric Therapeutics. Boston, Little, Brown, 1975
Isselbacher KJ: Metabolic and hepatic effects of alcohol. N Engl J Med 296:612–616, 1977
Jaffe JH: Drug addiction and drug abuse. In Gilman AG, et al: The Pharmacological Basis of Therapeutics, 6th ed. New York, Macmillan, 1980
Jellinek EM: The Disease Concept of Alcoholism. New Haven, College and University Press, 1960
Leiber CS (ed) Medical Disorders of Alcoholism: Pathogenesis and Treatment. Philadelphia, WB Saunders, 1982
Lishman WA: Cerebral disorder in alcoholism: Syndromes of impairment. Brain 104:1–20, 1981
Noble E (ed): Third Special Report to the U.S. Congress on Alcohol and Health from the Secretary of Health Education and Welfare. Rockville, National Institute on Alcohol Abuse and Alcoholism, 1978
Ritchie JM: The aliphatic alcohols. In Gilman AG, et al: The Pharmacological Basis of Therapeutics, 6th ed. New York, Macmillan, 1980
Pattison EM, Kaufman E (eds): Encyclopedic Handbook of Alcoholism. New York, Gardner, 1982
Thompson WL: Management of alcohol withdrawal syndromes. Arch Int Med 138:278–283, 1978
Vaillant GE: The Natural History of Alcoholism. Cambridge, Harvard University Press, 1983
Victor M, Adams RD: The effect of alcohol on the nervous system. Research Publications, Association for Research in Nervous and Mental Disease 32:526–573, 1952
Victor M: Neurologic disorders due to alcoholism and malnutrition. In Baker AB, Baker LH (eds): Clinical Neurology. Philadelphia, Harper and Row, 1984

Anna L. Stout and John F. Steege

14 Normal Human Sexuality and Psychosexual Disorders

This chapter will provide an overview of human sexuality and sexual functioning from the perspectives of physiology, psychology, and clinical treatment. The following areas will be reviewed: (1) male and female sexual physiology, (2) classifications of psychosexual dysfunctions, (3) treatment of psychosexual dysfunctions, (4) homosexuality, and (5) paraphilias.

Male and Female Sexual Physiology

Following the historic precedent of Kinsey, Pomeroy, and Martin, William H. Masters and Virginia E. Johnson expanded our understanding of human sexual physiology by their direct observations of sexual response in the laboratory. Many other investigators have followed, continually adding new information to our understanding of the psychophysiology of sex. For clinical purposes, however, the essential description of sexual physiology remains as it was described by Masters and Johnson.

Reduced to its physiologic minima, sexual response can be described as consisting of (1) changes in muscle tension and (2) changes in blood flow. Sexual arousal, although far more subjective, often follows the same time course as the muscular and vascular changes.

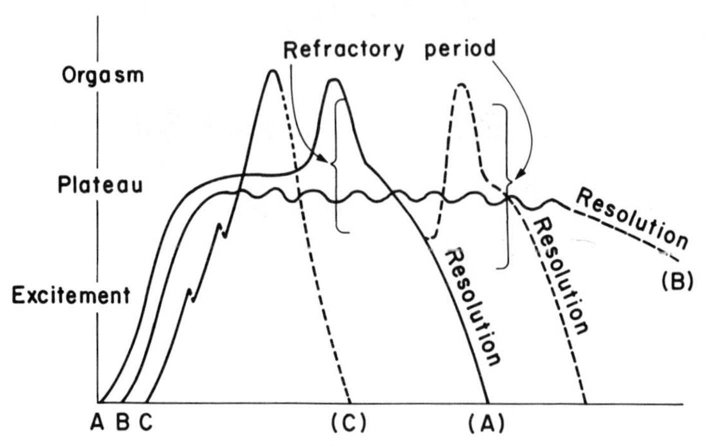

Figure 14-1. Male sexual response, including excitement, plateau, orgasm, and resolution phases. *Refractory period* is defined in the text. An individual man may experience any of these patterns during a particular sexual experience.

Masters and Johnson divided the sexual response cycle into four phases: excitement, plateau, orgasm, and resolution. We should recognize that these phases describe a continuum, and the boundary lines between them are often far from distinct. Nevertheless, they serve a useful framework for discussion.

Figures 14-1 and 14-2 describe these four phases in sequence. The abscissa of each graph does not contain time units, indicating that the duration of the sexual response cycle will vary dramatically among individuals, among different instances in the same individual, and over the course of a person's lifetime.

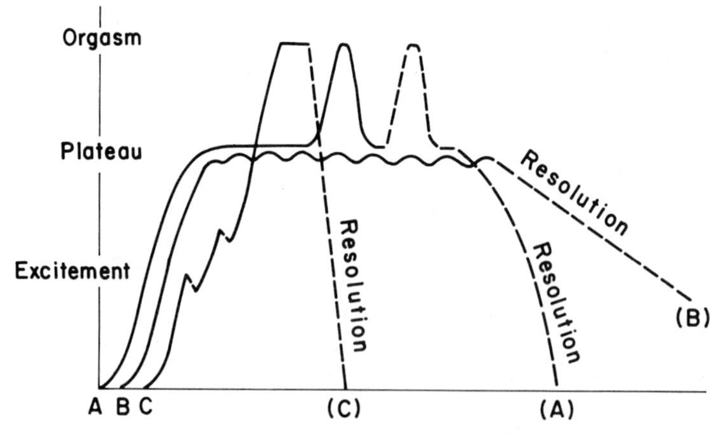

Figure 14-2. Female sexual response, including excitement, plateau, orgasm, and resolution phases. An individual woman may experience any of these patterns during a particular sexual experience.

When comparing the physiologic responses of men and women, one is struck by the frequent parallels between these responses. It would seem that many of the culturally accepted "differences" between the sexual responses of men and women may be superimposed by training and enculturation upon a common biological substrate. For example, Masters and Johnson discovered that under some circumstances women were capable of responding sexually in the laboratory just as quickly as men. The occasional differences in sexual response that do seem to exist between men and women will be pointed out in the following text, and even these are now subject to some question.

The Phases of the Sexual Response Cycle

Masters and Johnson's sexual response cycle phases will be discussed, comparing the responses of men and women during each of the phases. Some areas in which a misunderstanding of these response cycle phases may result in sexual miscommunication will also be pointed out.

Excitement Phase

Vasocongestion and a psychological feeling of sexual arousal are the major ingredients of this response phase. In the male, the first evidence of such vasocongestion is the filling of the corpus cavernosum following release of the *polsters* or vascular valves that control arterial supply to the penis (Fig. 14-3). In parallel fashion, the lubrication response occurring in the vaginal lining of the female seems to be the result of similar parasympathetic neurologic input. Masters and Johnson were the first to point out that the majority of vaginal lubrication is the result of the formation of a transudate through the vaginal walls and not the result of increased cervical mucus production or significant secretion by the greater vestibular (Bartholin's) glands. Although the presence of a beginning erection is obvious, often the vaginal lubrication may remain internal, depriving the woman and her partner of an observable physical cue to early arousal. This difference may lead both partners to perceive the female response as "slower."

Other evidence of vascular change during the excitement phase includes increases in testicular size in the male and congestion of the labia majora in the female. Muscle tension is evidenced by some increases in general myotonia throughout the body, as well as nipple erection in both male and female in about 60% of individuals, and scrotal elevation due to contraction of the cremaster muscle in the spermatic cord.

Many studies have been made of the erectile mechanism in men and are summarized in Figure 14-3. A sacral reflex erection can be produced even in the presence of a complete transection of the spinal cord in the lumbar region or at higher levels. Similar vasocongestive responses in neurologically impaired women have not been as extensively studied. In this situation, although vasocongestive responses may take place, no pleasurable genital sensations are perceived because of the interruption of the appropriate sensory tracts to the brain.

In a way that is similar to the increased myotonia of the scrotal sac, fine muscle fibers underlying the labia majora also contract and cause the vaginal introitus to widen late in the excitement phase. This response is much less prominent

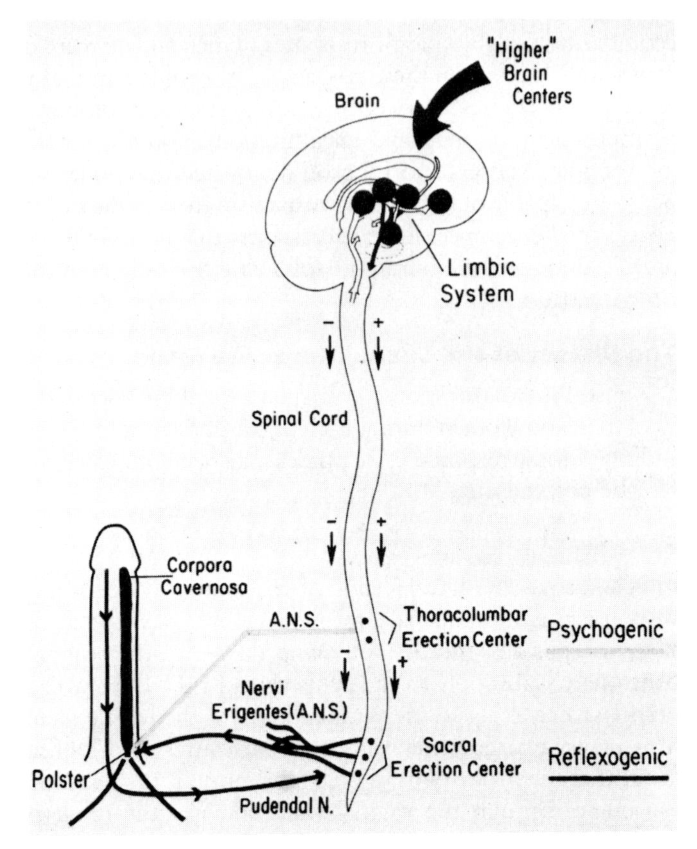

Figure 14-3. Psychophysiology of erection. Psychogenic stimuli, either facilitory (+) or inhibitory (−) may travel by way of either the thoracolumbar or sacral erection center to the polster valves. Reflexogenic erections involve only the sacral erection center.

after the vaginal delivery of a full-term child. A further vasocongestive response in the female is the increase in size of the labia minora.

Internal changes are more evident in the female than in the male. In women, the inner two thirds of the vagina will lengthen and distend, lengthening as much as 30% and nearly doubling in width at the apex. In the anteverted or midposition uterus, the uterus is elevated and the cervix therefore pulls away from the vagina. In the case of a retroverted uterus, vaginal expansion occurs along a more anteriorly directed axis, while the uterus remains in position occupying the cul-de-sac of Douglas.

Plateau Phase

Although the boundaries between the excitement and plateau phases are certainly indistinct, there are some changes that are peculiar to this latter phase. In terms of systemic changes, the *sex flush* described by Masters and Johnson, a "measles-like rash," may extend over the thorax and abdomen as well as the extremities late in excitement and throughout the plateau phase. This flush is present in perhaps 50% of individuals. Additional physiologic changes include hyperventilation and increased diffuse myotonia.

The genital changes also progress. In the male, the testicles increase further in size, reaching as much as a 50% increase over baseline. Cowper's gland secretions begin to collect in the posterior urethral bulb and be expelled through the distal urethra. These secretions may contain viable sperm. Vasocongestion of the corpus cavernosum increases further during this phase, allowing the penis to reach the fullest level of erection. Secretions from the seminal vesicle, containing sperm transported there by the vas deferens and secretions of the prostate gland (providing a nutrient environment for the maintenance and capacitation of sperm), accumulate in the posterior urethral bulb during the late plateau phase. As the end of plateau phase approaches, it is thought that the accumulated secretions in the urethral bulb, with this structure surrounded by perineal musculature, account for a psychologically perceived increase in sexual arousal. Ultimately, a point of *ejaculatory inevitability* is reached, or a point at which the response cycle would continue to orgasm even in the absence of further pleasurable stimulation. Masters and Johnson believed initially that this point of inevitability was unique to the male, and thus an example of one clear difference between male and female sexual physiology. However, a similar phenomenon has recently been speculated to exist in women.

In women, changes specific to the plateau phase include the development of an "orgasmic platform," or increasing vasocongestion and myotonia involving the mucosal lining of the outer third of the vagina and the surrounding musculature, providing a "grasping effect" upon the penis. Further vaginal expansion takes place and the uterus reaches a point of full elevation into the false pelvis.

Externally, late in the plateau phase, the clitoris in many women retracts beneath the clitoral hood, making it less accessible to direct stimulation. Since clitoral sensitivity increases dramatically during the plateau phase, sometimes to the point of discomfort, this retraction may provide a protective effect in some cases. The Bartholin's glands do secrete a small amount of fluid at this time, but again, this is unlikely to be a major portion of vaginal lubrication.

As diagramed in Figures 14-1 and 14-2, under response pattern B, both physiologic responses and a psychological sense of arousal may fluctuate during the plateau phase. This is especially true as people grow older, particularly in terms of fluctuating levels of erections. As described under Pattern C in Figures 14-1 and 14-2, both men and women are capable of completely bypassing a plateau phase and moving directly on to orgasm. This is a pattern most consistent with effective self-stimulation, since an individual is perhaps his or her own best feedback system regarding pleasurable sexual stimulation.

Orgasm Phase

Although the experience of the orgasm phase can certainly vary greatly at a psychological level, certain physiologic common denominators are present. Changes in muscle contraction are generally more prominent in this phase than changes in vascular congestion.

In the female the clitoris in general remains retracted under the clitoral hood. The urethral meatus may dilate, and in some women a small amount of urine may be emitted. There are no other characteristic external genital changes.

Internally, the uterus and vagina contract in a somewhat coordinated series of contractions beginning with an interval of 0.8 second and gradually spacing out in time as they continue for a total of 3 to 12 contractions. The contractions seem to travel in a wave from the fundus of the uterus down through the vaginal canal and including the musculature surrounding the vaginal introitus. In a strong contraction, the rectal sphincter may contract as well as the urethra. Recent investigations have suggested that there are many variations on this general pattern that may be reproducible from time to time in the same individual.

In the male, a very similar pattern of contractions occurs, again starting at a 0.8-second interval. The contractions involve the vas deferens, the seminal vesicles, the prostate and gland, the entire vulvar and penile urethra, and the rectal sphincter. The accumulated secretions previously described in the posterior urethral bulb are then expelled. Physiologically, the orgasm for men is often divided into the emission phase, which includes posterior urethral bulb filling, followed by the ejaculation phase, or the expulsion of semen through the urethra.

In both men and women, under normal circumstances, the bladder sphincter is closed by sympathetic input, making it impossible for a person to urinate during ejaculation. In cases of significant pelvic relaxation in women, this situation may be changed to the point that a significant volume of urine is expelled.

Recently, the possibility of a physiologic ejaculation for women has been raised. Several investigators have tried to film a female ejaculation, with results that to many observers look like the loss of urine rather than a unique fluid. Chemical assays of the ejected fluid have been described as being similar to prostatic secretions, but these results have not been repeated by other investigations. The same investigators have described the *Grafenberg spot.* Allegedly, this is an area along the anterior vaginal wall that appears during sexual response as a nodular and palpable area, which becomes the most sensitive area for sexual stimulation. While some writers have felt that this area may represent the female equivalent of the prostate gland, others have interpreted this to be an area of greater venous supply that becomes vasocongested during sexual response. This controversial "spot" is a current subject of investigation.

In the early 1970s, it became more widely known that women are capable of experiencing more than one orgasm in quick succession during the sexual response cycle. It is not yet known if this is a universal capacity of all women or the experience of a minority. Similarly, men seem to have the same potential, as diagramed in Figure 14-1. However, the male sexual response seems to include a refractory period during which a complete sexual response cycle is not physiologically possible. It is not clear whether the initial contractions experienced in a multiple male orgasm represent a complete orgasmic response or not. The refractory period increases in duration from several minutes or less during teenage years to as long as a day or several days in a person's seventh or eighth decade of life.

Resolution Phase

During resolution, the previously described changes in blood flow and muscle tension, as well as psychological feelings of sexual arousal gradually abate. In general, the psychological sense of arousal decreases first, followed soon thereafter with decreases in muscle tension. Vascular congestion may remain for longer periods of time, as evidenced by a gradually diminishing erection in the male and gradually diminishing pelvic sensations in the female. In men, the erections will first rapidly decrease to about a size roughly 50% larger than the resting state, and then return to the resting phase more slowly. The testicles decongest and return to baseline size, and the muscular fibers of the scrotum relax and together with relaxation of the cremaster muscle, allow descent of the testicle. In both men and women nipple erection disappears and the sex flush on the skin ebbs.

In the female pelvis, during resolution the orgasmic platform disappears, the vagina returns to its resting length, the cervix descends into the vaginal pool, and the uterus returns to its resting position in the true pelvis. It is not known whether the descent of the cervix into the vaginal pool has a specific function in promoting fertility.

In general, a prolonged resolution phase accompanies a cycle that has a longer excitement phase. Conversely, as demonstrated on curve C of Figures 14-1 and 14-2, a rapid excitement and orgasm phase is accompanied by a rapid resolution phase.

In both men and women, various symptoms have been ascribed to the failure to experience orgasm during a sexual response cycle. In men, congestion of the testicles and the prostate, colloquially called "blue balls," is alleged to be uncomfortable. The severity of this symptom is often overplayed, and there is no convincing evidence that the experience has any detrimental effect on libido, hormone production, or sperm viability. From a physiologic perspective, the female equivalent might be thought to be the pelvic congestion syndrome, which is described as persistent vasocongestion resulting in sexual arousal in the absence of orgasm. This syndrome is also said to occur as a nonspecific anxiety reaction, and has been the subject of much controversial discussion in the gynecologic literature in the last 40 years. The duration of pelvic aching and discomfort attributed to pelvic congestion syndrome has been described as lasting from several hours to several days in severe cases. In a way that is similar to that described for men, there has been no documented long-term effect of this phenomenon on fertility, and no known endocrinologic aberration has been connected with it.

Summary

The physiologic changes described in this section might usefully be thought of as the "bare bones" skeleton of human sexuality. The warmth, depth, and final form of the sexual experience are provided by the myriad elements of interpersonal communication, emotional sharing, and the development of intimacy. Although misunderstandings of physiology can contribute to sexual dysfunction, the most complete knowledge of sexual physiology is certainly no sure protection against difficulties in developing an emotionally and physically satisfying sexual relationship.

Classifications of Psychosexual Dysfunctions

The meaning of the term *sexual dysfunction* has changed over time and is greatly influenced by cultural and individual standards. For example, the ability to ejaculate quickly may have been regarded as desirable at one time from a biological perspective; whereas ejaculating too quickly was the most frequently reported "sexual dysfunction" reported by males in several surveys conducted in the late 1970s. Masters and Johnson in the early 1970s referred to women who did not experience orgasm through intercourse alone as dysfunctional; however, a number of subsequent surveys indicated that this condition may be so characteristic as to approach statistical normality. Any classification system of sexual dysfunctions implies some concept of normal sexual functioning that is based on societal expectations for a particular individual in a particular situation.

Historically, the two most frequently used classification systems for sexual dysfunction have been the systems of Masters and Johnson and Helen Singer Kaplan. Both systems designate dysfunctions as disruptions in the normal physiologic sequence of sexual response. The original Masters and Johnson model of the sexual response cycle started with the phase characterized by the physiologic markers of sexual excitement. Kaplan's model includes a desire phase that precedes the stage of physiologic arousal. Masters and Johnson refer to desire-phase problems as problems in initiating behavior rather than as sexual dysfunctions. Figure 14-4 illustrates how the two classification systems overlap.

At this time, the classification system of Helen Singer Kaplan appears to be the most comprehensive, and it has been adapted for inclusion in the *Diagnostic and Statistical Manual of Mental Disorders*, 3rd ed (DSM-III). The DSM-III defines psychosexual dysfunction as inhibition in the appetitive or psychophysiologic changes that characterize the complete sexual response cycle. A diagnosis of psychosexual dysfunction is not made if the specific complaint can be attributed entirely to organic factors, such as a physical disorder or a medication, or if it is an associated symptom of another mental disorder, such as clinical depression. The following classifications of psychosexual disorders are based on the criteria outlined in DSM-III.

Inhibited Sexual Desire

The diagnostic label of *inhibited sexual desire* refers to a persistent and pervasive condition that includes absence of fantasy, absence of initiating behaviors, or absence of physiologic arousal in the presence of sexual stimulation that is judged to be adequate. Females have sought treatment for this condition with greater frequency than males, but the condition can occur in both sexes.

Kaplan (1979) has offered the most extensive description of individuals experiencing inhibited sexual desire. In the group she studied by way of in-depth interviews, the lack of interest reported by the patient did not appear to reflect the complete absence of sexual desire, but to be related to a process in which the

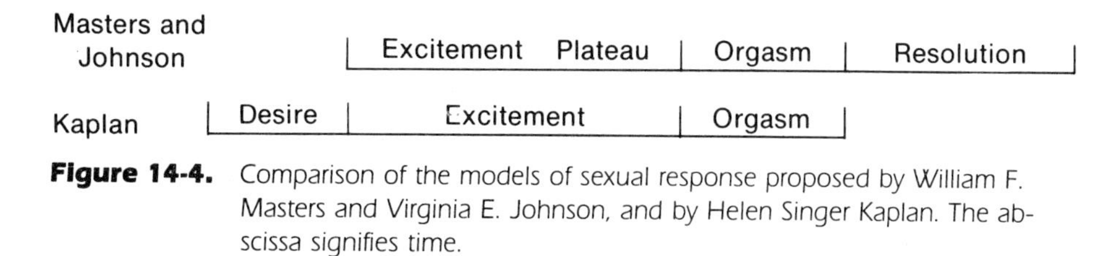

Figure 14-4. Comparison of the models of sexual response proposed by William F. Masters and Virginia E. Johnson, and by Helen Singer Kaplan. The abscissa signifies time.

individual "turns off" any sexual sensation. This suppression of sexual feelings is not an act of which the individual is thought to be actively aware, but may serve to reduce the negative feelings associated with sexual activity, such as fears of intimacy or commitment. An individual might also suppress sexual feelings because of issues related to the relationship; for example, a person harboring intense anger toward a partner understandably perceives the physical act of "making love" as incongruent with their feelings toward their partner. Reports exist of women who experience normal excitement or orgasmic phases when engaging in sexual activity despite the absence of sexual desire; however, the more usual case is for impairment in the desire phase to result in disruption of the sequence of excitement and orgasm.

Inhibited Sexual Excitement

Excitement phase disorders are defined by DSM-III criteria on a physiologic basis. In men, disruptions in this phase of the sexual response sequence are exhibited by the partial or complete failure to attain an erection or maintain an erection until orgasm, during sexual activity that is judged to provide adequate stimulation.

Before a psychosexual diagnosis is applied to the problem of inhibited sexual excitement, a thorough evaluation must determine that the disruption in the sexual response cycle does not appear to be due to organic factors such as diabetes, circulatory problems, or medications. A detailed behavioral assessment interview is essential to delineating possible etiology. A specific description of the erectile difficulty must be obtained. For example, Is the man unable to attain an erection? Can he attain an erection, but not maintain it long enough for intercourse to be initiated or completed? Can he only achieve partial erections? It is also important diagnostically to investigate situational determinants of the erectile difficulty. Does the problem occur with all partners? Is he able to achieve an erection under any conditions such as self-stimulation or erotic fantasy? Is he aware of experiencing nocturnal or early morning erections?

The presence of normal erections at any time, provides reassurance that the sexual physiology is intact without having to pursue extensive evaluation of organic factors, such as on awakening or with self-stimulation. The patient's lack of an awareness of normal erections does not mean, however, that his erectile difficulties are organically based. If a diagnostic interview fails to establish the occurrence of normal erections on any occasion, further evaluation by means of nocturnal penile tumescence (NPT) monitoring is valuable in the differentiation of organic and psychogenic factors. NPT monitors nocturnal erections that occur in association with rapid eye movement (REM) sleep in the normally functioning male. Negative psychological factors are presumably at a minimum under sleep conditions; however, there is some evidence that nocturnal erections may be affected by depression and severe stress.

Although the percentage of cases of erectile difficulty identified as having an organic component has increased with advances in the technology used for assessment, psychogenic factors remain the most common cause of erectile dysfunction, particularly in males under age 40. These psychogenic factors are frequently related to emotional factors operating in current sexual situations, particularly excessive anxiety about performance.

In women, inhibited sexual excitement is marked by the partial or complete failure to attain or maintain the lubrication–swelling response of sexual excitement while engaging in sexual activity that is judged to be adequate in focus, intensity and duration. To meet the criteria for this diagnostic label, the woman also must be judged to have adequate sexual desire. Relatively few cases of inhibited sexual excitement on a psychogenic basis have been reported in women. Psychophysiologic assessment of female sexual function has lagged far behind advances in the evaluation of male functioning, and no reliable indicator of female organic competency exists, although several methods of attempting to measure vaginal vasodilation are currently being investigated. Most cases of inadequate excitement phase response in the presence of adequate sexual desire appear to be related to estrogen deficiency, as in the case of menopausal or breast-feeding women. Participation in painful coitus associated with inadequate lubrication can, however, lead to secondary loss of sexual desire.

Inhibited Male Orgasm

In the male, inhibited orgasm is defined as a delay in or absence of ejaculation following an adequate phase of sexual excitement. This particular symptom can range in severity from those cases in which the man has never been able to ejaculate under any condition, to cases in which ejaculation is absent with specific conditions or particular partners. Lifelong absence of ejaculation is rare and usually appears to be related to psychogenic factors.

Ejaculation problems that develop after a period of adequate functioning have a greater risk of organicity, and a thorough medical evaluation is required because several medications and diseases can effect ejaculation. A differential diagnosis needs to be made between *retrograde ejaculation,* a condition in which semen is deposited in the urinary bladder rather than emitted from the penis, and *anejaculatory orgasm,* a condition in which normal orgastic contractions are experienced without the release of fluid. Retrograde ejaculation and anejaculatory orgasm are considered to be organic rather than psychosexual disorders.

Premature Ejaculation

The most commonly occurring sexual difficulty related to the orgasm phase in the male appears to be premature ejaculation. The DSM-III defines premature ejaculation as the condition in which ejaculation occurs before the individual wishes it, because of recurrent and persistent absence of reasonable voluntary control. Alternative attempts to define premature ejaculation have attempted to establish an adequate time interval between intromission and ejaculation, or sought to describe a percentage based on the number of times an erection is maintained long enough for a female partner to reach orgasm. Partly because of the obvious difficulties in applying these definitions, most diagnosticians have focused on the element of lack of control as the more meaningful description of the problem and as an appropriate target for treatment approaches. The causes of premature ejaculation are almost always psychogenic and are most commonly associated with anxiety or a deficit in the ability to recognize the physical sensations progressing to orgasm prior to the point of ejaculatory inevitability.

Inhibited Female Orgasm

Disorders of inhibited female orgasm are similarly defined by DSM-III as recurrent and persistent inhibition of the female orgasm following a normal sexual excitement phase during sexual activity that is judged by the clinician to be adequate in focus, intensity, and duration. Some women are able to experience orgasm during noncoital clitoral stimulation, but are unable to experience it during coitus in the absence of manual clitoral stimulation. There is evidence to suggest that in some instances this condition represents a pathologic inhibition that justifies this diagnosis, whereas in other instances it represents a normal variation of the female sexual response. It should be noted that the application of this diagnostic label assumes that responses of the desire and excitement phases are intact. Many loving and caring women report an enjoyable sexual relationship even though an orgasmic response is difficult or impossible to achieve.

Description of inhibited female orgasm as lifelong or acquired appears to be a meaningful distinction for treatment purposes. Studies suggest that couples in which the female develops inhibited orgasm after a period of normal functioning have greater marital distress than couples in which the female has never experienced an orgasmic response. Andersen (1983), in reviewing the literature related to orgasmic inadequacy, concluded that no personality variable appeared to be related to it except perhaps for marital "happiness." Hoon and Hoon (1978) contrasted groups of women with high and low orgasmic consistency and found that women with the lowest frequency had less frequent coitus and masturbation, found gently seductive rather than explicit activities more arousing, and were less aware of the physiologic changes accompanying sexual arousal.

Functional Vaginismus

The diagnostic label of *functional vaginismus* is applied when there is a history of recurrent and persistent involuntary spasm of the muscles of the outer third of the vagina that interferes with coitus. The condition may be situation-specific; for example, it may be present during sexual activity but not during a pelvic exam or vice versa. Functional vaginismus includes a continuum of symptoms that may range in severity from the case of the unconsummated marriage in which penetration is impossible to cases in which intercourse is possible but painful. The condition of vaginismus may arise from a natural protective reflex to pain originating from organic factors or from psychosocial factors. Repeated episodes of painful intercourse may produce a conditioned response so that even if the original precipitating cause heals spontaneously or is eliminated by proper medical treatment, the vaginismus may remain. Psychosocial factors associated with vaginismus include negative childhood conditioning to sexual activity and past history of physically or psychologically painful sexual experiences.

Functional Dyspareunia

Functional dyspareunia refers to the condition in either males or females in which coitus is associated with recurrent and persistent genital pain that cannot be exclusively attributed to a physical disorder, lack of lubrication, or functional vaginismus. Since many disease states can be associated with dyspareunia in both the male and female, a complete medical evaluation by a physician who is aware of the specific sexual concern in essential.

Treatment of Psychosexual Dysfunction

The publication of *Human Sexual Inadequacy* by Masters and Johnson in 1970 changed the approach to the treatment of psychosexual dysfunctions. Until then, psychosexual dysfunctions had been primarily conceptualized within a psychoanalytic framework that had been formulated at a time when much information about sexual physiology was lacking. Psychoanalytic and psychodynamic theorists viewed the treatment of psychosexual dysfunctions as lengthy and as having a relatively poor prognosis. Masters and Johnson introduced treatment techniques similar to approaches of behavior and social learning and began reporting much-improved success rates with relatively brief interventions.

It should be kept in mind that the patients accepted for treatment by Masters and Johnson were well screened and that the success of any of the specific treatment approaches depends on accurate assessment of the problem. Psychosexual dysfunctions occur within the context of a relationship, and assessment of the quality of that relationship is important because working on sexual difficulties requires a lot of cooperation and support.

A common feature of the therapy is the assignment of graduated tasks for couples or individuals to perform in the privacy of their own home. In general, treatment approaches to psychosexual dysfunctions are of two types: those aimed at treatment of an anxiety component of a psychosexual dysfunction and those directed at treatment of a skills deficit.

Sensate focus is a particular technique aimed at anxiety reduction that was introduced by Masters and Johnson in 1970. This particular technique is one of the most widely used in the field of sex therapy. Although Masters and Johnson did not explain their program on the basis of behavioral principles, their instructions for sensate focus strongly resemble *in vivo* desensitization procedures introduced by Joseph Wolpe. Sensate focus procedures include a temporary prohibition of sexual intercourse, which reduces the pressures to perform and allows natural sexual responsivity to emerge through instructions to enhance sensory awareness. Sensate focus exercises usually begin with nongenital massage and gradually progress to include genital stimulation exercises.

The focus of sensate focus exercises is on maximizing a relaxed, sensual interaction between partners. Couples with any type of sexual distress have frequently reduced any type of sexual contact to a minimum, and sensate focus exercises provide opportunities for relearning ways of relating sexually without demands for performance. The homework assignments of sensate focus serve as a model for exploring the interactions of the relationship so that difficulties couples have in completing the assignments are also productive for therapy.

In some cases of psychosexual dysfunction, it appears that a significant component of the problem may be a skills deficit. In addition to providing educational materials regarding sexuality, patients are frequently assigned a self-stimulation program to help them learn more about their own sexual responses. This information can them be shared with a partner during transition exercises if the patient desires.

Inhibited Sexual Desire

Empirical research in the area of inhibited sexual desire is limited; however, it is generally agreed that individuals in this category generally require longer treatment dealing with broader issues than sexuality and more issues from their past history. The treatment approach may also focus on helping the individual broaden his view of what is "sexual" and interrupting the performance-anxiety-avoidance cycle that is frequently an important part of inhibited sexual desire.

Inhibited Sexual Excitement (Male)

The primary goals in the treatment of psychogenic erectile dysfunction are decreasing performance anxiety, increasing stimulation, and restoring confidence. Zilbergeld (1978) outlines a treatment of erectile difficulties. Performance anxiety is decreased by instructions for a temporary prohibition of intercourse and de-emphasis on intercourse as the only pleasurable and satisfying way to relate sexually. Training is provided in refusal skills and the man is instructed not to attempt intercourse if he is not feeling aroused. Frequently, some cognitive restructuring may be needed to address myths, such as the idea that a man should be able to get an erection at any time under any condition. Sensate focus exercises and instructions to maximize awareness of physical sensations may be used to increase stimulation. Self-stimulation stop–start techniques for practice in losing and regaining erections can be assigned to help restore confidence.

Inhibited Sexual Excitement (Female)

Isolated disruption of the excited phase in the female related to psychogenic causes is unusual. For those cases in which an anxiety component can be identified, the sensate focus exercises may be helpful.

Inhibited Male Orgasm

The behavioral treatment approach for inhibited ejaculation involves a pattern of gradually shaping ejaculatory behavior, beginning with a condition in which ejaculation is likely to occur. The male with this psychosexual difficulty might be initially instructed to engage in self-stimulation alone to ejaculation (if he has been successful in that in the past), and a successive approximation procedure is used until he can ejaculate in his partner's presence. Partner stimulation may then be introduced and ejaculation shaped closer and closer to the vaginal entrance and then entry. Some suggestions concerning physiologic triggers that facilitate orgasm may also be helpful.

Premature Ejaculation

Following the DSM-III definition of premature ejaculation as the absence of voluntary control over ejaculation, most behavioral treatment techniques focus on fostering an increase in ejaculatory control through assisting the male to concentrate more fully on his preorgasmic sensations. One such approach is the stop–start or pause technique originated by Semans (1956). The female is instructed to stimulate her partner's penis manually until the male signals the physical sensations immediately preceding orgasm. At that point, stimulation is stopped until sensations subside. The sequence is repeated again and again until the male begins to develop ejaculatory control. The male is instructed to avoid any attempts at active control over ejaculation other than stopping stimulation at the proper time. The technique is then repeated with the addition of conditions that approximate intravaginal sensations. When the transition to intercourse is made, intercourse is recommended with the female above, with the male controlling movement. In some cases, stop–start techniques may be preliminarily applied with self-stimulation.

Masters and Johnson originated a modification of the stop–start technique in which the female partner places firm pressure with her thumb and first, second, and third fingers where the head and shaft of the penis join. This procedure, known as the "squeeze" technique, is applied in the same manner as the stop–start technique, and reduces ejaculatory tension.

Inhibited Female Orgasm

The empirical data to date indicates that the differentiation between lifelong or primary inorgasmia and situational or secondary inorgasmia is important for treatment purposes.

Self-stimulation or masturbation retraining are most effective for women who have not previously experienced orgasm and may have a skill deficit. Systematic desensitization, usually in the form of sensate focus, appears to be most effective when anxiety seems to be a component in secondary orgasmic dysfunction. In many cases, a combination of the two may be necessary. For example, a woman presenting with lifelong nonorgasmia may need sensate focus procedures to decrease anxiety, as well as the masturbation retraining techniques to learn about her own response patterns.

Relationship factors are more likely to affect secondary dysfunction, so often the inclusion of general relationship counseling or communication training is required. Educational material is useful with certain types of clients and may be a valuable component of therapy that might facilitate use of a therapist's time.

Functional Vaginismus

Treatment of vaginismus begins with the understanding that the condition is an involuntary reflex that is not currently under the woman's control. Firm rules are established with the patient and partner regarding terminating sexual activity with the occurrence of pain in order to provide the woman with an increased sense of control. The woman is then instructed in vaginal relaxation exercises using digital or dilator feedback. Transition is then made to doing the exercise in the presence of the partner or with the partner participating. When the woman feels comfortable, sexual intercourse may be resumed with instructions providing the woman with maximal control of the situation.

Functional Dyspareunia

The most common source of functional dyspareunia in the female is associated with attempts to engage in sexual intercourse without adequate arousal. Proceeding with sexual intercourse without physiologic arousal usually results in reports of vaginal irritation associated with inadequate lubrication. Reports of discomfort described as if "something is being bumped or hit" are frequently associated with penetration prior to the physiologic response of vaginal expansion and uterine elevation. In such cases, training in communication and refusal skills in combination with instructions not to engage in sexual intercourse without sexual arousal are appropriate. Sensate focus assignments are also beneficial in decreasing anxiety and enhancing stimulation that may increase arousal.

Reports of treatment of functional dyspareunia in males are too few to summarize a general therapeutic approach.

Homosexuality

An understanding of homosexual preference and behavior is an important facet of sexual medicine that will impinge upon the practices of the vast majority of physicians. This section will discuss the definition of homosexuality from several perspectives, as well as levels of sexual interest, sexual repertoire, and sexual problems encountered in homosexual men and women.

Many of the issues involved in homosexuality begin and end with the discussion of its definition. The American Psychiatric Association in 1980 brought this discussion to the greater attention of the public by omitting homosexuality from the DSM-III. This action was of course applauded by groups interested in gay rights and roundly condemned by many in religious and conservative circles. Although many groups view the question from a very straightforward perspective, it becomes very complicated when one considers exactly which behaviors one defines as homosexual.

Kinsey used a six-point scale to measure homosexual behaviors and homosexual feelings. The range of feelings and behaviors was graded from *0* for exclusively heterosexual to *6* for excusively homosexual. The various gradations in between describe large numbers of men and women who experience both homosexual and heterosexual feelings and may indulge in behaviors typical of both orientations. Kinsey estimated that approximately 10% of men and perhaps 5% of women would identify themselves as exclusively homosexual, but that the percentages occupying other places on the continuum are largely unknown. They observed that homosexual behaviors may be more common in younger individuals but may later be curtailed by a variety of social factors. Nevertheless, homosexual feelings may still persist despite the absence of overt behaviors in expressing these feelings.

A variety of other approaches to the definition of homosexuality have been employed, such as cultural stereotypes, biochemical differences, developmental differences, and the association of homosexual behavior with various forms of psychopathology. We will review each of these approaches briefly.

Bell and Weinberg's study is perhaps the most complete research project that describes the cultural stereotypes applied to homosexuality. Although the effeminate male and the "butch" or masculine female are glaring examples of stereotypes applied to homosexuals, many other more subtle stereotypes are widely held. For example, the stereotype that homosexual men are more prevalent among hairdressers, interior decorators, and ballet dancers is well known. Bell's detailed study pointed out very clearly that although examples of these stereotypes exist, the great majority of men and women with homosexual preferences are scattered among the many occupations and social roles in society. The stereotypic descriptions therefore provide only a caricature of homosexual expression.

Many researchers have explored the possibility that hormonal or chemical differences may explain homosexual expression. The underlying theme of this research is that a chemical "abnormality" may explain "abnormal" behavior. Although the research has been exhaustive, no clear consensus has emerged concerning any underlying biochemical difference between homosexual and heterosexual men and women. The occasional studies showing alterations of testosterone level or testosterone response to a variety of stimuli in homosexual men have been hampered by difficulties with subject selection and have been unable to answer the question of whether these changes are a primary chemical change leading to homosexual behavior or whether the prolonged experience of a homosexual lifestyle may modulate steroid hormone responses to heterosexual stimuli. From a clinical perspective, the search for hormonal changes to explain homosexual behavior, or the treatment of homosexual men and women with various hormonal preparations with the aim of eliminating homosexual behavior or converting it to heterosexual behavior is in general a useless enterprise.

Similarly exhaustive studies have been made of homosexuality from a psychological and developmental perspective. Bell points out that many of these studies are difficult to interpret because they tend to predominantly include homosexual individuals who have come to the attention of various helping agencies because their homosexuality has caused significant difficulty in their lives. It is therefore difficult to assess the role that homosexual preference plays in an individual psychopathology, as opposed to the role that cultural pressures and restrictions may play in promoting psychopathologic behavior and adjustment.

The Personal Definition of Homosexuality

Perhaps more important than the above considerations for the individual experiencing strong homosexual feelings, is the question of whether or not he or she chooses to define himself or herself as homosexual. While there are some instances in which a person wishes to make a radical feminist political statement by choosing homosexual expression and explicitly condemning heterosexual interaction, for the majority of individuals declaring homosexuality, or "coming out" as homosexual, the choice is an intensely personal one. A person making this choice is usually painfully aware of the many consequences and does so with only the greatest fear and trepidation.

On the positive side, many homosexual men and women find the coming-out experience a liberating one, reporting that they feel much more honest with themselves and with the people close to them. They find this feeling helpful in their efforts to maintain their personal relationships and their sexual lives in the face of continuous prejudice and opposition from most of society.

The next several sections will briefly describe some sexual aspects of homosexuality as described in the research literature.

Levels of Interest

It should come as no surprise that the level of sexual interest expressed by homosexual men and women, especially as described in Bell's studies, shows just as much variation as the level of heterosexual interest shown by heterosexual individuals and couples. A fraction of the homosexual world does conform to the stereotype of experiencing only multiple, fleeting, and emotionally uninvolved relationships. In general, Bell found this to be more prevalent among homosexual men than among homosexual women. He interpreted this pattern as being a response to the intense negative pressure put on homosexuals by a largely heterosexual society, but also acknowledged that this pattern of desperate searching for sexual experience may be an outgrowth of frustrations and lack of fulfillment in the professional and interpersonal lives of homosexuals. Certainly, a pattern of frenetic sexual behavior is not unknown in heterosexuals experiencing similar difficulties in developing intimate relationships and enjoying professional satisfaction.

At the opposite end of the interest scale, Bell points out that depression and anxiety aggravated by societal pressures may cause a decline in sexual interest. Again, this situation has its clear parallels in the lives of heterosexuals.

Sexual Repertoire

Bell's studies also described in some detail the preferred patterns of sexual expression employed among homosexuals. He reported that homosexual men most frequently begin with a pattern of mutual manual masturbation and go on to include fellatio. A minority come to include anal intercourse. However, he pointed out that the stereotypic description of "inserter" and "insertee" patterns is naive. Most men employing anal intercourse in their homosexual activity will enjoy either role at various times. In men experiencing both homosexual and heterosexual feelings, however, some who will act only in the inserter role maintain this preference in order to describe their behavior as involving a masculine role and therefore not really homosexual.

Bell's studies of female homosexuals revealed that the majority employ cunnilingus and mutual manual masturbation as their preferred sexual expressions, with a smaller percentage employing tribadism, or face-to-face genital contact in the fashion of simulated intercourse. An even smaller minority employ the use of penis substitutes or dildos in their sexual contacts.

Although he makes no claims for statistical validity, Bell's impression from his studies was that homosexual couples employing a relatively limited sexual repertoire also tended to have less emotionally intimate relationships. In evaluating the individual person, however, it would seem prudent to avoid applying this impression, as it may be simply another limiting stereotype.

Sexual Problems Experienced By Homosexuals

To the largely heterosexual society, which on occasion may view homosexuals as being "oversexed", it may come as a surprise that homosexual men and women experience all the levels of sexual interest, as well as all the physiologic varieties of sexual dysfunction that are experienced by heterosexuals. Following their studies of heterosexual difficulties, Masters and Johnson embarked on an ambitious study of the physiologic responses in homosexual interactions, as well as a study of the treatment of sexual dysfunction among homosexuals. The Masters and Johnson group very clearly established that the physiologic aspects of both male and female genital sexual response are identical, whether the sexual object choice is homosexual or heterosexual.

In their study of sexual dysfunction among homosexuals, Masters and Johnson defined successful homosexual function in terms of the individual's facility to respond to masturbation, partner manipulation, and fellatio/cunnilingus. Since anal penetration was a less frequent part of the desired repertoire, it was omitted from the definition of effective homosexual functioning. Just as in heterosexual dysfunction, erectile dysfunction was labeled as primary or secondary, and as situational or complete. In contrast to heterosexual dysfunction, the problem of premature ejaculation was not seen as an important one in the homosexual couples in Masters and Johnson's survey. They interpreted this as being due to the fact that neither man is dependent upon the other's ejaculatory control to achieve sexual satisfaction. Masters and Johnson's study did not include any experience with men who were unable to ejaculate in their sexual encounters. In working with 81 homosexual couples over a 10-year period, Masters and Johnson were able to resolve sexual dysfunction in approximately 75% of the cases, an overall result that is roughly parallel to their success figures in treating heterosexual dysfunction.

Masters and Johnson also treated a group of 54 men and 13 women who were dissatisfied with their homosexual feelings. Using a male–female cotherapy team in a 2-week intensive treatment format similar to that used for treating heterosexual dysfunction, approximately 65% of those treated succeeded in converting to exclusive heterosexuality. The applicability of these results to the general homosexual population is limited by the fact that couples were accepted only if they had either a committed or casual partner willing to cooperate with therapy.

Bell cautions that one must not interpret sexual difficulties as diagnostic of dissatisfaction with sexual preference. He notes that it would usually be erroneous to interpret dysfunction in a heterosexual setting as indicative of dissatisfaction with heterosexual orientation. Bell rather poignantly describes some of the ironies involved in homosexual relationships. The successful homosexual relationship, by virtue of its duration, is often more obvious to the involved couples's peers and families. This makes it progressively more difficult to avoid public acknowledgement of homosexuality. There is thus a strong social selection pressure against success or permanency in interpersonal relationships between homosexual men or women.

Summary

A single hypothesis to explain the existence of homosexual feelings and behaviors has failed to emerge. Investigations of possible biological, sociological, developmental, and psychopathologic etiologies have not allowed a consensus opinion. Psychiatric majority opinion has swung to the position that homosexuality is a normal aspect of sexuality in general. Treatment of sexual dysfunction can be carried out with homosexual couples in a manner similar to that applied to heterosexuals.

Paraphilias

Psychosexual disorders that are characterized by the necessity of unusual or bizarre imagery or acts for sexual excitement are classified by DSM-III as *paraphilias*. This subclass of disorders is frequently referred to as *sexual deviations* by other classification systems. According to DSM-III, the unusual imagery or acts tend to be insistently and involuntarily repetitive and generally involve either (1) preference for use of a nonhuman object for sexual arousal, (2) repetitive sexual activity involving real or simulated suffering or humiliation, or (3) repetitive sexual activity with nonconsenting partners. Many of the objects or images associated with the paraphilias are also related to sexual excitement in many individuals who do not have a psychosexual dysfunction; however, these arousal patterns are distinguished as pathologic when these objects or images become necessary and preferred. The DSM-III describes eight specific categories of paraphilias and includes an additional category, *atypical paraphilias,* to allow inclusion of arousal patterns that meet the criteria of a paraphilia but that have not been encountered or described with enough frequency to warrant a specific category. The eight categories of paraphilias described by DSM-III are as follows:

Fetishism

In *fetishism,* the use of inanimate objects (fetishes) is the repeatedly preferred or exclusive method of achieving sexual excitement. The diagnosis is not applied if the object is one specifically designed for sexual excitement, such as a vibrator. If the objects are limited to articles of female clothing used in cross-dressing, the diagnosis of *transvestism* is applied instead.

Transvestism

The condition of recurrent and persistent cross-dressing by a heterosexual male for the purpose of sexual excitement is described as *transvestism*. For the diagnosis it is also necessary that interference with the opportunity to cross-dress results in intense frustration for the individual. Although transvestism may evolve into transsexualism, transsexualism is distinguished from transvestism in that transsexualism includes a sense of discomfort with one's own anatomical sex to the extent of wishing to be rid of one's genitals. If the act of cross-dressing is not related to sexual excitement, as possibly in the case of female impersonators, the diagnosis of transvestism is not made.

Zoophilia

Zoophilia refers to the use of animals as the repeatedly preferred or exclusive method of achieving sexual excitement. This preference may be reflected through acts or fantasy, but the animal is preferred above other available sexual outlets.

Pedophilia

In the condition of *pedophilia,* the repeatedly preferred or exclusive method of achieving sexual excitement is the act or fantasy of engaging in sexual activity with prepubertal children. The difference in age between the adult and the prepubertal child is arbitrarily set by DSM-III as 10 years, although clinical judgment must be used in the case of late adolescents with this disorder.

Exhibitionism

Exhibitionism is characterized by repetitive acts of exposing the genitals to an unsuspecting stranger for the purpose of achieving sexual excitement, with no attempt at further sexual activity with the stranger. The diagnosis has been applied only to males in cases in which female children or adults have been the victims.

Voyeurism

The essential feature of voyeurism is repetitive looking at unsuspecting people, usually strangers, who are either naked, in the act of disrobing, or engaging in sexual activity, as the repeatedly preferred or exclusive method of achieving sexual excitement. This activity differs from that of watching pornography, in which participants are willingly and knowingly observed.

Sexual Masochism

The diagnostic criterion for sexual masochism is fulfilled when either of the following conditions exists: (1) the individual's preferred or exclusive mode of producing sexual excitement is to be humiliated, bound, beaten or otherwise made to suffer, or (2) the individual has intentionally participated in an activity in which he or she was physically harmed or his or her life was threatened, in order to produce sexual excitement. The DSM-III further specifies that the individual must have actually engaged in masochistic acts associated with sexual excitement, rather than merely masochistic fantasies. One episode of intentional participation in an activity involving physical harm or life threats in which sexual excitement did occur is sufficient for making the diagnosis.

Sexual Sadism

According to DSM-III, the diagnosis of sexual sadism should be applied whenever any one of the following conditions exists: (1) on a nonconsenting partner, the individual has repeatedly and intentionally inflicted psychological or physical suffering in order to produce sexual excitement, or (2) with a consenting partner, the repeatedly preferred or exclusive mode of achieving sexual excitement combines humiliation with simulated or mildly injurious bodily suffering, or (3) on a consenting partner, bodily injury that is extensive, permanent, or possibly mortal is inflicted in order to achieve sexual excitement. Some individuals with this disorder may commit rape; however, not all rape attempts are motivated by the desire to achieve sexual excitement by inflicting suffering.

Several reviews of the literature on treatment of paraphilias or sexual deviations have concluded that behavioral treatment approaches have demonstrated the greatest effectiveness with these disorders. In general, the focus of clinical treatment has been on the elimination of the undesired, or deviant, sexual arousal by application of aversion techniques. Further analysis of the problem has indicated, however, that "normal" sexual arousal patterns do not automatically appear when deviant arousal is suppressed. Most behavioral treatment programs for paraphilias include components directed at enhancing desired arousal patterns in addition to eliminating the undesired, or deviant patterns. Training in social skills may be a necessary component of a treatment package aimed at helping an individual develop and maintain more appropriate sexual outlets.

Bibliography

American Psychiatric Association: Diagnostic and Statistical Manual of Mental Disorders, 3rd ed. Washington, DC, American Psychiatric Association, 1980

Andersen BL: Primary orgasmic dysfunction: Diagnostic considerations and review of treatment. Psychol Bull 93(1):105–136, 1983

Bell AP, Weinberg MS: Homosexualities: A study of diversity among men and women. New York, Simon and Schuster, 1978

Hoon EF, Hoon PW: Styles of sexual expression in women: Clinical implications of multivariate analyses: Arch Sex Behav 7:105–116, 1978

Kaplan HS: Disorders of sexual desire. New York, Brunner/Mazel, 1979

Kinsey AC, Pomeroy WS, Martin CE: Sexual Behavior in the Human Male. Philadelphia, WB Saunders, 1948

Kinsey AC, Pomeroy WS, Martin CE: Sexual Behavior in the Human Female. Philadelphia, WB Saunders, 1953

Masters WH, Johnson VE: Human Sexual Response. Boston, Little, Brown & Co, 1966

Masters WH, Johnson VE: Homosexuality in perspective. Boston, Little, Brown & Co, 1979

Semans JH: Premature ejaculation: A new approach. South Med J 49:353–358, 1956

Zibergeld B: Male Sexuality. New York, Bantum Books, 1978

Jack W. Barber

15 Psychosomatic Disorders

Medical and psychiatric conditions may interact in a wide variety of ways, ranging from the contractures and muscular atrophy that develop over the course of a long-standing conversion disorder to a brief reactive psychosis or major depressive episode following myocardial infarction or diagnosis of cancer. Medical conditions may present with psychiatric symptoms, and emotional stress is a frequent cause of exacerbations in medical illnesses such as ulcerative colitis, hypertension, and rheumatoid arthritis. Psychosomatic does not mean "it's all in the head," as is commonly believed. Rather it is descriptive of a number of diseases or syndromes in which the constellation of personality factors, responses to emotional stress, and organic symptomatology is more tightly clustered and consistent than in other medical–psychiatric interactions. Over the course of this chapter you will gain some familiarity with these disorders, their respective psychiatric and organic components, how these components are linked physiologically and symbolically, and what implications there may be for treatment or long-term management.

Historical Perspective

The interaction between mind and body has been a major concern through the ages and has generally reflected the philosophical outlook of the particular culture involved. In primitive societies as well as in later Babylonian and Assyrian civilizations and the Middle Ages, diseases were felt to be the result of spiritual powers or sins, and were treated with religious and spiritual rituals involving exorcism, trepanation, and suggestion. Early Egyptian medicine combined both magical rites and more rational methods such as surgery, massages, ointments, or prescribed recipes, depending on the affliction. In the Greek civilization of Socrates and Hippocrates it was felt that both the body and the soul required treatment, an idea not far removed from modern approaches to psychosomatic conditions. During the Renaissance and later in the 19th century, the dualism that separated the mind and body became more prominent, aided by the work of Louis Pasteur and others in infectious diseases. The concept that mental processes had no significance, as put forth by such scientists as Thomas Huxley, anticipated the medical model of treating the disease rather than the whole patient. The work of Sigmund Freud had some effect in restoring this split by elucidating the role of emotions and unconscious conflicts in physical processes; however, Freud's work has never been more than incompletely accepted in the general medical community.

Franz Alexander (1934, 1950), Flanders Dunbar (1947), and others began to explore the relationships between personality features and psychosomatic conditions, while W. B. Cannon (1932) and Hans Selye (1950) began systematic investigations into the physiologic concomitants of emotional stress and the mediating roles of the autonomic nervous system and the endocrine system. Since that time, much has been written about the physiologic effects of stress and their relationship to physical disorders. The cardiovascular, gastrointestinal, respiratory, immune, and endocrine systems all manifest responses to stress and have important implications for the development of pathology. Modern concepts of psychosomatic disorders feature an interactional model involving genetic and constitutional factors, personality, and emotional stress. We will turn briefly to the current theoretical concepts of psychosomatic medicine before reviewing the specific psychosomatic conditions.

Current Theoretical Concepts in Psychosomatic Medicine

Modern psychosomatic medicine and consultation–liason psychiatry are based largely on George Engel's biopsychosocial model (1977). This model is an application of general systems theory that states that organizations have different hierarchical levels interconnected in such a way that changes on one level necessarily produce changes in other levels. Engel felt that the standard biomedical model was inadequate because it failed to consider the wealth of evidence demonstrating that emotions, conflicts, and attitudes not only affect patients' reactions to illness, but also the illness itself. Failure to attend to psychological and social factors may result in inadequate or misapportioned treatment plans, noncompliance, and overall treatment failure.

Biological Factors

The biological sphere includes not only the pathophysiologic processes involved in disease and their medical or physical consequences, such as reduced cardiac output following a myocardial infarction, but also the physiologic concomitants of stress and their effects on the endocrine, immune, gastrointestinal, and autonomic nervous systems. In addition, genetic and constitutional factors are included. Modern research has yielded a great deal of knowledge regarding the physiologic consequences of stress, such as increased catecholamine release and cortisol secretion resulting in increased heart rate and blood pressure, changes in gastric motility, distribution of blood flow to major organs, and immune reactivity. Another interesting aspect of this area is that certain visceral responses such as diastolic blood pressure or blood flow to organs such as the stomach can be conditioned in a classical or operant model. The implications of such data have not been fully worked out, but they may have importance for conditions such as peptic ulcer disease, asthma, hypertension, ulcerative colitis, and others.

Psychological Factors

Psychological factors include personality traits, characteristic ways of handling particular conflicts or stress, and the types of defense mechanisms used. A great deal of qualitative and subjective data exist in this area, but quantifying personality factors and concepts such as repressed hostility or dependence has proved difficult. More demonstrable entities such as anxiety and depression have been more easily quantified, but their relationship to patients' psychosomatic complaints may be limited. The work of Alexander (1934, 1950, 1968) and Dunbar (1947) still stand as landmark conceptualizations in this area. Alexander defined the "holy seven" psychosomatic disorders: hypertension, hyperthyroidism, bronchial asthma, peptic ulcer disease, ulcerative colitis, rheumatoid arthritis, and neurodermatitis; and he related particular conflicts and repression to autonomic nervous system overactivity and the development of pathology. Dunbar postulated personality patterns that were specific for particular psychosomatic conditions (*e.g.*, the overambitious, driven man who develops coronary artery disease).

Social and Cultural Factors

The family, social environment, and culture make up the important variables in the social realm. Family and other social relationships may be salubrious and sustaining or they may be detrimental. Conditions of loss and separation are especially relevant to exacerbations of some skin disorders, asthma, and ulcerative colitis. The life change scale of Holmes and Rahe (1967) has allowed more systematic study of the role of stressful events in aggravating the course or occurrence of events such as myocardial infarctions. Cultural differences in the expression of pain and depression, the meaning of symptoms, and the acceptance of medical treatment may all be important. For example, in many cultures it would be considered normal for depression to present with somatic complaints such as abdominal pain; and certain religious groups may not accept medical treatments, such as Jehovah's Witnesses not accepting blood transfusions.

Summary

The key concept in current psychosomatic medicine involves the interaction between the various biopsychosocial components relevant to a particular patient. This interaction will determine the course of his illness and his adaptation to it; therefore, simply treating the disease or the symptoms is likely to be inadequate for many patients. This is especially true for patients with psychosomatic disorders. As more information regarding the mechanisms mediating the effects of stress becomes available, the relationship between personality factors and organic symptomatology may become clearer. This information may allow a more precise selection of treatment interventions on each level and better overall patient care. With this general outline in hand we will now proceed to a more detailed description of some prominent psychosomatic conditions.

Cardiovascular Disorders

Cardiovascular disorders represent the major cause of death in this country and appear to be related to risk factors that are significantly affected by social and cultural determinants. Diets high in saturated fat and cholesterol, elevated serum triglyceride and cholesterol levels, medical conditions such as diabetes mellitis or renal disease, personal habits such as smoking or overeating, psychosocial factors such as personality patterns and stress, and hereditary factors all appear to be important. Emotional states such as fear, anger, and excitement can produce changes in heart rate and rhythm, cardiac output, and arterial blood pressure. The rich interconnections between the limbic system and the hypothalamus mediate neuroendocrine processes such as cortisol secretion and the activity of the autonomic nervous system, both of which play important roles in these effects. Beyond its physiological importance, the heart is also imbued with a wealth of symbolic meaning that may account for the frequency of cardiac complaints in hypochondriacal patients or those with phobic or conversion disorders. Psychosocial factors are not etiologic by themselves, but interact with others factors to contribute to the development of cardiovascular problems.

Hypertension

Essential hypertension affects one out of every five Americans and, while generally asymptomatic, is associated with an increased risk for myocardial infarction, congestive heart failure, stroke, and renal failure. It is more common among blacks, in conditions of overcrowding or poverty, and in occupations involving a high level of stress. Proposed mechanisms have centered on the renin–angiotensin–aldosterone system and central-nervous-system (CNS) induced excesses of sympathetic outflow, but an interactional model involving each of these systems and their various components is probably more accurate.

Alexander (1950) proposed that people with hypertension had conflicts resulting in the inability to express hostile or aggressive feelings, leading to excessive sympathetic discharge and elevated blood pressure. Other personality descriptions have included passive–dependent, guilt-ridden, insecure, tense, and compulsive; however, no specific personality type has been elucidated. Meaningful psychological stimuli resulting in stress or excitement have been shown to increase renin secretion in normotensive people and may be important in some cases. Fear, anxiety, and anger may all lead to elevated blood pressure, more so in hypertensive patients than in normotensive controls. Elevated blood pressure has been noted in the survivors of major disasters, soldiers in combat, men who have recently lost jobs, people in crowded living conditions or poverty, and people in highly stressful occupations, such as air traffic controllers.

Treatment must be aimed at reduction and control of blood pressure through medication, behavioral changes with regard to smoking, inactivity, and diet, and the reduction of stress (where applicable and possible). The treatment program must begin with a stable and supportive physician–patient relationship. Education regarding the illness and medication must be included and should involve the family as well as the patient. Relaxation techniques involving daily rest, periodic vacations, biofeedback, behavioral modification, or meditation have been helpful in selected patients. Psychotherapy alone has not been helpful, but may be a necessary adjunct for some cases. In all of these modalities, strict attention must be paid to compliance, which is the most significant problem in managing hypertension once it is detected. Better compliance may be facilitated by frequent, scheduled, follow-up visits to one physician, who can provide the necessary encouragement and support while monitoring the blood pressure itself. It should be kept in mind that some antihypertensive medications (*e.g.*, reserpine, methyldopa, clonidine, guanethidine, and propranolol) may cause depression in some patients.

Coronary Artery Disease

Coronary artery disease is the leading cause of death in this country and carries considerable additional morbidity in terms of disability, restricted lifestyle, and general reduced quality of life. A number of risk factors have been found, which include diets high in fat and cholesterol, obesity, lack of physical activity, smoking, elevated serum triglyceride and cholesterol levels, a positive family history, and psychosocial factors such as Type A personality, high occupational stress, and marital discord. Many of these factors are culturally bound to Western societies and may represent side effects of rapid industrialization and change in these cultures.

No one group of psychosocial factors can be thought of as etiologic in the development of coronary disease; however, personality type and psychosocial stresses have been associated with an increased risk of morbidity and mortality. Friedman and Rosenbaum (1974) coined the term *Type A personality* to describe a behavior pattern of ambitiousness, competitiveness, impatience, time urgency, inability to relax without guilt, tendency to multiple commitments, and a general preoccupation with success. Such a personality is associated with an increased risk of coronary artery disease and its complications. Increased serum cholesterol and triglyceride levels, increased diurnal secretion of norepinephrine, accelerated clotting, and more marked blood pressure responses to challenging tasks have been found in patients with Type A personality. These people have two to three times the risk of developing coronary heart disease than do people without these characteristics (Type B personality).

Psychosocial factors, including occupational stress and significant life changes such as moving, switching jobs, separation from spouse, or retirement, may result in an increased risk of mortality from coronary heart disease. Divorced, widowed, or never-married individuals have higher death rates than those who are married.

While the exact mechanisms involved are not clear, these environmental factors seem to have some role in the development and course of this disease.

The prevention of coronary artery disease has been initiated on a nationwide scale. More attention is being paid to efforts to decrease smoking and eating, increase exercise, and increase compliance with hypertension control measures. Behavior programs aimed at stress management, relaxation, and avoidance of extremely competitive situations are all useful in some patients.

Myocardial Infarction

While certain behavioral patterns and chronic stress may be important in the development of hypertension and coronary artery disease, more acute psychosocial stressors have been implicated in cardiac events such as angina, myocardial infarction, and sudden death. Sudden-death victims have higher life change indices than survivors. These life changes can include increased responsibility, anxiety, depression, business or domestic problems, increased activity, and moving. Acute anxiety, excitement, anger, and fear can all precipitate myocardial infarctions in susceptible individuals.

Immediate responses in patients suffering myocardial infarctions fall into several patterns, but commonly they include fear or an attempt to minimize the danger. Both such responses can result in fatality due to lethal arrhythmias or delay in seeking help. Once heart disease is known to be present, patients may either realistically accept the condition and begin appropriate rehabilitation, become excessively dependent and fearful, deny the significance of the illness and live as if it never occurred, or use the illness to manipulate others. The type of coping strategies or behavior patterns that occur are influenced by the patient's general medical status, premorbid personality patterns, and the influences of the family. Additional problems that may occur in the aftermath of a myocardial infarction include depression, anxiety, inability to work, financial losses, and changes in the roles of family members if the patient becomes significantly disabled.

The goal of rehabilitation is to reach the highest degree of premorbid functioning that is possible, given the extent of the ischemic damage and resulting cardiac function. Unfortunately, anxiety, depression, fear of another attack, and stresses in the social or family setting frequently retard or preclude meeting this goal. The infarction represents an existential crisis for both the patient and the family, which varies in its severity. If domestic problems coincided with the heart attack, guilt may lead to overprotection of the patient and may block rehabilitation efforts. As the ability of the spouse to accept and adjust is an important factor in determining the success of the recovery process, education and support must be extended to the spouse as well. Brief psychotherapy for the patient during the recovery period may improve later rehabilitation progress, allay anxiety and depression, and shorten hospital stays. It may prevent the development of maladaptive coping strategies as well. As a general rule, tricyclic antidepressant medications should be withheld for a period of several months following an infarction.

Congestive Heart Failure

Congestive heart failure describes a condition in which the heart is no longer able to pump blood sufficiently to empty the venous inflow into the arterial system, resulting in dyspnea, fatigue, and edema. It can result from any type of heart disease and may be aggravated by psychosocial factors such as anxiety, depression, anger, and intense arousal. Psychosocial stresses are frequent antecedents to acute decompensations requiring hospitalization.

Treatment generally involves diet restrictions and medications such as digitalis and diuretics. Noncompliance remains a significant problem. This may result from an inability to accept the illness or an attempt to maintain the sick role and its secondary-gain components; or it may be a manifestation of depression or suicidal ideation. Physical restrictions may necessitate behavioral changes that are frequently difficult for patients. This is especially so for those who maintain their self-esteem largely through work or physical activities that they may no longer be able to pursue. Supportive psychotherapy with education may help the patient maintain self-esteem, repair damaged self-concept, and develop behavior patterns and activities that he is capable of and that provide personal satisfaction.

Respiratory Disorders

Because breathing is necessary for life, any compromise in respiration may result in varying degrees of fear and helplessness. In addition, sighing, coughing, crying, gasping, and yawning are respiratory maneuvers connected to emotional states of despair, sadness, surprise, and boredom. Thus, the relationship between respiration and the psyche is an intimate one. Difficulties with breathing can be a result of primary lung disease, or they may be sequelae from other conditions such as obesity, increased intracranial pressure, or metabolic derangements. While the mechanisms responsible for producing the relationship between respiration and emotion are not well understood, it is known that attacks of bronchial asthma and hyperventilation are frequently related to emotional stress and psychological factors. In addition, chronic obstructive pulmonary disease is a common and severely limiting condition frequently associated with adjustment problems for those afflicted.

Bronchial Asthma

Bronchial asthma represents a condition of small-airway hyperreactivity to a variety of allergic, chemical, physical, or emotional factors resulting in bronchoconstriction, mucosal edema, and excessive viscous secretions into the airways with subsequent obstruction, wheezing, and dyspnea. The "extrinsic" type tends to affect children and adolescents, is associated with elevated IgE antibodies, eczema, allergic rhinitis, food allergies, and a positive family history, and is typically outgrown by adulthood. An "intrinsic" type affecting middle-aged and older people may be associated with eosinophilia, nasal polyps, sensitivity to drugs suppressing prostaglandin synthesis, and may be caused by a viral illness. The latter type may become unresponsive to medications.

While many potential precipitants may exist for a given patient, no one agent will be responsible for every episode of asthma, and it is best to consider and manage the condition as one that is multidetermined. Emotional stress is an important precipitating factor in many acute cases, perhaps through the activation of parasympathetic pathways to the lungs. In some patients an attack can become a conditioned response to a given setting, whether the original inciting agent is present or not. Thus, the alleviation of stress may profoundly improve the clinical course of some patients.

While no single personality type exists for patients with asthma, many have strong wishes for dependency and protection. The dependency of a child or adolescent is greatly increased and prolonged by asthma due to the need for readily available caretakers in the event of respiratory distress. This dependency may foster fears of independent functioning, loss, or separation, and may at times produce a general retardation of emotional development. Asthmatic children may be timid, overly dependent, and emotionally immature with poor impulse control, little tolerance for separation or frustration, and occasional explosive behavior or temper tantrums.

Asthmatic adolescents may be overly sensitive to rejection or disappointment and may be anxious about physical activity, sexual excitement, or socially stressful situations that could precipitate an asthma attack. Some may become withdrawn and depressed, while others become rebellious and temperamental due to frustration over their illness and its limitations. Adults with asthma or those who had severe asthma when they were younger may also be overly dependent, shy, and immature in their coping strategies and relationships. They may become depressed and hopeless when there is little support from those around them.

In all cases, asthma may become a significant part of the personality and how the patient relates to others, and thus be used for the procuring of all manner of needs or as a vehicle for obtaining secondary gain in the form of reduced responsibility for independent functioning in all spheres of life. The management of dependency and fear of loss may be critical to the overall development of a child or adolescent as well as the emotional and physical well-being of the adult.

The aim of treatment is to facilitate the best physical and emotional development and functioning possible. This involves avoidance of known offending agents, the maintenance of adequate hydration, hyposensitization therapy when indicated, and medications such as bronchodilators, β-adrenergic agonists, and at times, corticosteroids.

Psychologically, attention must be directed toward providing consistent emotional support, both to reduce fear of loss and separation, and to prevent the development of a pattern of caretaking based solely on asthmatic attacks and physical infirmity. Encouragement of age-appropriate activity and independent functioning in the context of emotional support can be vital to the child's development. Similar principles apply to adult patients; that is, consistent support, reduction of secondary gain for "sick" behavior, and positive reinforcement for appropriately independent behaviors.

Hyperventilation

Hyperventilation involves rapid deep breathing for a period of several minutes with consequent lightheadedness, tingling of the perioral area and extremities, palpitations, epigastric discomfort, apprehension, and panic. Fainting may occur. Because hyperventilation is a manifestation of acute anxiety, fear, or pain, it can potentially affect almost anyone in these circumstances; however, it more typically affects people with anxious or "hysterical" personalities, or those with phobic or panic disorders. Acute treatment consists of holding one's breath or breathing into a paper bag, but psychotherapy or anxiolytic medication directed at the underlying cause is generally required for long-term management.

Chronic Obstructive Pulmonary Disease

Chronic obstructive pulmonary disease is a situation in which the mechanical properties of the lung have been compromised, occurring most often in primary lung diseases such as chronic bronchitis, emphysema, or chronic asthma, though it may occur in systemic conditions such as polyarteritis nodosa. It may result in severe limitations on usual activities such as work, recreation, or sexual functioning, and may create difficult adjustment problems for these patients. They may become anxious about activities that aggravate their breathing problems and may therefore withdraw into inactivity. Inability to accept one's limitations may result in depression, which may be manifested as noncompliance, or alternatively, overactivity with frequent exacerbations of their illness. In some patients, the reality of their limitations may lead to suicidal ideation, which may be acted on directly or carried out passively by noncompliance. The loss of the ability to breathe normally and the fear of suffocation may escalate dependency needs and fears of separation or loss. They may be unable to express their frustrations because they fear others will abandon them.

The best management involves a solid and empathic relationship with the primary physician, who can provide education, recommend activity suited to the patient's capability, listen to frustrations, and provide the appropriate medical care. Educating the family with regard to the condition may help prevent the patient from regressing into passive inactivity.

Gastrointestinal Disorders

The gastrointestinal system is so richly endowed with psychological significance that it has been referred to as the "sounding board of the emotions." In the infant, hunger and satiety are intimately tied to emotional warmth and nurturance. During the period of toilet training, developmental opportunities for autonomy, control, and approval go far beyond the matters of proper bowel evacuation. On a physiological level, anger and excitement may cause vascular engorgement, hypermotility, and gastric secretion with indigestion, "butterflies," nausea, gas pains, and diarrhea. On the other hand, emotional withdrawal and depression may lead to decreased gastric secretion and motility. Both the rich gastrointestinal symbolism in our language and the wealth of autonomic innervation and endocrinologic responsiveness point to the substantial relationship between "psyche" and "soma" in this area.

Vomiting and Esophageal Reflux

While vomiting is the border between voluntary and involuntary control, patients with psychogenic emesis typically have conflicts related to incorporation and dependency resulting in the symbolic rejection of food through vomiting. The idea of being dependent may be so contaminated with feelings of being controlled or losing one's sense of self that everything from the outside, including food, may be rejected symbolically. Food may also be rejected because of unconscious guilt over primitive aggressive wishes. Vomiting may be a feature of either anorexia nervosa or bulemia.

Esophageal reflux has been related to psychogenic vomiting in the past by psychodynamic theorists, but the comparison is probably inadequate. This is a relatively common condition that has a variable association with hiatal hernia and results from the reflux of gastric contents through the lower esophageal sphincter into the esophagus. Emotional stress may decrease the sphincter pressure, causing or aggravating this condition. Reflux may serve as a mask for states of anxiety or depression.

Peptic Ulcer Disease

Peptic ulcers are erosive lesions in the gastric, or more commonly, the duodenal mucosa, resulting in clinical symptoms of epigastric aching or gnawing, typically when the stomach is empty. Acid and pepsin are required for ulcer formation, which may result from excessive secretion of acid or by a decrease in mucosal resistance. The capacity to secrete acid and pepsin appears to be genetically determined and can be measured by serum pepsinogen levels. A defect in the feedback inhibition of acid secretion may be relevant in the etiology of duodenal ulcers but is of unclear importance in gastric ulcers.

Patients with peptic ulcer disease typically show elevated pepsinogen levels, a greater increase in acid secretion during stress than seen in non-ulcer patients, and have a pattern of acid secretion that is much more continuous than the normally episodic patterns of non-ulcer patients. While there is no prototypical ulcer personality, these patients appear to have a rigid denial of dependency needs, or dependency needs clearly in excess of that which can be reasonably gratified. Franz Alexander (1950) theorized that these patients manifest a psychological hunger, paralleling the continuous pattern of gastric acid secretion, that is functionally insatiable. Mirsky and colleagues (1952) proposed that the genetic predisposition toward greater acid production resulted in increased demands for feeding in infancy, resulting in maternal frustration, which could be perceived by the child as rejection. Such interactions contribute to a lifelong personality pattern of excessive needs for nurturance and dependency that are frustrated. In many cases these patients fail to express their anger and frustration because they fear further rejection or deprivation. This frustration manifests itself in the form of ulcer formation. Thus, ulcer patients combine a genetic predisposition and repressed or excessive dependency needs with a tendency to inhibit the expression of anger. This makes them vulnerable to ulcer formation during times of prolonged insecurity, uncertainty, or unexpressed resentment.

Medical treatment may involve antacids before and after meals, frequent small feedings, or histamine receptor antagonists such as cimetidine, which inhibit acid secretion. The best management, however, requires attention to the underlying psychological makeup of the patient as well as the illness itself. A stable and empathic relationship with the primary physician is important, and supportive or insight psychotherapy may also be needed in some cases. A subpopulation of these patients tend to seek competitive, independent life situations as part of their attempt to deny underlying dependency needs, which result in conditions of chronic stress. Thus, lifestyle modifications may be important. A nonthreatening, supportive relationship may strengthen a patient's confidence, allow him to be less anxious in the face of uncertainty, and afford him more freedom to express his frustrations and resentments, thus decreasing the likelihood of recurrence.

Ulcerative Colitis and Crohn's Disease

Ulcerative colitis is a serious illness of the colonic mucosa, associated with diarrhea and bleeding that can be life threatening in severe cases. It follows a pattern of exacerbations and remissions, the overall prognosis varying roughly with the severity. Complications include liver disease, hematologic and thromboembolic disorders, renal problems, arthritis of the large joints, and anal fissures, fistulas, or abscesses.

Relatively consistent personality patterns have been elucidated for these patients. They include compulsive traits such as neatness, perfectionism, obstinacy, and conformism, as well as pronounced needs for love and affection and a marked dependency on parents or parental substitutes. Such patients may be extremely sensitive and feel both rage and vulnerability when separated from important figures in their lives. Indeed, the events typically associated with exacerbations are those involving separations or losses. At these times, patients react with depression, childlike behavior, and rage, which are all inhibited and expressed through their colonic symptomatology. The mechanism by which these affective states are translated into disease exacerbations is unclear, but it may involve both vascular and immunologic factors.

Individual psychotherapy with environmental manipulation and family therapy may be quite effective for the majority of patients, and may reduce the number of exacerbations, the degree of symptomatology, and improve the condition of the colonic mucosa. The goal of psychotherapy is to improve the capacity of higher ego functions while decreasing the potential for psychological regression, which may require support, ventilation, suggestion, and in some cases, more formal insight psychotherapy. It is important that the psychiatrist work continuously with the primary physician, because intermittent crisis-oriented psychiatric consultation is rarely productive in the long term.

Crohn's disease, or regional enteritis, is an inflammatory disease of the small intestine and less frequently, the colon. It involves discontinuous segments of bowel, and produces abdominal pain, diarrhea, perianal lesions, and enteric fistulas or sinus tracts. Though closely related to ulcerative colitis, Crohn's disease is distinguished by the occurrence of granulomata and segmentally distributed lesions. From a psychological perspective the two diseases are quite similar, sharing compulsive personality traits, excessive dependent features, and exacerbations paralleling losses of significant others or self-esteem. While less work has been done using psychotherapy in patients with Crohn's disease, they appear to respond positively to approaches similar to those used for patients with ulcerative colitis.

Irritable Bowel Syndrome

This condition, called *mucous colitis, irritable colon, spastic colitis,* and many other names, refers to a syndrome of abdominal pain or cramping with diarrhea or constipation. It is characterized by sudden or gradual exacerbations and accounts for as many as 50% of patients presenting to physicians with gastrointestinal complaints. It typically has its onset in adolescence or young adulthood and tends to recur during times of emotional stress. While it may be readily treated in the short term with antianxiety or antispasmodic agents, it generally becomes chronic and recurrent.

There is no distinctive personality type for these patients, but they have been described as compulsive, overconscientious, dependent, anxious, hypersensitive, and unassertive. Typically they do not have the narcissistic or borderline features present in patients with ulcerative colitis or Crohn's disease, but are more likely to be psychiatrically disturbed than the normal population.

Generally, successful treatment in the short term may prevent many patients from pursuing a long-term solution to this problem. However, for those who are so motivated, behavioral programs can be developed based on precipitants, responses, and consequences for the individual. Also, intensive insight-oriented psychotherapy may be helpful for some patients otherwise suitable for this modality.

Obesity

By the simplest definition, obesity is the excess accumulation of fat in the body, resulting in a weight greater than 20% above the standard listed on height–weight charts. It is a risk factor for diabetes mellitis, degenerative joint disease, alveolar hypoventilation syndromes, and cardiovascular disorders such as hypertension, stroke, and coronary artery disease. Less than 5% of cases have an organic cause, and it is generally more common in women and lower socioeconomic classes. While obesity constitutes an important health problem, much remains to be understood in terms of mechanisms, etiologies, and treatment.

Pathophysiology

It is relatively clear that body weight is maintained within well-regulated limits in the animal kingdom and in non-obese humans. A biological "set point" has been postulated and appears to be consistent with Kleiber's rule that animals use energy in proportion to their normal body weight. In animals that weigh above or below their normal weight, this relationship does not seem to hold; energy use and intake may become progressively more unbalanced, leading to a vicious cycle of weight gain or loss. A high-fat diet, abnormalities in the dietary fat content, or the number of fat cells may raise this biological set point to the extent that normal weight seems biologically too low in some obese people. Thus, an abnormality in weight regulation appears to be important in the development and maintenance of obesity.

Genetic factors in obesity may involve a propensity for an increased number of fat cells or a relationship to somatotype. Ectomorphy appears to be protective against the development of obesity and is more hereditary than obesity itself. The number of fat cells present is related to two major periods of proliferation: (1) during the first two years of life, and (2) during puberty. In addition to genetic predisposition, overnutrition in these critical periods is probably involved. Once fat cells are present, they remain throughout life. Obesity may develop from an increased number of fat cells (*i.e.*, hyperplasia), or from hypertrophy of existing fat cells, as is most common in adults. (Some increase in cell number may occur outside the critical periods, under certain conditions.) There is some suggestion that with significant weight loss, fat cell size can become subnormal and may increase nutritional demand. While the overall significance of this finding is unclear, it may represent part of the reason that obese people have difficulty maintaining weight loss once it has occurred.

Energy output has three main components: basal metabolic rate, specific dynamic activation of food, and physical activity, which is under voluntary control. Physical activity is an important aspect of weight control due to its direct expenditure of energy and its indirect role in lowering relative caloric intake. Obese people tend to be sedentary and this inactivity may cause a relatively high caloric demand through as-yet-undefined mechanisms.

Emotional Factors

Emotional factors have long been considered to be important in the development of obesity, but most careful studies have revealed little difference in psychopathology between obese and nonobese populations. There is no prototypic personality profile of obese people. Significant numbers of obese people do tend to view their bodies with hostility and contempt, which are closely related to problems in social functioning due to self-consciousness and low self-esteem. This characteristic does not apply to all overweight people, but tends to be more important in those who have been obese since adolescence or childhood. Some obese people tend to be more susceptible to external cues for eating than people of normal weight, at times overriding the internal cue of hunger. Others may have difficulty in restraining from eating, which makes dieting and the maintenance of a lower weight problematic. Some patients may eat more in response to feelings of depression, rejection, frustration, or anger. Two stress-related overeating syndromes that have been described are the binge-eating syndrome, which is present in only a small percentage of obese persons, and the night eating syndrome, usually involving young women of middle and upper socioeconomic backgrounds.

Treatment

The treatment of obesity is challenging and has been the subject of innumerable diet plans and special programs, most of which have failed to produce any lasting benefit. Three basic methods of treatment have been developed: behavioral modification, protein-sparing modified fast, and surgical bypass.

Behavioral modification involves documenting the eating behaviors to be changed, identifying stimuli that seem to produce the behaviors, developing ways to alter the behavioral responses, and changing the consequences of the behavior by rewarding desired behaviors. Typical points include using a prepared list for grocery shopping, keeping only small amounts of food in the home, always eating in the same place (generally away from the bedroom or television), and eating more slowly. Rewards can range from buying clothes, books, or other desired objects to activities the person enjoys. This program appears to be most effective for those people who are only mildly obese and can be administered by both physicians and lay persons or organizations.

The protein-sparing modified fast has been used for patients who are moderately obese. Complications of renal or hepatic impairment and cardiac dysfunction have made its use controversial. It involves the use of high-quality protein and potassium supplementation, with salt, minerals, and vitamins added to a fluid intake of more than 1500 ml per day. Patients receive less than 700 kcal per day and are essentially anorectic with ketonemia and ketonuria. Weight loss of up to 18 kg may be expected, after which behavioral programs may need to be instituted to prevent regaining the weight. While this program may be carried out on an outpatient basis, close supervision by a physician is essential.

Surgical bypass procedures are restricted to patients who are severely obese (more than 100% overweight), have been so for longer than 5 years, have developed sequelae such as diabetes or hypertension, and have failed with other forms of treatment. Gastric bypass involves isolating a small pouch of stomach and attaching it to the jejunum, leaving the remainder of the stomach essentially nonfunctional. Weight loss, better eating patterns, and improved psychosocial functioning occur with regularity. Jejunoileal bypass has more complications, such as diarrhea and malnutrition, and involves attaching the jejunum directly to the ileum, effectively stopping substantial amounts of absorption that normally occur in the small intestine.

Anorexia Nervosa

Anorexia nervosa is a condition that primarily affects women in adolescence or young adulthood and involves profound weight loss, preoccupation with ideas related to food and weight, behavioral disturbances, distorted perceptions of body image, and problems related to self-concept and personal identity. It was described as "nervous atrophy" by Richard Morton in 1689 and was given its current name in 1874 by William Gull. Secondary problems that may develop during the progression of the illness include metabolic, endocrinologic, and neurologic disturbances. In fact, the condition carries an eventual mortality rate of up to 15% of those cases reaching treatment. However, it is not a uniform condition, having a variety of manifestations and degrees of severity, and may occur in association with affective, psychotic, or personality disorders.

Clinical Features

Anorexia nervosa has been increasing in frequency over the past 20 years with 80% to 85% of cases occurring between the ages of 15 and 25, with women accounting for approximately 95% of cases overall. The condition is associated with middle and upper socioeconomic class, and an increased incidence of affective disorders is seen in relatives of patients. Although an association between anorexia nervosa and

Turner's syndrome has been noted, as well as an increased morbidity risk for sisters of anorectic patients, the role of heredity is unclear.

The diagnosis of anorexia nervosa is made when the patient (1) has lost 25% of her original body weight or has fallen 25% below the expected norm for age and height, (2) manifests an intense fear of becoming obese, (3) has a disturbance of body image such that the patient's own body is perceived as being "fatter" than it is, (4) does not have a medical condition that would account for the weight loss, and (5) has amenorrhea (in women). It should be noted that the term *anorexia* is actually a misnomer because the patients do not suffer from a lack of appetite. In fact, as many as 50% engage in recurrent episodes of binge eating, typically involving sweets or other fattening foods.

In addition to markedly reducing their intake of calories, these patients may engage in excessive and usually ritualistic exercise programs that may be clandestine. They may use diet pills, emetics, laxatives, and diuretics to aid them in losing weight. There is an intense and frequently secret desire for thinness and a more-or-less continual preoccupation with food, calorie counts, recipes (which they may collect), and the preparation or serving of food to others, (*e.g.*, these patients are typically those most involved in cooking for outings in the home or hospital). They may hide food in their rooms, carry candy bars and cake with them, and be preoccupied with arranging food on the plate. They typically see themselves as "fat," an image that usually worsens as the condition progresses. Compulsive personality traits such as desire for neatness and order, overattention to detail, a strong sense of duty or obligation, and rigid principles regarding moral or ethical issues. Although they manifest a conscious desire for independence, they remain acutely sensitive to the opinions of others and may attempt to please others, including their therapists. However, when anxious or pressured, these patients may become obstinate, expressing their anger directly or indirectly through passive–aggressive means.

Common defense mechanisms of anorexia include isolation, reaction formation, intellectualization, projection, displacement, splitting, and denial (of appearance, hunger, fatigue, and anger). The encouragement of others to get them to gain weight may be regarded as a threat to their own fragile sense of self-control. Typically, these patients were well behaved, polite, compliant, and successful children. Nevertheless, they have unrealistic fears of failure, poorly formed self-concepts, and doubts concerning their own self-worth and competence. Projective psychological testing may demonstrate an abundance of oral–aggressive themes and a marked ambivalence toward mother figures.

In women, amenorrhea frequently occurs prior to significant weight loss and may be the presenting complaint. Once malnutrition has developed, a reversion to prepubertal patterns of luteinizing hormone (LH) secretion occurs with low LH, low estrogen serum levels, and an impaired LH response to gonadotropin-releasing hormone. Although these abnormalities correct with weight gain, the amenorrhea itself may continue for a prolonged period of time, which is probably related to an abnormality in the positive feedback release of LH in response to estrogen secretion.

Physical manifestations of prolonged starvation and weight loss include bradycardia, hypotension, hypothermia, and dependent edema. Metabolic changes include thyroid abnormalities, incomplete dexamethasone suppression of cortisol, hypercholesterolemia, and hypercarotenemia. Hypokalemic alkalosis may result from vomiting or diuretic abuse. Electrolyte abnormalities may lead to electrocardiographic changes such as T-wave inversion or flattening, prolongation of the QT interval, and ST segment depression. Electroencephalographic abnormalities include diffuse background slowing, paroxysmal dysrhythmias, and decreased rapid eye movement (REM) sleep in some cases. Leukopenia with a relative lymphocytosis, bone marrow hypocellularity, low erythrocyte sedimentation rate, and reduced plasma fibrinogen levels occur in some patients.

Causes

Anorexia nervosa develops during periods involving increased expectations of independent or mature functioning in social or sexual roles. During adolescence or young adulthood, when it is appropriate to move outward from the realm of the family, long-standing feelings of personal ineffectiveness, lack of control, and poor sense of identity become intensified. The rigid restriction of diet and rigorous pursuit of thinness become a way to establish a personal autonomy, a sense of control (over weight and eating behavior), and a way to identify oneself. This behavior and associated defiance of others results not from a sense of strength, but from a fear of losing oneself and losing control in the face of new expectations. It becomes a solution, albeit an extreme and maladaptive one, to the sense of inner deficit and lack of effectiveness or control. By becoming "small" they can avoid dealing with important adolescent matters of independence, sexuality, and identity. Thus, they revert to a more childlike way of behaving, just as their LH and estrogen secretion patterns revert to a prepubertal state.

While early psychoanalytic writers felt that the condition represented a repudiation of wishes to become pregnant based on fantasies of oral impregnation, others have seen it as a phobic avoidance response either to eating or to social and sexual demands through starvation and malnutrition. Alternate theories include a dependent but seductive relationship to a passive father, with ambivalence toward the mother based on guilt over aggressive urges, and the blocking of self-concept formation due to overprotection and deprivation in the oral stage. A useful formulation based on the work of Hilde Bruch (1982) is that these patients were required to meet the emotional demands of the mother in order to have their own basic needs met. As a result they become extremely sensitive to what others expect of them, but develop a defective sense of their own bodily and emotional needs, and self-concept. They become model children but harbor extreme rage inside that frightens them and causes them to avoid emotions in general. At times when increased demands are placed upon them, their rage may be turned against themselves, resulting in starvation and suppression of hunger and fatigue, or may be directed toward others through passive–aggressiveness, obstinacy, and the induction of guilt and anxiety in those who watch the patient slowly starve herself.

Although it has not yet been fully elucidated, there may be a biological link between the affective disorders and anorexia nervosa. Family history, similar responses to neuroendocrine challenge tests such as the dexamethasone suppression test, and the response of some patients to tricyclic antidepressant medications such as imipramine seem to support this notion. However, these patients typically manifest a much more complicated pattern of psychopathology than would seem to be accounted for by an atypical depressive disorder.

Treatment

Anorexia nervosa is a complicated disorder that requires a prolonged and generally difficult period of treatment. While there have been few controlled studies on the many approaches taken, some useful guidelines are as follows: (1) establishment of adequate nutrition, (2) correction of abnormal eating behaviors, (3) disengagement from the overly tight involvement with the family, and (4) resolution of the patient's identity confusion and sense of personal ineffectiveness.

The importance of the first step must not be overlooked because the physical and metabolic consequences of cachexia, vomiting, and diuretic abuse may not only be fatal, but may compromise the patient's ability to use the treatment program. In extreme cases tube feedings or parenteral nutrition may be required even though these regimens may be threatening to the patient's sense of control and effectiveness. Behavioral programs, based on positive reinforcements such as increased privileges or physical activities for weight gain, and negative alternatives for weight loss or vomiting, may be effective in settings where sufficient monitoring is possible.

For some patients, pharmacotherapy may be effective in abetting weight gain and improving some of the affective and eating behavior manifestations of this disorder. Antidepressant medications such as imipramine or amitriptyline have been effective in 50% to 60% of cases in some reports. Antipsychotic medications such as chlorpromazine have been useful in some cases and may be indicated for more disturbed patients. Cyproheptidine, an antihistamine, has been used effectively as an appetite stimulant in some cases and has fewer side effects than the other agents mentioned. Electroconvulsive therapy (ECT) has been used effectively in a few cases that were unresponsive to other modalities.

Disengaging the patient from the tight involvement with the family may be approached in a number of ways. The patient's family must allow the patient a realistic level of independent functioning and control. This may require simple supportive work, but more commonly it necessitates intensive family psychotherapy. Frequently, the patient's weight has become the central controlling feature in the family setting, and altering this focus is essential to the treatment.

In individual psychotherapy, the patient must feel that she is treated as a person of importance and that her thoughts and feelings will be listened to carefully. Existing strengths should be reinforced while uncovering the addressing basic deficiencies in her personality. The patient's sense of ineffectiveness and vulnerability, lack of trust, marked dependence, and underlying anger beneath the passive and cooperative facade must be kept in mind. The patient must gradually experience a sense of genuineness, autonomous identity, and personal effectiveness.

Patients who are older, have had a longer duration of illness, reach a lower weight, and have had problems with social adjustment prior to the onset of the illness have a poorer prognosis. It is important to keep in mind that anorexia nervosa is not a uniform condition, and some flexibility in selecting the type and timing of the various treatment modalities must be maintained.

Endocrine Disorders

Brain regions prominent in the regulation of emotional states, such as the limbic system and hypothalamus, are intimately involved in the regulation of hormone secretion by way of hypothalamic releasing factors and multiple feedback loops from the pituitary gland and peripheral organs. The relationship between emotions and the endocrine system is one in which hormones can both exert influences on sexual, aggressive, and social behaviors, and be affected by emotional states such as fear or anxiety. Such relationships have been used to develop biological parameters (*e.g.*, the dexamethasone suppression test) for primary psychiatric disorders such as major depression. While the role of emotional stress and other psychosocial factors in the etiology of endocrine disorders has not emerged, many primary endocrine conditions may present with psychiatric symptoms of depression, anxiety, or psychosis.

Hyperthyroidism

Hyperthyroidism may present with complaints of nervousness, inability to relax or slow down, insomnia, or irritability, as well as emotional lability with crying spells or euphoria, decreased attention span, and impaired recent memory. In severe cases, the patient may be floridly psychotic or delirious. Other clinical features include palpitation, tachycardia, shortness of breath, weight loss despite increased appetite, fine rhythmic tremor of the hands and tongue, exophthalmos, lid lag, and elevated basal temperature. Once the condition is suspected, laboratory tests of thyroid function should be obtained and endocrinology consultation requested. It is important to keep in mind that the condition may be precipitated by acute emotional stress or shock, which may complicate the initial diagnostic assessment. Premorbid personality characteristics may include premature assumption of responsibilites, martyrdom, and suppression of dependency needs with an exaggerated fear of death or injury. The relationship between these characteristics and the condition itself is not at all clear. Treatment is directed at the underlying cause and may include antithyroid drugs or surgical ablation. Propranolol provides symptomatic relief.

Hypothyroidism

Hypothyroidism results from insufficient thyroid hormone synthesis secondary to loss of functioning thyroid tissue or inadequate stimulation from the hypothalamus or pituitary gland. It develops slowly, except when secondary to surgical ablation. A significant number of patients show mental disturbances. These include slowed mentation and speech, decreased initiative, slowed comprehension, and impaired recent memory. Fatigue and drowsiness may occur. Some patients appear to be depressed, while others may develop *myxedema madness,* a psychotic condition with paranoid ideation, auditory hallucinations, and evidence of organic dysfunction. Other findings include thickened skin, dull expression, hair that is brittle and dry with loss of the lateral margins of the eyebrows, husky voice, thickened tongue, cold intolerance, constipation, decreased appetite with weight gain, and the slow return of deep tendon reflexes. Treatment involves appropriate replacement of thyroid hormone.

Addison's Disease

Addison's disease is primary adrenal insufficiency resulting in decreased levels of circulating cortisol, aldosterone, and androgens. It has an insidious development with early changes in personality and behavior such as apathy, fatigue, depression, poverty of thought, and decreased initiative. The patient may be irritable, socially withdrawn, psychomotor-retarded, and have reduced cognitive capabilities. In an Addisonian crisis, delirium may develop with delusions and hallucinations, and this may proceed to coma and death. Physical signs of Addison's disease include weight loss, hypotension, weakness, loss of appetite, diffuse pigmentation of the skin, nausea and vomiting, and abdominal pain. Primary treatment is glucocorticoid and mineralocorticoid replacement. Idiopathic atrophy has replaced tuberculosis as the most common etiology of Addison's disease.

Cushing's Syndrome

Cushing's syndrome results from a chronic excess of circulating cortisol. Psychiatric symptoms may be the presenting complaint in up to 50% of cases. These include depression, insomnia, loss of libido, irritability, acute anxiety, inability to concentrate, and short-term memory deficits. Some patients may become confused and disoriented, and a small percentage may develop paranoid ideation and hallucinations. Physical findings include central obesity with a "buffalo hump," moon facies, muscle wasting and weakness, abdominal striae, impaired glucose tolerance, and osteoporesis. Etiologies include: (1) adrenal hyperplasia, adenoma, or carcinoma: (2) an adrenocorticotropic-hormone (ACTH)–secreting tumor in the pituitary (Cushing's disease), and (3) exogenously administered glucocorticoids. Treatment is based on the underlying cause.

Hypopituitarism

Patients with hypopituitarism demonstrate the effects of adrenal, thyroid, and gonadal deficiencies secondary to lesions in the anterior pituitary. These lesions include infections, tumors, head trauma, and postpartum necrosis (Sheehan's syndrome). Most if not all patients develop psychiatric symptoms such as depression, lethargy, apathy, indifference, fatigue, and loss of libido. Cognitive deficits are not uncommon and some patients may develop delusions. Delirium may develop in the context of an Addisonian-type crisis. The skin has an alabaster appearance and may be finely wrinkled around the mouth and eyes. Pubic and axillary hair is lost as is the pigmentation of the areolae and the capacity to tan. Treatment consists essentially of replacement therapy and may lead to dramatic results, though a few patients have some residual apathy and fatigue despite treatment.

Menopause

Menopause is generally defined as the cessation of menses for one year, usually occurring between the ages of 45 and 50. Symptoms include anxiety, irritability, depression, emotional lability, dizzy spells, changes in libido, hot flashes, headaches, and atrophic changes in mucous membranes. Many of these symptoms are related to decreasing estrogen levels, but androgens and luteinizing hormone may also be involved. For women with a chronic problem of low self-esteem, especially those whose self-esteem has depended on child rearing, the involutional period may be one of particular stress. The loss of childbearing ability and changes in physical appearance and capabilities may have both symbolic and real implications for women during this period. The use of hormone replacement therapy is somewhat controversial, but is generally accepted for the short-term relief of physical symptoms. Psychotherapy is focused on helping the patient find satisfying new activities and interests, and working through the grieving process for lost capabilities and time, in some cases. The individual needs and social context must always be kept in mind.

Premenstrual Syndrome (PMS)

Premenstrual syndrome includes a number of physical and psychological symptoms occurring to a greater or lesser degree in many women during the 3 to 5 days prior to the onset of menses. Symptoms include anxiety, depression, emotional lability, irritability, fatigue, changes in appetite and food preferences, fluid retention, and gastrointestinal complaints, among others. Criminal acts, psychiatric admissions, and suicide attempts have all been noted to be increased during this time. Diuretics may be helpful in decreasing fluid retention, and education concerning the syndrome may also be useful. Supportive or insight-oriented psychotherapy may be indicated for some women with premenstrual symptoms, but not solely on the basis of premenstrual syndrome.

Other Endocrine Disorders

Psychogenic amenorrhea refers to the cessation of menses without demonstrable organic cause in premenopausal nonpregnant women. It occurs in psychiatric conditions such as anorexia nervosa, pseudocyesis, and massive obesity, and may also occur under conditions of severe and persistant stress. In most women, cycling will return without intervention, though in some the use of birth-control pills or psychotherapy aimed at the underlying cause may be indicated.

Hypocalcemia secondary to hypoparathyroidism may produce anxiety, depression, emotional lability, fatigue, and in more extreme cases, delirium or psychosis. Hypercalcemia secondary to hyperparathyroidism may produce apathy and depression, problems with concentration and short term memory, and occasionally delirium. Hypoglycemia may produce an array of psychiatric symptoms ranging from anxiety, sweating, tachycardia, and feelings of panic or doom, to delirium with disorientation, marked confusion, and psychosis. The most common cause is overdose of exogenous insulin, but a number of medical conditions may be responsible, including chronic alcohol abuse.

Diabetes mellitis represents a substantial and chronic stress on the patients afflicted. Their ability to follow the dietary and medical regimens is dependent on their personality structure and relevant psychosocial factors. Patients may resist treatment indirectly through dietary indiscretions or general noncompliance based on an inability to accept the restrictions imposed by the illness. Key factors in long-term management include the physician–patient relationship, the social support systems available, and the patient's ability to maintain his self-esteem and identity in the face of this chronic condition.

Skin Disorders

The skin serves important functions as a protective barrier, a point of contact between people, and a regulator of fluid and temperature status. It may translate certain emotional states into visible reactions, such as blushing with embarrassment, turning red with fury, or becoming pale with fear. The psychosomatic skin disorders include (1) exaggerations of normal cutaneous functions, (2) conditions in which the patient harms the skin secondary to an underlying psychiatric disorder, (3) conditions that are aggravated or precipitated by emotional stress or anger, and (4) chronic conditions in which there is disfigurement, creating secondary psychiatric problems.

Pruritis

The sensation of itching, which may occur in a variety of dermatologic and systemic conditions, is conveyed centrally by the same slow-conducting afferent fibers responsible for pain and tickle. From a psychiatric perspective, guilt, unexpressed anger, or unacceptable sexual wishes may all be responsible for itching, which becomes the avenue of expression of these repressed emotions. Itching usually leads to scratching, and this sequence may represent a cyclic process linked psychologically as follows. Guilt, anger, and repressed wishes to be held, caressed, or loved may give rise to itching. When these desires are thwarted, anger and frustration may be turned against the self in the form of scratching, which becomes a compromise solution for these unexpressed impulses. *Pruritis ani* and *pruritis vulvae* are localized conditions that develop after an organic condition in these areas has been treated. The two conditions are felt to be related to conflicts regarding sexual wishes and prohibitions.

Urticaria

Many physical, chemical, and biological factors may cause urticarial eruptions. While an allergic etiology can usually be found in the acute case, the etiology of chronic cases is seldom determined. Afflicted patients have been characterized as having repressed hostility over the loss of love or having unfulfilled wishes to be loved, which "erupts" into the typical "wheal and flare" manifestations of urticaria. The condition thus represents a compromise between the wish to be loved and attended to and the rage against resulting frustration that creates a sense of guilt over these aggressive impluses. The lesions draw attention in an exhibitionistic way, and when combined with scratching, gratify the rage by turning it against the self and the guilt by way of self-punishment and an unattractive appearance.

Rosacea

This condition can be thought of as an exaggerated blush response and involves an increased vascularity over the blush region of the face and upper chest, with associated papule formation. Most investigators believe that a constitutional tendency exists in these patients because they also have an increased vascular response to heat or spicy foods. Typically, these patients have an abnormally inflated self-esteem that is overly dependent on positive feedback from others, making them quite sensitive to even minor disapprovals or slights. They demand perfection from themselves and typically have a restrictive code of morals, associated with a strong sense of guilt, shame, and deep-seated feelings of unworthiness or failure. The skin condition develops in response to transgressions against their moral prohibitions and serves as an outlet for unacceptable erotic or aggressive impulses, while preserving their rigid psychological exterior. For example, a young woman with strong prohibitions against sex and vulgar language may blush on hearing a leud comment. This way, she maintains her appearance of being innocent while demonstrating that on another level she understood the comment and may have derived some gratification of unconscious wishes through it. This mechanism is thought to operate excessively in patients with rosacea and combines with constitutional factors to produce the condition.

Psoriasis

Psoriasis is a relatively common inflammatory skin disease affecting all ages, and is notable for it's chronicity and variable severity. Clinical features include large red plaques covered with thick white scales, commonly occurring over the knees and elbows as well as other areas. Although the disease appears to have a recessive inheritance pattern, there are a number of aggravating factors, especially emotional stress, which frequently precedes both the onset and exacerbations of the illness. There is evidence of increased skin temperature and hyperemia in response to stress in these patients. Although there is no prototypic personality for psoriasis, it has been proposed that these patients have strong needs for contact and security. The skin condition reflects repressed hostility secondary to frustration of these wishes, which is then turned against the self.

It must be kept in mind that psoriasis can be a very disfiguring condition that may cause these patients to feel repulsive to others. Supportive psychotherapy aimed at improving the patient's self-concept and reducing their social isolation may be helpful. Finding alternative means for handling stress, through problem-solving or relaxation techniques, may also be beneficial.

Atopic Dermatitis

Originally described as *neurodermatitis* by Brocq and Jaquet in 1891, this common skin condition is essentially a form of endogenous eczema, the cause of which is multiply determined and involves both immunologic and emotional factors. The skin is erythematous and dry, with papules, vesicles, hyperkeratosis, exudation, and crusting. These patients are noted to have intense longings for physical closeness, which is perhaps related to inadequate maternal contact early in life, and thus they chronically seek attention and contact in an effort to restore this deficit. Relapses or exacerbations are usually related to personal losses or events that constitute a loss of love or contact. The scratching that is invariably present provides an outlet for tension and self-punishment for hostile feelings toward those who "rejected" them. It is not known how these personality factors and psychological responses to losses interact with immunologic factors to produce this condition.

Alopecia Areata

This is a condition of sudden patchy hair loss, most frequently seen in childhood, and identified by the short, stumpy "exclamation mark" hairs that are present. Although an autoimmune reaction has been suggested, no mechanism has been identified. Characteristic features involve an early symbiotic loss such as the birth of a sibling, real or threatened abandonment, or traumatic weaning followed by a period of partial adjustment that breaks down in the face of an event recreating the early loss. Interestingly, and for unknown reasons the hair loss occurs approximately 2 weeks following the precipitating trauma. The hair usually grows back quickly, and any treatment beyond brief supportive measures is rarely required.

Hyperhidrosis

Perspiration in humans is of two types, thermoregulatory and emotional, with the latter mediated by the eccrine sweat glands on the palms, soles, and axillae. Patients complaining of hyperhidrosis, or anxious perspiration, frequently have a preoccupation with their appearance in general, and concern over their own offensiveness may reach delusional proportions. They may have sexual concerns or exaggerated social anxiety that may require psychotherapeutic or behavioral treatment.

Acne Vulgaris

This condition occurs with such frequency in puberty and adolescence that it may be viewed as a normal part of growing up. It may be exacerbated by emotional stress, however, and may lead to anxiety and avoidance in some teenagers, at a time when appearance and social interactions are very important. While no one would suggest that psychological factors alone are responsible for acne vulgaris beyond adolescence, Wittkower (1953) proposed that in adults with acne vulgaris, there has been a failure to develop emotionally beyond the time of puberty, leading to a high frequency of frigidity and sexual disturbance in these patients. Good dermatological care with support may be sufficient for adolescents, but more intensive psychotherapy may be a useful adjunct in adults.

Other Dermatologic Conditions

Dermatitis artefacta results from scratching and may occur in patients with inadequate psychosexual development who may be demanding and dependent. These patients, like those with *trichotillomania* (the impulse to pull out one's own hair), have an unconscious wish to make themselves unattractive, perhaps as a punishment for sexual wishes or arousal. Another unusual condition presenting to dermatologists has been called *delusional parasitosis,* which is a condition primarily affecting women in middle to late life, who complain of having small insects in their skin, which they can feel crawling around. One must rule out an organic psychosis in these patients.

Rheumatoid Arthritis

Rheumatoid arthritis is a chronic systemic disease involving inflammation of synovial joints that leads to pain, disability, and gradually debilitating deformities such as ulnar deviation, in some patients. Women are afflicted three times more frequently than men. Rheumatoid arthritis typically has its onset in middle age and follows a variable course in terms of severity, punctuated by periodic exacerbations that are frequently associated with emotional stress or turmoil. Alexander (1950) included rheumatoid arthritis in the "holy seven" psychosomatic diseases and proposed that the condition represents the indirect expression of repressed or inhibited hostile impulses.

Clinical Features and Pathogenesis

The onset of rheumatoid arthritis is frequently preceded by symptoms of fatigue, malaise, weakness, weight loss, and fever, followed by the development of inflammation and pain in the knees, elbows, and proximal interphalangeal joints of the hands. Morning stiffness, subcutaneous nodules, and extra-articular manifestations such as pericarditis or pleuritis may develop. Laboratory findings include positive rheumatoid factor and poor mucin clot formation in the synovial fluid. An underlying immunological disorder in which an immunopathic response to an unidentified antigen occurs is felt to be involved, but the exact mechanism is unknown. Rheumatoid factor, immune complexes, and complement accumulate in the synovial tissues. Lysosomal enzymes released from phagocytes appear to account for much of the damage to cartilage and synovium, leading to joint destruction.

Psychophysiology

There are several ways in which emotional stress may contribute to the arthritic process in this disease. Connective tissue synthesis regulation and immune system reactivity may be altered by hormones, such as corticosteroids, which are known to be affected by emotional stress. Ligaments, joint capsules, and synovia are richly supplied with autonomic nerve supply and may be affected by the large sympathetic outflow that can result from fear, anxiety, or excitement. Muscle tension can result from anxiety and may play a role in the production of joint deformation. Finally, immunoglobulin levels may be associated with elevated life-change indices. The degree to which any of these mechanisms are involved etiologically is not known. They represent interactions between psychosocial, emotional, and physiologic processes that potentially affect the course of the condition.

Personality

Alexander (1950) postulated that arthritic-prone children are restricted from expressing hostility and instead discharged their aggressive impulses through activity. When the level of activity could not match the level of hostility, increases in muscle tone produced or exacerbated arthritic symptoms. The idea of repressed hostility remains a common one. These patients tend to have conflicts regarding the expression of angry or aggressive feelings, resulting in attempts to control these emotions that are sometimes rigid. Rheumatoid arthritis patients have been described as more compulsive, masochistic, self-conscious, and depressed than nonarthritic patients. Men patients tend to be hostile, rigid, and depressed, while women seem to be more preoccupied with somatic concerns, control, and the repression of angry or hostile feelings. Many have underlying or overt dependent traits, and exacerbations have been noted to occur at times of loss or separation from caretaking figures. It should be noted that no single personality profile exists for these conditions, despite some general tendencies related to issues of control, dependency, and the expression of anger. The disease is rare in prison populations and almost never occurs in patients with schizophrenia.

Rheumatoid arthritis is a chronic, disabling, and at times disfiguring condition wrought with pain. It may seriously limit social and occupational functioning as well as damage the patient's self-concept and self-esteem. Moldofsky and Chester (1970) found increasing levels of depression with increasing complaints of pain in most of their patients. Fortunately, some patients will respond to antidepressant medications with improvement of mood and pain symptoms. Nevertheless, coexisting depression and the inability to cope or adjust to functional losses present significant obstacles in the treatment of many of these patients.

Treatment

The goal of treatment is to establish a program that will reduce pain and inflammation, prevent or correct deformities, and maintain optimal functioning, given the restrictions of the disease. A consistent and supportive relationship between the patient and the primary physician is important, and the physician's responsibility involves coordinating the treatment program and providing education for both the patient and the family. Medications such as aspirin, phenylbutazone, indomethacin, naproxen, and steroids in the setting of an acute exacerbation may be used. Physical therapy may be needed to help establish an appropriate exercise program aimed at maintaining range of motion and strength. Orthopedic surgery may be required to correct deformities.

Psychotherapy for rheumatoid arthritis patients has been most beneficial for those having good ego strength and impulse control. It may be of little benefit, however, in those patients with poor premorbid functioning, little psychological insight and poor impulse control. Supportive psychotherapy should be directed toward maintaining self-esteem and self-concept, allowing the expression of angry or hostile feelings, and preventing the patient from reaching the point of helpless dependence and despair. It may be necessary to teach the family to give positive reinforcement for appropriate patient activities while reducing secondary gain from overly dependent or independent activities. The use of antidepressant medication for symptoms of pain and depression may be helpful in some patients.

Headache

Headache is one of the most common problems dealt with in medical practice. When chronic, it can result in numerous visits to family physicians, internists, neurologists, and psychiatrists, at great expense and frustration for the patient. There are a variety of potential etiologies including muscle contraction or tension, vascular spasm, increased intracranial pressure, tumor, inflammation, sinus conditions, and hypochondriacal or conversion disorders. In many cases, stress or other emotional factors are important in the precipitation of a headache, in which case a thorough evaluation must include both physiologic and psychological parameters. This section will focus on the types of headaches that involve emotional factors most consistently, such as muscle contraction, migraine, and those headaches associated with psychiatric conditions such as conversion disorders, delusions, or hypochondria.

Migraine or Vascular Headache

Clinical features of migraine headaches include visual or neurological deficits preceding the onset, pain lateralized to one side that is initially intense and throbbing, nausea and vomiting, and for some patients, ophthalmoplegia, speech abnormalities, and mood disturbances. Variants of this type of headache include facial cephalgia, cluster headaches, and headaches associated with the premenstrual syndrome or menses. The etiology is unknown but may involve abnormalities in brain-stem serotonergic pathways. Many factors trigger migraine attacks, but common ones include anxiety, stress, fatigue, lack of sleep, hunger, temperature changes, certain foods and alcohol, as well as menstruation or oral contraceptive use.

Although there is no one personality type that is predisposed to migraine headaches, these patients as a group are perfectionist, ambitious, and controlling, with tendencies to suppress or control anger. They are vulnerable to migraine development during times in which their ambitions are thwarted, or when the level of stress reaches the point that their control mechanisms are less useful. Treatment generally revolves around the removal or avoidance of triggering factors and the use of medications. Ergotamine continues to be the main treatment for the acute attack, although aspirin or codeine may abort the headache if taken quickly enough. Methysergide continues to offer the greatest chance for a headache-free existence, but its side effect (involving connective tissue proliferation in the heart, kidneys, and lungs) may limit its usefulness. Other more benign agents, including ergonovine, propranolol, and amitriptyline, may be used alone or alternated monthly. A supportive physician–patient relationship in which there is reassurance and emotional contact is important, and psychotherapy may be helpful in some cases by modifying behavior patterns that create stressful situations. Psychotherapy alone, however, has not been shown effective in treating this condition. For some patients, relaxation techniques may be helpful in moderating stress and preventing some stress-related migraine attacks.

Muscle-Contraction Headache

This type of headache is generally described as bilateral, dull, aching, of variable severity and duration, and typically involving the suboccipital region, where the muscles may be tense and tender, or less frequently, the parietotemporal regions may be involved. There are no visual or neurological prodromata and nausea is rare. While these headaches are generally mild in severity and responsive to simple therapeutic maneuvers such as aspirin or acetaminophen, they may become chronic and debilitating. Although early investigators of this disease believed that the pain resulted from prolonged contraction of the skeletal muscles of the neck, scalp, face, and shoulders, the exact physiologic mechanism remains to be elucidated. Emotional stress, fatigue, glare, frustration, and loud noises, however, may cause some degree of headache in the majority of people.

People with persistent anxiety are the most frequent sufferers of chronic headaches of the muscle-contraction type, and may additionally be irritable, unable to sleep, overly dependent on the opinions of others, or depressed. Headache may be the presenting problem in major depressive disorder; it also may be used as a vehicle for the gratification of otherwise unmet dependency needs. The use of denial of their own frustration and hostility may produce tension and somatization in the form of tension headache in these patients.

Initial treatment is aimed at the relief of symptoms through pharmacologic approaches or behavioral techniques such as relaxation or biofeedback. Antianxiety agents and muscle relaxants have been useful for many patients. Supportive or insight psychotherapy may be effective, depending on the patient's personality structure and the underlying cause.

Headaches Associated With Primary Psychiatric Disorders

Headache may be the presenting complaint of patients with schizophrenia or major depressive disorder. In patients with schizophrenia, it may represent a persistent delusion or, in some cases, a way of initially describing other symptoms related to thought disorder. A severe depressive state may be somatized with headache as the major complaint. Thus, assessing the patient with regard to sleep, appetite, energy, libido, and interest may be revealing.

Hypochondriacal patients frequently have headache as a prominent symptom, usually associated with poor sleep, concentration, memory, and other complaints. These patients have longstanding preoccupations with their bodies and usually have problems with intense dependency needs that go unmet, creating hostility that is repressed and manifested as somatic complaints. These somatic complaints may exempt the patient from more independent functioning, and thus result in secondary gain that can be difficult to alleviate. Altering the contingencies of dependency gratification through family therapy may be effective in these patients.

Treatment of Psychosomatic Disorders

The key tenet in the treatment of psychosomatic disorders is that the patient, rather than the disease, is the focus of the physician's interest. While fear, anxiety, anger, and frustration may lie at the root of the patient's problems, the complaints are likely to be somatic ones, with variable physiologic manifestations. Premature suggestions that the symptoms are the result of emotional problems may not only be erroneous, but will more often than not entrench the patient in seeking help for his "real" complaints. The primary physician must be alert to the psychosocial factors involved, but must also address the physical symptoms while providing emotional support. Care must be taken to prevent the patient's misunderstanding *psychiatric consultation* to mean his symptoms are "all in his head," or that the primary physician is abandoning him. This can be a very delicate situation because somatic complaints may represent some of the most rigid characterologic defenses, in which the patient translates his emotional conflicts into physical symptoms or exacerbations of chronic illnesses and presents them for "cure." The patient's passive dependent stance and strong investment in organic symptoms may quickly result in a situation in which the physician becomes frustrated, which may then lead to an increase in the patient's dependency and hostility. In the context of a supportive physician–patient relationship, emotional factors that the patient can accept will usually emerge. Reassurances that the patient is not regarded as "crazy" and that his complaints are legitimate and the object of concern may be necessary. Explanations regarding the physiologic components of stress and their effects on particular conditions are useful. Even in the best of circumstances, some patients will refuse psychiatric consultation and must be managed solely by the primary physician. A consultation between physicians may be important in some of these cases regarding the management of symptoms and personality patterns. For example, with extremely dependent patients, the physician may require frequent brief visits from the patient to gratify the patient's dependency needs and prevent him from using physical complaints to receive caretaking.

Psychotherapy with psychosomatic patients obviously varies depending on the particular conditions, but generally must proceed slowly with much support and reassurance. Frequently, the patient must be allowed to maintain his passive dependent or overcontrolling stance early on to prevent premature rejection of treatment due to perceived rejection or fears of being controlled. Care must be taken not to interpret the patient's symptoms too quickly, and thus overburden his ego with fear or anxiety, which are then further defended with somatic complaints. Indeed, "removal" of the validity of physical symptoms too quickly may precipitate a severe depression or psychosis. Proceeding cautiously, the patient may gradually develop more mature ways of handling stress or obtaining necessary gratification.

The overwhelming majority of patients with psychosomatic disorders requiring intervention by a psychiatrist will need supportive rather than insight-oriented psychotherapy. The psychiatrist should (1) take a more active stance, at times making suggestions and giving advice, (2) be more overtly concerned and supportive, and (3) attempt to strengthen existing defenses while gently reinforcing the development of higher-level defenses where more primitive ones exist. Family consultation and therapy may be needed to alter reinforcements of somatic complaints, and thus reduce secondary gain while maintaining overall support. Medications and nonpsychotherapeutic modalities such as biofeedback and relaxation techniques must be used when indicated.

The management of patients with psychosomatic disorders requires greater-than-usual sharing of responsibility and regular communication between physicians. The psychiatrist must maintain familiarity with the patient's medical condition, and the primary physician needs to be aware that the expression of somatic symptoms may reflect the emergence of underlying conflicts. When patients require hospitalization for medical reasons, the psychiatrist should maintain contact with the primary physician and the patient, and be willing to help in situations where management problems may develop.

It must be kept in mind that a significant number of patients with psychosomatic disorders may not stand to benefit from direct psychiatric intervention. These may be patients who refuse such alternatives or who require supportive therapy that for a number of reasons may be most appropriately performed by the primary physician. For these patients, it is the responsibility of the primary physician to manage the treatment program. Several general principles are relevant in this situation. First, the physician–patient relationship is the foundation for any intervention. It needs to be stable and supportive, with the physician manifesting a willingness to try to help the patient in the best way he can. Second, psychosomatic disorders are, for the most part, chronic problems for which management, rather than cure, is the goal. Patients may see the physician as someone who will "make their problems go away" by some means. After careful evaluation that includes an assessment of pertinent psychosocial factors, this goal of management may need to be communicated to the patient, along with the physician's willingness to continue to follow the patient's progress. Care must be taken to attend to the patient's needs while avoiding becoming involved in the patient's expectations that all his suffering be relieved, an expectation that may lead to a futile search. Finally, treatment interventions must be presented to patients in a manner consistent with the patient's personality. Some patients view the physician as "someone who knows best" and will respond best to a paternal manner. Others wish to maintain some control, and they respond best to recommendation, rather than being told what to do.

Consultation–Liaison Psychiatry

Psychiatric consultation for medical and surgical services began in the 1920s, but the term *consultation–liaison psychiatry* was coined, in the 1960s, to more fully describe the role of psychiatrists in the general hospital setting. This role includes formal consultations, teaching, working with the primary-care team, staff and administrative duties, and, in some cases, becoming involved in activities such as support groups for staff or patients. Psychiatrists may be consulted for the presence of psychiatric symptoms such as anxiety, depression, psychosis, drug withdrawal, emotional stress, formal psychosomatic disorders, or the suspicion of a psychiatric disorder presenting with somatic complaints that have no apparent organic basis. Patients who become management problems for other services due to psychotic or delirius behavior, suicidal ideation, uncooperativeness, hostility, or failure to make progress toward leaving the hospital, may result in a consultation request as well.

Disposition problems, patients with a past psychiatric history, or questions regarding psychotropic medications account for other consultation requests. Occasionally, psychiatrists will be asked to make a determination regarding a patient's mental competency to make decisions about his treatment.

It is important for the consulting psychiatrist to clarify the question asked by the requesting physician or service. Many failures to comply with recommendations are due to the consultant's failing to answer the requesting service's fundamental question. For example, the consultant may find evidence of a personality disorder that is impeding treatment. He may then suggest certain ways of interacting with the patient to facilitate compliance, which may go unheeded because the real question was whether the patient needed to be transferred to the psychiatry service, and whether he needed antidepressant medications or treatment for drug withdrawal. Obviously, once the consultant has seen the patient, he may have important recommendations that go beyond the original question, but it is essential to understand the needs of the requesting service.

The consultation itself should be pursued on the basis of the biopsychosocial model. The patient's organic disease, medications, and current medical status should be reviewed as well as the expected treatment course and prognosis, where applicable. The presence of psychiatric illness should be evaluated with attention to possible interventions such as medications, follow-up, or transfer. Personality factors and general responses to stress should be noted, as should the patient's understanding of and acceptance of his medical condition, the role of his family, and the social, occupational, and recreational implications for the patient. Once these factors have been assembled, interventions may be made that will address the pertinent problems for a given patient. Interventions must be practical in terms of time, motivation, and resources available on the part of the patient, staff, and family. Examples of interventions might include (1) prescribing antidepressant medication for a major depressive episode and arranging psychiatric follow-up once the patient is discharged from the hospital, (2) prescribing a minor tranquilizer for situational anxiety related to an upcoming operation, (3) short-term psychotherapy to help a patient work through a sense of guilt or damaged self-esteem following an injury or operation (*e.g.*, mastectomy), (4) helping a family adjust their respective roles in the face of an illness or disability in the patient, or (5) arranging a vocational rehabilitation evaluation for a patient whose medical or surgical condition will necessitate his finding a new occupation. Once the evaluation is completed, recommendations should be discussed with the primary physician, at which time questions can be answered, responsibilities delineated, and follow-up care established. This last step is very important in terms of implementing suggestions, and for education of nonpsychiatric staff or physicians.

Beyond the formal evaluation and recommendations for a particular patient, formal and informal liaison relationships with other services may permit the psychiatrist to provide some education to the medical or surgical physicians or nursing staff. This may include formal teaching rounds on topics such as major psychiatric disorders and their typical symptoms, adjustment difficulties that are typical for certain conditions (*e.g.*, end-stage renal disease and dialysis), or ways to manage hostile or uncooperative patients, as well as informal teaching around individual consultations. It is important when teaching in this context to be clear and pragmatic, avoiding the use of complicated and unfamiliar psychiatric language (this is also true for written consultations).

The liaison psychiatrist may also be involved in leading support or stress-management groups for staff involved in specialized care facilities such as intensive care units or hemodialysis centers. These types of counseling services may reduce the anxiety and pressure present in these settings, preventing staff "burnout" and aiding in problem-solving, which may result in improved patient care and staff satisfaction.

Bibliography

Alexander F: Psychosomatic Medicine—Its Principles and Application. New York, WW Norton, 1950

Alexander F, French TM, Pollack GH: Psychosomatic Specificity. Vol 1: Experimental Study and Results. Chicago, University of Chicago Press, 1968

Bruch H: Anorexia nervosa: Therapy and theory. Am Psychiatry 139:1531

Cannon WB: The Wisdom of the Body. New York, WW Norton, 1932

Dunbar F: Emotions and bodily changes, 3rd ed. New York, Columbia University Press, 1947

Engel GL: The need for a new medical model: A challenge for biomedicine. Science 196:129, 1977

Engels WD (ed): Dermatologic disorders. Psychosomatics 23:1209, 1982

Freidman M, Rosenbaum RH: Type A Behavior and Your Heart. Alfred A Knopf, New York, 1974

Halmi K: Anorexia nervosa and bulemia. Psychosomatics 24:111, 1983

Holmes TH, Raye RH: The social readjustment rating scale. J Psychosom Res 11:213, 1967

Kaplan HI, Freedman AM, Sadock BJ: Comprehensive Textbook of Psychiatry, 3rd ed. Baltimore, Williams & Wilkins, 1980

Keesey RE, Corbett SW: Metabolic Defense of the Body Weight Set Point. Psychiatric Annals 13:839, 1983

Latimer PR: Irritable bowel syndrome. Psychosomatics 24:205, 1983

Lipowski ZJ, Lipsitt DR, Whybrow PC: Psychosomatic Medicine: Current Trends and Clinical Application, New York, Oxford University Press, 1977

Martin MJ: Muscle contraction headache. Psychosomatics 24:319

Mirsky IA, Futterman P, Kaplan S: Blood plasma pepsinogen. Part II: The activity of the plasma from "normal" subjects, patients with duodenal ulcer, and patients with pernicious anemia. J Lab Clin Med 40:188, 1952

Moldofsky H, Chester WJ: Pain and mood patterns in patients with rheumatoid arthritis. Psychosom Med 32:309, 1970

Powers PS: Obesity: Psychosomatics 23:1023, 1982

Raskin NH: Migraine headache. Psychosomatics 23:897, 1983

Rosenbaum M: Ulcerative colitis. Psychosomatics 24:515, 1983

Selye H: The Physiology and Pathology of Exposure and Stress. Montreal, ACTA, 1950

Stunkard AJ (ed): Obesity: Basic mechanisms and treatment. Philadelphia, WB Saunders, 1978

Taylor CB, Fortman SP: Hypertension. Psychosomatics 24:433, 1983

Wittower ED, Russell B: Emotional Factors in Skin Diseases. New York, Harper 1953

Wolf S: Peptic ulcer disease. Psychosomatics 23:1101, 1982

Wyngaarden JB, Smith LH (eds): Cecil Textbook of Medicine, 16th ed. Philadelphia, WB Saunders, 1982

James E. Lee

16 Child Psychiatry

Children and adolescents require psychiatric evaluation for a number of reasons: developmental problems, disturbed behavior, interpersonal difficulties, psychotic disorders, and emotional turmoil. Diagnosis and treatment of the common childhood emotional problems will follow a brief description of child development.

Normal Development

Development spans the entire life cycle and consists of identifiable phases. Each phase influences and is influenced by preceding and succeeding phases of development. At each stage of development, basic physical, cognitive, and emotional tasks arise that must be accomplished (Table 16–1). This section will discuss these tasks along with the developmental theories and observations of Freud, Erikson, Mahler, and Piaget.

Infancy

Bonding with the mother becomes strikingly visible immediately following birth. For brief moments, the newborn is in an alert inactive state with wide-open eyes that fix on a point and follow it. By 3 months, the infant begins to discriminate between caretakers and strangers, reinforcing a psychological symbiosis with the mother. Around this time the social smile develops as the infant responds to the

(Text continues p. 333)

Table 16–1
Developmental Tasks

Age	Phase	Motor and Cognitive Functions	Psychosexual Stages	Object Relations	Predominant Defenses	Psychosocial Stage
1 month		Roots, sucks, and grasps		Bonding		
2 months						
3 months		Social smile			Projective identification	
4 months					Incorporation	
5 months		Sits and grasps objects			Projection	
6 months	Infancy		Oral–incorporative	Symbiosis	Primitive denial	Basic trust vs mistrust
7 months		Crawls (6–8 mo)				
8 months		Stranger anxiety		Separation–individuation—differentiation		
9 months		Separation anxiety				
10 months		Object permanence				
11 months		Walking (10–14 mo)				
12 months						
13 months						
14 months				Separation–individuation—practicing		
15 months		Imitation				

16 months						
17 months	Toddler					
18 months		Talking (few words)				
19 months		Preoperational thought				
20 months						
21 months						
22 months		Toilet training	Anal–retentive	Separation–individuation—rapprochement	Splitting	Autonomy vs shame
23 months					Early reaction formation	
24 months						
30 months				Separation–individuation—object constancy		
36 months						
42 months						Initiative vs guilt
4 years	Preschool			Oedipal		
5 years			Immature genital			
6 years		Shift to verbal memory			Repression	
7 years		Concrete operational thought		Latency relationships	Identification	Industry vs inferiority
8 years	Latency		Relative latency		Reaction formation	
9 years						

(Continued)

Table 16–1
Developmental Tasks (*Continued*)

Age	Phase	Motor and Cognitive Functions	Psychosexual Stages	Object Relations	Predominant Defenses	Psychosocial Stage
10 years						
11 years	Preadolescence			Second separation–individuation	Regression	
12 years		Formal operational thought		Mourning of childhood loves	Displacement	
13 years					Reversal of affect	Identity vs identity diffusion
14 years	Adolescence		Mature genital		Identification	
15 years						
16 years						
17 years						
18 years						

human face, particularly the mother's face. During infancy the rudimentary oral functions are well developed and loving, and aggressive impulses are expressed by sucking and biting. Freud called this period of psychosexual development the oral stage. To Erikson, the main psychosocial task of infancy is the establishment of basic trust.

Margaret Mahler, in studying normal child development, noticed that children progressed through certain stages as they gradually separated from the close emotional bond with the mother. Mahler called this separation process the separation–individuation phase of development and divided the phase into four overlapping subphases: differentiation (6 to 12 months); practicing (9 to 18 months); rapprochement (15 to 24 months); and object constancy (24 to 36 months), leading up to a stable emotional sense of self as separate from others.

At 6 to 12 months of age, the *differentiation* subphase, the infant's capacity to discriminate between the mother and strangers matures and stranger anxiety develops, reaching a peak at 8 months. The baby also begins to understand separateness and can remember the mother in her absence; consequently, separation anxiety—distress in response to separation from the parent—appears. Favorite pastimes during the differentiation subphase include peek-a-boo and comparison of the mother's face and hair with the infant's own. Motor development accelerates and the baby is able to creep, crawl, and standup, using the whole body in its initial limited forays into the world away from the parent.

Toddler Stage

With the first steps at 11 to 13 months, the toddler moves into the practicing subphase of *separation–individuation*. The toddler actively practices rapidly improving locomotor skills, venturing away from the mother, absorbed in a "love affair with the world" and relatively oblivious to external danger.

One-and-a-half to two years of age marks the *rapprochement* subphase of separation–individuation. With the onset of language, the ability to remember, and the capacity to form mental images of the mother, the child becomes more aware of his separateness and vulnerability when away from the mother. Each bump or fall shatters the child's illusion of omnipotence, and the child longs for maternal protection, while at the same time wishing for more independence. This ambivalence is demonstrated by clinging, demanding behavior alternating with moving away from the mother. This ambivalence intensifies at 18 to 22 months, the peak of the rapprochement crisis. At this point, the toddler tends to swing rapidly between "all-hating" and "all-loving" feelings with a split of intrapsychic representations into believing the mother to be "all good" on occasions and "all bad" at other times. This splitting is a defensive process that protects the good parent image from imagined destruction by the toddler's aggressive feelings. Internal representations of the self are similarly split. As the child matures, love mollifies aggression, and the good and bad images and the corresponding feelings are gradually integrated into one stable mental representation of the mother and a separate, stable sense of the self.

Rapprochement coincides with the anal phase of psychosexual development. Toilet training becomes an arena of conflict as the toddler expresses opposition to the mother's wish for an unsoiled and dry diaper. Gradually, the child counters the urges to mess by taking pride in toilet training accomplishments. To Erikson, learning toilet training leads to autonomy, and failure leads to shame; hence the psychosocial task for this stage is autonomy vs shame and doubt.

Object constancy at 24 to 36 months, the final subphase of separation–individuation, witnesses a consolidation of trends already underway: The child perceives others as dependent and reliable (object constancy) and thinks of himself as a worthy individual (stable sense of the self). The recognition of the anatomical differences between the sexes by the age of 2 contributes to the formation of gender identity, which is consolidated by the age of 3.

Preschool

The preschool period, ages 3 to 6, is characterized by rapid physical growth and nervous system maturation. By the age of 5, over 90% of the central nervous system (CNS) is myelinated, including cortical and subcortical structures. The vocabulary exceeds 1000 words; the child develops an improved sense of time, space, and causality; and reasons on a basis of configurations and comparisons, which Piaget, the "father of learning theory," called preoperational thinking.

The preschool child, according to Freud, falls in love with, and wishes to marry and mate, the parent of the opposite sex, while feeling jealous rivalry toward the parent of the same sex. This triangular configuration is known as the Oedipus complex in boys and the Electra complex in girls, in reference to the mythical Greek figures.

The murderous wishes create a dilemma for the child: First, the smaller child fears that the rivaled parent will retaliate and injure him; secondly, the hostile feelings conflict with the feelings of love that the child has for the parent. A variety of defensive maneuvers solve the struggle. The child pushes the oedipal wishes into unconsciousness (repression) and decides to become like the parent instead of trying to eliminate him. Consequently, the child identifies with the parental prohibitions, norms, and morals, leading to the formation of the conscience or superego. The loving aspect of the conscience approves initiative and enhances happiness, while the critical component of the superego prohibits incestuous and hostile wishes and produces feelings of guilt. To Erikson, this preschool period is the psychosocial stage of initiative vs guilt.

Latency

The latency-age child, aged 6 to 11, learns to channel aggressive and sexual feelings into work and play, establishes social relationships beyond the family, and continues cognitive development. To Erikson, latency is the time for industry vs inferiority. Classifications of objects, and the understanding of basic mathematical concepts are achieved when the 7 to 8-year-old develops the capacity for what Piaget calls *concrete operations*.

Adolescence

Adolescence, a time of transition from childhood to adulthood, marks a resurgence of sexual feelings that accompanies puberty. Affectionate ties are displaced from the parents to other persons outside the family and intense peer group loyalties develop. Rapid swings of mood are common: from love to hate and optimistic elation to pessimistic depression and despair. Behavior is also unpredictable and often fluctuates between opposing extremes.

Cognitive growth helps adolescents cope with their emotional vicissitudes. After 12 years of age, the young adolescent enters what Piaget calls the stage of *formal operations* and develops a capacity for abstract thought.

Adolescents plan for their futures in terms of jobs, further education, marriage, and so forth; thus, to Erikson, adolescence is a time for identity consolidation vs identity diffusion.

Modery society with its changing expectations, higher education demands, and changing marital conventions prolongs adolescence. The attainment of emotional stability, appropriate self-esteem, social responsibility, and a stable sexual identity indicates entry into the adult phase of development.

Adjustment Disorders

Adjustment disorders, maladaptive reactions to stress, are usually self-limited. If the stress persists, the conflict may produce a more serious and less reversible emotional disorder. Age-specific adjustment disorders will be discussed here.

Adjustment Disorder of Infancy

Reactive attachment disorder of infancy, also known as *failure to thrive,* results from overstimulation or understimulation of the child. Sometimes the mother is depressed, as illustrated in the following case:

> ☐ Cathy, a 4-month-old infant, presented to the emergency room with a history of persistent vomiting and weight loss. On examination, Cathy was lethargic and apathetic; she had an expressionless face; and there was an absence of cuddliness, playfulness, eye contact, and visual tracking. All vocalizations and cries were weak and sporadic. The history revealed that soon after Cathy's birth her father had unexplainedly left home. Her mother became increasingly isolated, withdrawn, and depressed; Cathy was left in her crib without human contact throughout most of the day and night. After Cathy's mother had been treated for depression, an appropriate mother–daughter relationship was established. Cathy's vomiting cleared and development proceeded normally.

The restitution of a normal parent–infant relationship will generally reverse the failure-to-thrive syndrome. Substitute parental figures may be necessary in cases of parental death or severe, untreatable parental psychopathology. Without adequate restitution, the infant may develop a full-blown depression with catatonia, excessive developmental delays, and increased susceptibility to infection, marasmus, and death.

Adolescent Adjustment Disorders

An estimated 10% to 15% of all adolescents experience a maladaptive adjustment disorder at some time during adolescence. Symptoms range from anxiety and depression to severe withdrawal or antisocial behavior. Middle to late adolescents are particularly susceptible to an identity disorder characterized by severe anxiety and concerns about sexual identity, morals, and career choices. Their doubts about "Who am I?" lead to impaired academic, job, or social functioning. During moments of extreme anxiety, they may experience depersonalization, confusion, and suicidal or aggressive ideation. Treatment of adolescent adjustment disorders promotes the reintegration of successful coping mechanisms and reestablishment of adaptive functioning. Short-term supportive psychotherapy facilitates this process.

Adjustment to Illness and Hospitalization

Illnesses and accidents are common stressors that every child experiences. Younger children, with their tendency toward magical thinking, may misinterpret their illness as a punishment. Illness depletes energy, thereby inducing regression, especially in younger children: Increased demands for attention may alternate with social withdrawal. Other children fight against the fearful regressive pull and oppose what they feel is humiliating treatment: Battles over diet and medicine may ensue.

Body image changes secondary to illness may contribute to low self-esteem and depression. Young children often display feeding, sleeping, and motoric disturbances as depressive equivalents. Older children and adolescents may demonstrate apathy, withdrawal, or dysphoric mood. Adolescents are especially sensitive to changes in body image brought on by illness.

Hospitalization magnifies adjustment difficulties. Children younger than 4 years of age may have intense separation anxiety with protest and despair in response to any separation from the parents. Preoperative disturbances in feeding, sleeping, and speech; as well as tics, enuresis, encopresis, and prolonged dependency have been observed in children undergoing surgery. Surgery serves as a focus for fears of mutilation; any procedure requiring anesthesia also brings about fears of loss of control, a prominent anxiety in early adolescents.

Education and special play opportunities can help children understand their illnesses, hospitalizations, and surgical procedures. Adolescents often benefit from patient groups. Such groups not only offer support, but they can provide positive models for identification and strengthen self image. Active participation in treatment and hospital ward activities also minimizes passivity and regression.

Adjustment to Chronic Illness

An estimated 30% to 40% of all children suffer from chronic physical illness, mental retardation, visual, speech or hearing disability, learning disorder, or behavioral disorder. Poor adaptation to chronic illness can result in a wide spectrum of personality disturbances: from an overdependent, overanxious, passive, withdrawn, and overprotected child; to an overindependent, aggressive, and risk-taking child.

Children who use cognitive flexibility, compensatory physical outlets, appropriate emotional release, and realistic dependency tend to adjust to chronic illness better. Adaptation is enhanced by parents who can master their fear and guilt, overcome their tendency to overprotect, and come to accept their child's limitations.

Mental Retardation

Mental retardation is defined by an intelligence quotient (IQ) of less than 70. Further subgroupings of mental retardation are: mild mental retardation, with an IQ of 50 to 70, comprising 80% of all mental retardation; moderate mental retardation, with an IQ of 35 to 49, comprising 12%; severe retardation, with an IQ of 20 to 34, comprising 7%; and profound retardation, with an IQ of less than 20, comprising less than 1% of the total.

Prevalence estimates of mental retardation range from 1% to 2% of the total population. Twenty-five percent of all mentally retarded children and adolescents have a definitive biological abnormality. Somatic chromosomal abnormalities (*e.g.*, Down's syndrome) and metabolic defects (*e.g.*, phenylketonuria [PKU], leukodystrophies, or gangliosidoses) produce moderate to profound retardation. Prenatal cytomegalic or rubeola viral infections, maternal malnutrition, maternal alcoholism, and toxemia in pregnancy can result in mental retardation. Prolonged and complicated labor with fetal distress and anoxia, as well as prematurity, increase the risk of developing mental retardation secondary to brain damage. Finally, a variety of postnatal events can bring about mental retardation: CNS infections, head trauma, lead poisoning, hypothyroidism, hydrocephalus, spina bifida, myelomeningocele, and craniosynostosis.

The remaining 75% of retarded people have no discernable biological etiologies. A large proportion of this group are of lower socioeconomic status; and because of a familial tendency, it is hypothesized that this type of mental retardation may be attributable to genetic as well as to cultural and environmental factors. These children tend to be mildly mentally retarded, hence they are often not diagnosed until they enter school.

Children with mental retardation have a higher incidence of attention disorders and movement disorders than children with normal intelligence. A large percentage of the mentally retarded manifest some sort of behavioral disturbance, such as severe temper tantrums, disorganized behavior, and self-mutilating acts. Because of his intense desire for peer acceptance and his poor judgment, the mentally retarded child or adolescent may readily volunteer for or take the blame for delinquent acts.

Profound mental retardation is chronic and unremitting (Table 16–2). These children will generally need constant structure and supervision throughout their lives. The severely mentally retarded can learn simple words and limited self-care tasks; the moderately retarded are trainable and capable of autonomous functioning; and the mildly mentally retarded are capable of minimal self-support. The following case represents the management of a person with moderate mental retardation:

☐ Bobby, a 6-year-old, was referred for psychiatric evaluation because of behavioral problems in school. A developmental history revealed that following an uncomplicated gestation period and birth, Bobby appeared to develop normally until the age of 9 months, when his parents noted that he failed to "pay attention." Later he began to throw temper tantrums when he couldn't get his way. His kindergarten teacher had recommended the evaluation when his behavior could not be controlled on the first day of school.

Table 16–2
Classification of Mental Retardation

Subtypes	IQ on Stanford–Binet Scale	Academic Potential	Social and Work Skills
Mild	70–50	Sixth grade by late teens (educable)	Minimum self-support
Moderate	35–49	Second grade by late teens (trainable)	Unskilled work under sheltered conditions
Severe	20–34	Able to communicate; trainable in elementary health habits	Partial self-maintenance under complete supervision
Profound	Below 20	Totally dependent	None (needs nursing care)

(From American Psychiatric Association: Diagnostic and Statistical Manual of Mental Disorders, 3rd ed. Washington, DC, American Psychiatric Association, 1980

Physical examination revealed triangular-shaped eyes with mild epicanthal folds, pronated feet, abnormal palmar creases, and mild hypertonia. In the psychiatric interview, Bobby exhibited a short attention span, little control over his aggressive impulses, and an increased activity level. His speech was that of a 3-year-old. Intelligence was estimated at 3 years and 2 months by psychological testing. An electroencephalogram (EEG) revealed a mild diffuse encephalopathy that was believed to have been present since birth.

Treatment involved a coordinated, multidisciplinary approach. Special education was designed to meet Bobby's particular needs and abilities, and behavioral therapy helped modify the temper tantrums. The parents received short-term psychotherapy to help them deal with the emotional impact of having a mentally retarded child. Reassessments and modification of treatment plans were necessary during crisis periods. Following completion of formal schooling, Bobby was able to live in a minimal-care home and work as a janitor.

Attention-Deficit Disorders

Attention-deficit disorders (ADD) can be divided into those with and those without hyperactivity. Hyperactivity is a symptom that occurs in a wide variety of childhood psychiatric disorders, including ADD. ADD with hyperactivity is characterized by overactivity, inattention, impulsiveness, and poorly organized behavior. Associated features include negativism, low frustration tolerance, poor peer relationships, lability of mood, and specific learning disabilities.

Prevalence estimates for ADD with hyperactivity range from 3% to 5% of prepubertal children; the disorder is 4 to ten times more common in males than in females. There is an increased incidence of alcoholism and antisocial behavior in laden precipitating stressor. At times anxiety may so overwhelm the person that certain aspects of the personality become dissociated from each other, causing a sudden temporary alteration in the normal integration of consciousness, identity, memory, and behavior. DSM-III describes four types of dissociative disorders: psychogenic amnesia, psychogenic fugue, depersonalization disorder, and multiple personality.

Psychogenic Amnesia

Psychogenic amnesia is defined in DSM-III as "a sudden inability to recall important personal information that is too extensive to be explained by ordinary forgetfulness, and which is not due to an organic mental disorder, including states of drug intoxication and withdrawal."

Four types of memory disturbance have been described. In the most common type, *localized amnesia,* the memory disturbance involves an inability to recall all events occurring during a circumscribed period of time. Most frequently this involves a period of several hours immediately following a very traumatic event.

A less common type of memory loss is *selective amnesia,* where the individual experiences an inability to recall some but not all of the events occurring within a circumscribed time period. The least common types of transient psychogenic memory loss are *generalized amnesia,* in which the failure to remember encompasses an individual's entire life, and *continuous amnesia,* in which the individual cannot recall events occurring after a specific time up to and including the present.

☐ DF was a married 48-year-old man brought to the emergency room one evening by police. He had been found wandering the streets and disturbing the peace by breaking street lights and overturning garbage cans. He was withdrawn and he mumbled incoherently. There was no evidence of trauma or any significant physical abnormalities. Laboratory evaluation revealed no electrolyte or other metabolic abnormality, and a toxicologic screen was negative. An electroencephalogram and head computed tomography (CT) scan were also normal.

The patient was held overnight for observation, and by the next morning he was alert, oriented, and able to communicate coherently. He denied any recollection of the events of the previous 18 hours, stating that the last thing he remembered was returning home from work the previous afternoon. Memory functions were otherwise intact. With the patient's consent, a series of interviews using sodium amobarbital (Amytal) were performed. Under the influence of Amytal he revealed that his wife had confronted him with her desire for a divorce the evening before, and was able to recall wandering through his neighborhood venting his anger. Later, when DF was no longer under the influence of Amytal, this information was reviewed with him and served as the beginning of what was to be a productive course of brief crisis-intervention psychotherapy.

The case of DF outlines many of the salient features of psychogenic amnesia, including the necessity of excluding possible organic etiologies as well as the potential diagnostic and therapeutic utility of the "Amytal interview." Other functional fathers of hyperactive children; as well as increased incidence of histrionic personality in their mothers. ADD with hyperactivity is more common in family members than the general population.

A significant proportion of hyperactive and distractible children exhibit evidence of constitutional or neurological involvement. These hyperactive children often display soft neurological signs, a history of delayed developmental milestones, electrophysiologic abnormalities, impaired body image, and perceptual processing deficits with specific learning disabilities.

One popular theory used to explain the distractability and overactivity of neurologically based ADD implicates an immature or dysfunctional anterior reticular activating system that is ineffective in filtering sensory input or inhibiting motor output. Another theory postulates a dysfunction of the cerebellar–vestibular complex. A variety of environmental toxins have been implicated as causative factors in ADD, including lead intoxication and food additives. The studies linking food additives with hyperactivity, however, have been inadequately designed and poorly controlled.

There are three main outcomes of childhood ADD with hyperactivity: The symptoms may disappear at puberty; the hyperkinesia may gradually diminish in adolescence but leave residual symptoms such as low frustration tolerance and poor self-image; or symptoms may persist into adulthood. Factors involved in predicting outcome are difficult to ascertain, but children with higher IQs appear to have a more favorable prognosis.

A multimodal treatment approach can be effective in ameliorating academic, behavioral, family, and emotional problems. Treatment modalities include psychopharmacotherapy, behavior modification, remedial education, and individual and family psychotherapy.

Stimulants can be helpful by specifically enhancing attention and decreasing motor restlessness so that the child can perform in school and benefit from therapy. Stimulants enhance dopaminergic and noradrenergic activity within the CNS, leading to the postulation that they strengthen the anterior reticular activating system's filtering ability. More than 500,000 children in the United States take stimulants, most commonly methylphenidate and pemoline, and less commonly, amphetamines. A response is generally noted in 1 to 2 weeks. Methylphenidate is generally initiated at a dose of 5 mg before breakfast and lunch and gradually increased as necessary up to a maximum of 1.7 mg/kg/day. During summers and on weekends during the school year, the medicine may be discontinued. As in all medications, the lowest possible dose that achieves symptomatic results should be used.

Initial side effects of anorexia and sleep disturbances generally disappear by the fourth week of administration. A few children will develop hypersensitivity, eosinophilia, tic disorders, choreoathetosis, acute behavioral deterioration, and psychosis when treated with stimulants. Because high doses may retard growth, the height and weight of children taking stimulants should be monitored. Not all hyperactive children respond to stimulant therapy, particularly those children whose hyperactivity has a strong emotional etiology. Antidepressants, such as imipramine 25 mg to 75 mg/day, are also used to treat ADD.

Individual psychotherapy and family therapy help the child and his family deal with the emotional components of ADD. Family dynamics may need to be addressed in cases where the symptoms fulfill a scapegoat role. Behavior modification can be used to reverse the maladaptive behavioral patterns that have been established in school and at home. Finally, educational therapy is necessary to relieve accumulated education deficits and treat any associated learning disabilities. The following case represents the multimodal treatment approach used with hyperactive children:

> ☐ Justin, a 7-year-old boy, was referred by his first grade teacher for restlessness and misbehavior in school. His mother reported that Justin had always been overly active, even in his sleep. He broke his crib at the age of 2½; he could not sit still in a movie or when he was watching his favorite television shows; and he would run up and down the aisles at church. In the interview, Justin displayed an extremely short attention span and high activity level—he did not remain engaged in any play activity for more than a minute. Play themes centered around sexual excitement and anxieties. Psychological testing indicated a learning disorder, revealing a full-scale IQ of 83, a performance IQ of 93, and a verbal IQ of 73. Additional interviews revealed that Justin's mother unconsciously encouraged some of his maladaptive behavior—she would laugh at his pranks and tease him rather than set reasonable limits on his behavior. Justin's father, a traveling salesman, appeared smugly indifferent to the problem. When his father was away from home, Justin's mother would frequently crawl into bed with him. Justin was started on methylphenidate and began a special reading program at school; his mother was helped to act more appropriately toward Justin's misbehavior, and she learned that sleeping with Justin increased his hyperactivity; Justin's father assumed a more active role in rule setting. Justin's hyperactivity gradually abated.

Learning and Developmental Disorders

Learning disorders, generally defined as a 1-to-2-year lag in school achievement, are the most common reason for psychiatric referral of school-age children.

Learning disorders arise from a wide spectrum of biological, emotional, and environmental etiologies. Inadequate intellectual stimulation, poor teaching, psychological trauma, neurologic deficits, and maturational lags contribute to the development of learning disorders. Emotional causes for learning problems include psychoses, neuroses, and personality disturbances. Unresolved sexual or aggressive conflicts may also contribute to learning disabilities.

Reading and Arithmetic Disorders

Children with developmental reading disorder, or dyslexia, constitute more than half of all learning-disabled children. Dyslexic children can exhibit faulty reading with word omissions, deletions, and additions; difficulty in word naming, spelling, and writing; a performance IQ greater than the verbal IQ; difficulty in symbolic arithmetic tasks; disturbances in right and left directionality; finger agnosia; and dominent hemispheric electrophysiologic adnormalities. A much smaller group, arithmetic underachievers, have deficits in nonverbal functions; difficulties in orientation; problems with arithmetic and constructional tasks; difficulties with visual motor integration; atypical speech prosody; poor visual memory; a verbal IQ greater than the performance IQ: and frequent nondominant hemispheric electrophysiologic abnormalities.

The above syndromes and mixtures thereof may be associated with both gross and fine motor coordination problems. A large proportion of learning-disabled children display hyperkinesia, distractability, or ADD. Any learning disability may induce secondary emotional problems.

A multimodal treatment approach to learning disabilities involves collaboration between an educational therapist, a family therapist, and a child therapist. Special educational help is necessary to ameliorate any maturational lags; when indicated, individual psychotherapy can deal with the secondary emotional conflicts; medication may be used to treat hyperactive symptomatology; and family therapy is crucial in cases where the child's learning difficulty fulfills a scapegoat role within the family.

The outcome is negatively related to the initial severity of the learning disability and is positively related to the child's compensatory strengths and cognitive endowments. For example, up to one fourth of mildly reading-disabled 7-year-olds (one grade behind), when given treatment, can be expected to read at grade level by the age of eleven, as compared to only 6% to 9% of all severely reading-disabled 7-year-olds.

Speech Disorders

Developmental speech disorders include articulation disorders, stuttering, and delayed speech. Articulatory errors of omission, substitution, and distortion of vowel and consonant phonemes usually disappear by the age of 7 or 8, but persist in 6% of grade-school boys and 3% of grade-school girls. This "baby talk," or dyslalia, may be accompanied by emotional immaturity. Speech therapy is an effective treatment of articulation disorders; psychotherapy may also be helpful.

The peak onset of stuttering occurs between 4 and 5 years of age, with boys outnumbering girls four to eight times. Stuttering displays a familial tendency and probably represents a complex interaction of neurophysiologic and emotional factors. Stuttering may intensify in anxiety-provoking situations and may stem from unconscious aggressive conflicts. Stuttering usually disappears with neurophysiologic maturation, although it persists in 1% of the population. Psychotherapy in conjunction with speech therapy may be helpful in severe or persistent cases of stuttering.

Delayed speech may be secondary to inadequate environmental stimulation, infantilism of the child, or regression following psychological trauma (*e.g.*, separations or sibling births). Children with deafness, infantile autism, and mental retardation frequently manifest impaired or delayed speech development. Specific neurologic deficits result in expressive aphasias in 0.1% of children, and receptive aphasias in 0.05% of children. Early treatment of delayed speech is important because stimulation is most beneficial during the exponential phase of linguistic growth, from 20 to 40 months.

Stereotyped Movement Disorders

Stereotyped movement disorders, called *tics,* involve repetitive, involuntary, and rapid motor movements or vocal utterances. The most common tics involve the facial muscles. Tic disorders generally begin between the ages of 2 and 15, display a familial tendency, and are more common in boys. It is hypothesized that each tic disorder arises from an interaction of emotional stress with a variable degree of neurophysiologic dysfunction. Tics may also be a symptom of neurotic, charactero-logic, psychotic, or organic disorders.

Transient tic disorders last less than 1 year and are estimated to occur in 12% to 23% of children. The intensity of tic disorders may wax and wane, depending on the level of stress; any tic can be voluntarily suppressed for varing amounts of time.

Gilles de la Tourette's syndrome is a chronic tic disorder that involves vocal as well as motor tics. Incidence rates vary from 0.1% to 0.01%. Tourette's syndrome may start early in life with a single facial tic and slowly develop to include vocal tics as well. Coprolalia, the repetitive utterance of obscene words, is pathognomic of Tourette's syndrome and develops in 60% of the cases. Some of these children also imitate other people's speech (echolalia) or movements (echokinesia), or exhibit obsessive compulsive stereotypes.

Approximately one half of Tourette's syndrome cases have discernable CNS pathology, as evidenced by neuropsychological testing, nonspecific EEG abnormalities, soft neurological signs, or a history of perceptual difficulties. This group shows a good response to the dopamine-blocking agent haloperidol. Futhermore, dopamine-releasing stimulants, such as methylphenidate or amphetamines, have been known to precipitate Tourette's syndrome. Consequently, it is postulated that Tourette's syndrome may involve dopaminergic hyperactivity in the corpus striata.

Roughly one half of Tourette's syndrome patients will spontaneously outgrow their tic disorder. A favorable outcome is related to higher IQ, good academic performance, and minimal CNS pathology.

Disorders of Arousal

Disorders of arousal include *pavor nocturnus* (night terror), somnambulism (sleep-walking), and somniloquy (talking while asleep). Sleep disturbances display a familial tendency and are more common in boys. Some investigators hypothesize that these disorders arise from a CNS developmental lag. Disorders of arousal tend to remit spontaneously at times of neurologic maturation, for example, upon transition into latency and at puberty.

Sleepwalking and Talking

Persistent somnambulism occurs in 1% to 6% of children. The episode generally occurs in the early hours of sleep when the sleeper is shifting, or arousing, from prolonged deep sleep (stage 3 or 4 sleep) into rapid eye movement (REM) sleep. REM sleep is normal. During the episode, which may last as long as 30 minutes, the child exhibits automatic behavior such as walking, talking, or urinating; and does not respond to people. The child will not remember the event. Unlike adult

Table 16–3
Characteristics of Dream Disturbances

	Night Terror or Nightmare Syndrome	Dream Anxiety
Onset	Early in night	Late in night
Autonomic arousal	High	None
Dream recall	Usually absent; if present, it is for an isolated single hallucination	Excellent, vivid
Sensorium during attack	Confused	Lucid
Stage of sleep	3 and 4	REM sleep
Etiology	Disorder of arousal	Possible emotional disturbance
Treatment	Diazepam	Psychotherapy

(Adapted from Walker JI: Clinical Psychiatry in Primary Care. Menlo Park, California, Addison–Wesley, 1981)

somnambulists, childhood sleepwalkers do not manifest an increased incidence of personality disorders. Severe and persistent somnambulism may be treated with diazepam, which suppresses both stage 4 sleep and REM sleep.

Sleep Terrors

Pavor nocturnus, or night terrors, may occur at any age. During the episode, the child screams, stares, and manifests signs of autonomic arousal. Stress, antidepressants, or neuroleptic medication may increase the frequency of sleep terrors. Diazepam 0.2 mg to 0.3 mg/kg/day may be helpful in severe cases.

Nightmares, in contrast to sleep terrors, are anxiety dreams that occur during REM sleep (Table 16–3). Young children are more prone to have nightmares because their dream defenses against unacceptable impulses are not well established. In severe cases of fears or anxieties about dreams or sleep, psychotherapy may be indicated.

Pervasive Developmental Disorders

Pervasive developmental disorders, occurring in children under the age of 12, involve developmental distortions or retardations of basic cognitive, psychological, and psychosocial functions. These disorders, in conjunction with childhood schizophrenia, are also known as the childhood psychoses.

Infantile Autism

Autism, consisting of impaired attention, social relatedness, and linguistic abilities, afflicts from 0.02% to 0.04% of children under the age of 10. Attention to auditory and visual stimulae is unpredictable and variable. Insensitivity to pain may be noted. Empathic human attachment and social interaction, which have usually been deficient since birth, are replaced by aloofness or withdrawal. Autistic children often have an intense attachment to certain odd objects (*e.g.*, rubber bands or strings) and are preoccupied by unusual functions of the object, for example, spinning.

Verbal and nonverbal communication are defective in autistic children. When they are not fully mute they exhibit echolalia and abnormal speech melody (dysprosody). They may have a strong interest in music. Perseverative, ritualistic, and compulsive behaviors are common in autistic children. They have a compulsive need to preserve the sameness of their environment and routine. Ritualistic self-stimulatory stereotypes include rocking, twirling, and head rolling.

> ☐ Teddy, age 3, was referred for a psychiatric evaluation after a medical work-up that included audiometric testing had failed to demonstrate an organic cause for his delayed speech. Teddy's mother recalled that he was an "especially good baby," who, unlike his brothers, never fussed or demanded any attention. However, his parents felt like they had never known Teddy. He never smiled or looked knowingly at them, and he never cuddled or displayed affection. He spent most of his time in his room playing with his toys. His favorite pasttime was sitting for hours watching the platter turn on his record player. The family had moved when Teddy was 2½, at which time he uncharacteristically threw a temper tantrum until he was allowed to rearrange his room exactly as it had been at his old house.
>
> During the interview, Teddy twirled on his tiptoes in a corner of the room, oblivious to the presence of the interviewer or his mother. He was unresponsive to verbal comments and appeared deaf. His affect was flat. When his mother opened a candy wrapper, he quickly ran to her and stared at the candy, his favorite treat. Teddy spent the remainder of the hour spinning a toy airplane propeller.

Prenatal and postnatal traumas, metabolic disturbances, and neurologic disorders may contribute to the autistic syndrome. Approximately one in ten cases of congenital rubella manifests the autistic syndrome. Mental retardation is frequently associated with infantile autism: 70% of autistic children have an IQ of less than 70 and half these children have an IQ below 50. The disorder is three to four times more common in boys than girls.

Infantile autism is 50 times more prevalent in siblings of autistic children than in the general population. The concordance rate of autism of monozygotic twins is 36%. These statistics indicate that at least a few types of infantile autism involve a polygenic inheritance mode. Recently, one type of infantile autism has been found in a sex-linked, recessive, fragile X-chromosomal syndrome.

Approximately one sixth to one third of all autistic children grew up to succeed in an occupation and lead independent lives, even though they remain egocentric and socially awkward. The remainder, generally those children with moderate to severe mental retardation and severe language deficits, remain seriously handicapped.

Treatment programs attempt to gradually break through the individual child's isolation and promote the development of language, adaptive behavior, social skills, autonomy, and, when possible, academic functioning. Behavior modification techniques are frequently used and may employ alternative communication channels such as singing, sign language, or pictures. Conservative doses of haloperidal (0.02 mg–0.03 mg/kg/day) are occasionally used to reduce autistic withdrawal and facilitate learning.

Childhood-Onset Pervasive Development Disorder

Childhood-onset pervasive development disorder (COPDD), marked by grossly impaired social relationships beginning after 30 months of age and before 12 years of age, has, according to the *Diagnostic and Statistical Manual of Mental Disorders*, 3rd ed, (DSM-III), at least three of the following characteristics:

1. Excessive anxiety
2. Inappropriate affect
3. Resistance to environmental change
4. Oddities of movement
5. Unusual speech patterns
6. Sensitivity to sensory stimuli
7. Self-mutilation

There are several types of COPDD. Symbiotic psychosis results from an overly intense parent–infant symbiotic relationship. Threat of separation may produce a full-blown psychosis with panic reactions, temper tantrums, loss of reality testing, and intense, inappropriate clinging. Another type of pervasive developmental pscyhopathology is known as *borderline psychosis* because these children rapidly shift between a reality-oriented state and a psychotic state. Borderline children have not mastered the rapprochement subphase of separation–individuation. They are unable to modulate or integrate thoughts or feelings, they overuse magical thinking, and they display poor frustration tolerance. Other children may incompletely internalize the characteristics of a psychotic parent.

Prognosis for childhood-onset developmental disorders is guarded. Treatment is lengthy, and is tailored for the child's specific needs. The common goal is to gradually help the child separate psychologically from the parents and develop autonomy. Simultaneous supportive psychotherapy for the parents is necessary.

Childhood Schizophrenia

Childhood schizophrenics, similar to infantile autistics, manifest impaired behavior, communication, perception, affect and social relatedness. In addition, schizophrenics demonstrate disordered thought. Schizophrenic children speak in incomplete and fragmented sentences with loose associations, disturbed grammar, and neologisms. Thought content may include a morbid preoccupation with aggression and bodily functioning. Delusions in early childhood schizophrenia may include bizarre introjections, for example, animals or machines are felt to be within the body. As the child grows older, persecutory delusions become more common. Affect is also inappropriate: There may be hebephrenic-like giggling, intense panic, rage, or apathy. Interpersonal relatedness varies from intense clinging to excessive distancing and autistic-like withdrawal. Hallucinations occur in older schizophrenics and are most commonly auditory. Approximately one fourth of all schizophrenic children have an IQ of less than 70 and one tenth have an IQ of less than 50.

> ☐ Sally, age 7, was seen in emergency evaluation because she was refusing to eat or drink: She felt there was "a snake in my belly" that she didn't want to feed. She was afraid that the snake would grow bigger and "eat her up." Although her affect was mostly flat, she would occasionally giggle inappropriately and glance from side to side. Her thought processes were loose and difficult to comprehend. At one point, for no apparent reason, she curled up in a fetal position and became mute.

Childhood schizophrenia has a genetic predisposition that is similar to adult schizophrenia. The course of childhood schizophrenia may be marked by exacerbations and remissions. From 70% to 95% of childhood schizophrenics manifest schizophrenia as adults and more than half of these patients are chronically institutionalized. The prognosis is more hopeful if the child has a higher IQ and intelligible speech, a history of good premorbid functioning, and is older at the time of onset. Schizophrenia with an acute onset has better prognosis than insidious-onset schizophrenia.

Supportive psychotherapy promotes mature defenses and adaptive functioning. In addition, the family often benefits from understanding the nature of their child's disorder. Antipsychotics may be used to treat severe agitation, aggressiveness, hallucinations, and delusions. Dose ranges from 0.05 mg to 0.15 mg/kg/day of haloperidol or its equivalent. The dose should be as low as possible to prevent acute and chronic side effects, such as seizures, a condition that develops in some childhood schizophrenics. Residential treatment may be necessary for schizophrenic children with severe behavior problems.

Adolescent Psychoses

Psychotic reactions constitute approximately 10% of all adolescent psychiatric hospital admissions. One third of these acute psychotic reactions present as an early adult schizophrenic disorder; the remainder are attributable to drug reactions, CNS pathology, affective illness, or brief reactive psychoses.

Brief reactive psychoses develop suddenly in response to a loss or psychosocial stressor. A brief reactive psychosis may be characterized by any of the following: labile affect; loose, disorganized, and confused speech; and bizarre and uncontrollable sexual, suicidal, and aggressive behavior. The delusions and hallucinations in brief reactive psychoses, in contrast to the persistent thought disorder in schizophrenia, do not last longer than 2 weeks.

Hospitalization is indicated when a pathologic family or home environment provides little support or when the adolescent displays seriously disturbed behavior. Hospitalization can promote immediate reconstitution or can permit further regression before reintegration occurs. Antipsychotics may be helpful in hastening reintegration. Following hospital discharge, supportive psychotherapy can help prevent relapse.

Organic Brain Syndromes

Children and adolescents with organic brain syndromes (OBS) suffer from some degree of permanent or temporary brain dysfunction due to neuronal destruction or metabolic disturbance. This dysfunction is generally due to an identifiable cause, unlike the subtle or undefinable organic dysfunctions that are postulated as etiologies for some of the other childhood disorders (*e.g.*, ADD or infantile autism).

Organic brain syndromes are a heterogeneous group of disorders that impair cognition and perception, and affect modulation or behavior. Subtypes of OBS include delirium, dementia, amnesia, organic hallucinosis, organic delusional syndrome, organic affective syndrome, organic personality syndrome, and substance intoxication and withdrawal. The wide variety of etiologies of organic brain syndromes in children and adolescents can be categorized as traumatic, infectious, metabolic, neurologic, or toxic. Organic disease has been discussed in greater detail in Chapter 8.

Affective Disorders

Infants and preschoolers react to separations and losses with protest and despair. Early loss makes a child more likely to become depressed when losses are experienced later in life. A reactive attachment disorder of infancy (see Adjustment Disorders) can develop into an anaclitic depression. These infants may become catatonic and die.

Unresolved, internalized conflicts can produce a heterogenous group of depressions known as *dysthymic disorders*. Children with chronic and pervasive dysthymic disorders often have chaotic family backgrounds and have suffered lifelong, repeated traumatic separations. In the first 2 years of life, these characterologically depressed children may have unconsciously identified with a depressed parent or developed self-deprecatory feelings by internalizing a hateful family conflict.

The symptom complexes of dysthymic disorder and major depression are qualitatively similar, but the symptoms of major depression are more severe. Children with either major depression or dysthymic disorder often exhibit a sad demeanor or hypactivity. They complain of loss of pleasure in their usual activities. They may have intensified separation anxieties, along with social and academic withdrawal. Sleep or appetite disturbances may be present, particularly in a major depression.

Occasionally, depressed children will present with somatic symptoms: headaches, abdominal complaints, pruritis, or dizziness. Other defensive attempts to avoid the painful depressive affect include hyperactivity, provocative behavior that elicits guilt-assuaging punishment, clowning in an attempt to cover up sadness, or obsessive–compulsive behaviors. Suicidal ideation may be present in depressed children. Children with major depression may demonstrate delusions of personal inadequacy, guilt, death, or nihilism.

A significant proportion of children with major depression, like biologically depressed adults, have a strong familial history of major affective disorder and alcoholism. Approximately one half do not suppress cortisol in response to dexamethasone.

Signs of depression in adolescents may include hypochondriacal concerns, somatization, psychophysiologic disturbances, sexual or aggressive acting out, delinquency, apathy, social withdrawal, school failure, drug abuse, and running away. Prolonged depressive signs and symptoms help differentiate a depressive disorder from the depressive mood swings that normally occur in adolescence.

☐ Jane, age 17, was seen for depression and intense suicidal ideation. At age 13, her twin sister had been killed in an auto accident. At age 15, Jane was diagnosed as having leukemia. She had suffered nausea, vomiting, and hair loss from chemotherapy and had become socially isolated, requiring a home tutor. Following remission of her illness, Jane began to feel guilty, depressed, and suicidal. She spoke to her psychiatrist of the anger, helplessness, and loss of control she felt in response to her life-threatening illness. Themes of loss and guilt were prominent. When she thought of her deceased twin sister, anger, survivor guilt, and reunion fantasies emerged. Jane was angry at her sister for dying; she unrealistically felt she was to blame both for her sister's death and her own illness. Psychotherapy softened her harsh conscience and allowed her to mourn the death of her sister and come to terms with her illness.

Bipolar disorder is extremely rare before puberty. In adolescents, the course and nature of the manic–depressive disorder approximates that of the adult illness (see Chapter 7).

Treatment of affective disorders depends on the diagnosis. Dysthymic disorders may respond to psychotherapy. Children or adolescents with mania, severe depression, or persistent suicidal ideation often require hospitalization. Antidepressants have been used successfully to treat major depression in latency-aged children and in adolescents. Lithium, in a dose to maintain the serum level at 0.6 mEq/L to 1.2 mEq/L, is used to treat bipolar disorder.

Eating Disorders

Pica

Pica, a rare disorder, is characterized by the persistent eating of nonnutritive substances such as paint, hair, dirt, cloth, or plaster. Ingestion of paint may result in lead poisoning. Pica generally begins in the second year of life and usually remits before the age of 6 or 7. It is most common in mentally retarded and neglected children.

Anorexia Nervosa

Anorexia nervosa is characterized by fear of fatness, weight loss of at least 25% of normal weight, refusal to maintain normal weight, and, in girls, amenorrhea. Anorexics have a disorted body image that may reach delusional proportions—they "feel fat" even when emaciated. Some anorexics use laxatives, self-induced vomiting, and extensive exercising to maintain emaciation. Onset usually occurs in adolescence, with a peak age at 17. Ninety-five percent of all cases are girls. Prevalence estimates run as high as one case per 250 girls between the ages of 14 and 19.

The self-imposed starvation may represent an attempt to avoid one or more of the following: separation from the family, adult sexuality, a loss of control, or a loss of identity. These conflicts may be precipitated by leaving home to attend college, a sexual encounter, parental death, or parental divorce. Families of anorexics tend to be enmeshed and overprotective and to have difficulty expressing feelings openly. Often, the adolescent's anorexia serves to diffuse family tensions.

☐ Belinda, age 15, was admitted to the hospital with a 6-month history of anorexia and progressive weight loss. The youngest of eight children, she had been an honor student until the onset of her symptoms. Belinda was obsessed with food and exercise: She talked often about recipes and restaurants, and would frequently cook elaborate meals for her family while eating nothing herself; she swam 2 to 3 hours every day to maintain her slimness. Her mother, an extremely controlling person, required that, before bed, Belinda and her older sister come to her room and relate all of their day's activities; there were no secrets. Her mother was devastated by Belinda's anorexia. Her father, who was distant and had workaholic tendencies, believed that Belinda would "grow out of" her illness. In the hospital, Belinda was started on a behavioral program in which swimming time was given for caloric intake and weight gain. Belinda became more cooperative when her parents were able to work out some of their anger toward each other and present a united commitment to treatment. In individual therapy, Belinda began to talk of her need to control her rage toward her mother. Aggressive conflicts and then sexual conflicts were addressed. Family therapy focused on the controlling family patterns and helped Belinda establish a sense of individuality and autonomy.

Anorexia can be an intractable disease. Approximately half of all anorexics continue to experience eating or psychological difficulties, and mortality rates range from 2% to 10%. An integrated treatment approach involves individual, family, milieu, and behavior therapies. Hospitalization is often necessary to reverse the life-threatening cachexia. A poor response to treatment is related to the presence of bulimia, premorbid obesity, poor peer relations, and symptom duration longer than 3 years.

Bulimia

Bulimia is marked by episodic binge eating accompanied by a realization that the eating pattern is abnormal, and a fear of being unable to voluntarily stop eating. The majority of bulimics are women in their late teens or early twenties. Similar to anorexics, they display an abnormal preoccupation with their weight and body image and think they are fat, even though their weight is normal or below normal.

During an eating binge, the bulimic eats out of control and will often terminate the overeating by vomiting. Following eating binges, the bulimic becomes depressed, feels guilty, and has self-deprecating thoughts. A significant proportion of bulimics display biological markers of depression (dexamethasone suppression test [DST] non-suppression and a blunted thyrotropin [TSH] response to thyrotropin-releasing hormone [TRH]) and a family history of affective illness. Imipramine and other antidepressants have been used, with some success, to treat bulimia. Other treatment modalities may include individual psychotherapy and cognitive behavioral therapy.

School Phobia

School phobia, a type of separation anxiety disorder, is marked by an intense, conscious, and morbid fear of school. The school phobic's anxiety and fear emanate from intrapsychic conflict and will not respond to a change in classroom or school. Physical complaints often accompany the fear of school and the child complains of gastrointestinal (GI) upsets, headaches, or other illness. If the child is allowed to remain at home, the anxiety and somatic complaints subside rapidly.

School phobia must be distinguished from the refusal to attend school, which may occur in other conditions such as conduct disorder, learning disability, ADD, depression, or in a wide variety of anxiety states that range from adjustment disorders to psychoses. Transient school refusal in response to environmental or developmental stresses usually remits in a day or so if the parents are supportive, firm, and clear in their expectation that the child return to school. School refusal lasting more than a few days requires a thorough evaluation to rule out school phobia or any other serious psychiatric disorder or physical illness.

Incidence rates of school phobia vary from 0.07% to 1.7%; the disorder is equally common in both sexes. Onset is most common from nursery school through the third grade; rates slowly taper after the third grade except for an increase in preadolescence and early adolescence. School phobia is most prevalent in families that place a high premium on education and achievement.

According to psychodynamic theory, school phobia arises from an intense hostile–dependent relationship between the child and parent. Typically, the parents have unresolved unconscious infantile conflicts about aggression that are reactivated by the infant or child. The ambivalence and hostility that the parent unconsciously feels toward the child produce parental anxiety and guilt. The parent attempts to assuage the guilt and deny the hostile feelings by excessively gratifying and overprotecting the child. Hostility and resentment accumulate in both the child and parent, and they displace, externalize, and project the unconscious hostile feelings onto the school. Through this mechanism, the school is both feared and hated. Consequently, the parent and child feel that they must stay together to protect each other and ward off the projected and externalized hostility.

Two general types of school phobia predominate. Younger children tend to have acute, discrete, and well-encapsulated school phobias, which are frequently precipitated by an emotional event that occurs at school. For example, minor accidents or humiliations may be perceived by the child and parent as a dangerous loss of control, and acute symptoms erupt. Prognosis in these cases is generally good because the acute symptoms force conflict resolution and growth.

Older school phobics tend to have more severe character disturbance and poorer prognoses. These children often present with a lifelong history of chronic, insidious, and subclinical separation and dependency difficulties that have seriously interfered with development. Throughout grade school, the child marginally attends school while the family implicitly agrees that there will be no development or growth. However, this equilibrium or pact is destabilized by the development push toward separation that accompanies puberty, and the youngster experiences acute panic and massive regression with overt school refusal.

☐ Claudia, age 11, was seen in consultation for school refusal and nonorganic nausea, vomiting, headaches, abdominal pain, and fainting spells. Claudia's parents were divorced when she was 3, and since that time she had had difficulty separating from her mother. Nine months prior to psychiatric consultation, Claudia had had a medulloblastoma resected, with subsequent chemotherapy and radiation therapy. Her symptoms kept her from attending school regularly, requiring her mother to stay home from work to care for her. In the first interview, Claudia spoke of her worries that kept her awake at night; she feared that she would fall down the stairs at school or that her mother would die in an accident on the way to work. These fears had been present most of her life, but had intensified since the cancer had been discovered. In psychotherapy, Claudia ventilated her anger and rage at her mother for supporting treatment and returning to work. Eventually, she was able to connect the rage with her fears as she talked of her fear that she would "become possessed and kill my mother." At night, she would touch her sleeping mother to make sure she was still alive. Eventually, Claudia was able to master her irrational fears and return to school.

Acute school phobia is viewed as a psychiatric emergency. To prevent the establishment of secondary gain and chronic incapacitation, acute refusal should be reversed as soon as possible. Behavior modification techniques, such as gradual desensitization of the child to the anxiety-provoking school situation, have been used to help reverse the symptom. Close cooperation between the therapist and the school is essential for handling the child's reintegration into the school and strengthening coping capabilities. Treatment must continue after the child returns to school in order to work with the underlying psychopathology and prevent the development of chronic difficulties. Combined family and individual psychotherapy are necessary to deal with the classical phobic dynamics. Excellent treatment outcomes are obtained when the parents are able to work through their residual conflicts that are being expressed through the child's phobic symptoms. Imipramine has been used to enhance the treatment process in school phobia because it is postulated to modify or decrease the separation anxiety.

Overanxious Disorder

Children with overanxious disorder or anxiety neurosis, experience pervasive and excessive anxiety and irrational fear. The anxiety originates from psychological conflict and is not attributable to any particular stressor. These anxieties are often present in one or both parents, and are unconsciously transmitted to the child. Nightmares, enuresis, nail biting, hair pulling, and hypochondriasis are common findings in these children. In some cases, psychotherapy can help resolve the conflicts. Short-term anxiolytic medication may be indicated for acute anxiety reactions that interfere with sleep or school attendance.

Enuresis

Nocturnal enuresis, or bedwetting, is a relatively common disorder. An estimated 5% to 15% of youngsters between the ages of 3 and 15 suffer from this condition. Boys outnumber girls two to one. Functional enuresis must be differentiated from enuresis that is secondary to organic causes such as diabetes, genitourinary pathology, and epilepsy.

Nocturnal enuresis tends to remit spontaneously either at the age of 7 or 8 or at puberty. Enuresis that persists past the age of 7 may result from unconscious psychological conflict. Other causes that have been postulated include a small bladder capacity, delayed central nervous system (CNS) development, and a disorder of arousal.

The parents of an enuretic child of any age need guidance to help them understand the nature of the disorder and avoid power struggles that tend to perpetuate the symptom. Behavior modification techniques are helpful in treating enuresis: The child can be conditioned to awaken when the bladder is full by using a moisture-sensing mattress pad that rings a bell with the first drop of spilled urine; the child can be rewarded with a star system, tokens, or money for dry nights. Older children should be expected to change and wash the bedsheets. Psychotherapy may help reduce the shame that accompanies enuresis. Imipramine, given 6 to 8 hours prior to bedtime, has been used with some success to treat severe, intractable enuresis.

Encopresis

Encopresis is defined as fecal soiling that persists past the age of 3. Approximately 1% of 5-year-olds have this disorder; boys are four to five times more likely to be encopretic than girls. One third of these children also have enuresis. A child that presents with fecal soiling needs a full medical work-up to rule out organic causes such as megacolon or leakage around an impaction.

Encopretic children tend to be immature and passive. Separation, divorce, or serious marital tensions are frequently found in families of encopretics; the father may be passive and distant, the mother domineering, intrusive, and controlling. Mother and child may get locked into perpetual struggles, and the child may be afforded little autonomy. The child then feels defeated and expresses anger through soiling. The mother cannot control the soiling, feels defeated, and strives for control. The long-term outcome is closely related to the resolution of family conflict. Untreated encopresis generally remits at puberty.

Conduct Disorder

A youth with a conduct disorder repeatedly violates the basic rights of others. In the past, these children and adolescents have been termed *delinquent*, *sociopathic*, or *antisocial*. Prevalence rates range from 2% to 7%. Boys are found to have conduct disorder 4 to 12 times more commonly than girls. The conduct disorders are

Table 16–4
Characteristics of Conduct Disorders

Conduct Disorder	Behavior Violates Norms of Society	Aggression is Characterized by Physical Violence or Thefts Involving Confrontation With Victims	Normal Social Attachment to Others is Demonstrated by Friendship, Trust, and Concern
Aggressive undersocialized disorder	Yes	Yes	No
Aggressive socialized disorder	Yes	Yes	Yes
Unaggressive undersocialized disorder	Yes	No	No
Unaggressive socialized disorder	Yes	No	Yes

(Adapted from Walker JI: Clinical Psychiatry in Primary Care. Menlo Park, California, Addison–Wesley, 1981)

categorized according to the presence or absence of socialization and aggressivity (Table 16–4).

Treatment of conduct disorder is very difficult and requires consistent limit-setting by the parents, school, and courts. Clear consequences for actions must be established. In some cases, residential treatment may be necessary. The less guilt a child feels for his actions, the poorer the prognosis.

Child Abuse

Child abuse and neglect are prevalent in modern-day society. Abuse may result in injury or death. Certain patterns have been observed in abuse cases, and they involve factors that are attributable to the parent, child, and environment.

Abusive parents often repeat the abuse, neglect, or deprivation they received at the hands of their own parents. They may have never experienced a satisfying parent–child relationship and are unable to establish one with their own child. Many abusing parents have a lifelong poor self-image, poor impulse control, and intense dependency needs. Alcoholism, psychoses, and chronic illness are commonly associated with the abusing symptom.

The majority of child abuse cases begin in the first 2 years of life, a time when the child is fully dependent. The parent may feel angry and rejected because his dependency needs aren't met by the child. The parent then projects his feelings of self-worthlessness onto the child, identifies with his own aggressive parent, and abuses the child. Anger from current and past sources is unleashed.

Physically or neuropsychiatrically defective children may be most vulnerable to projection and scapegoating. Prematurity may increase the risk of subsequent abuse. Stepfamilies have an increased incidence of abuse.

Child abuse should be suspected in every child suffering from unexplained injuries, including the following:

Multiple burns
Bruises on buttocks and lower back
Injuries at different stages of healing
Ruptured spleen or liver
Subdural hematoma

If abuse is suspected, the clinician's first duty is to protect the child by reporting cases to the Child Protection Service Division of the Department of Health and Human Services. In cases of developmental disturbance or ongoing abuse, hospitalization or temporary foster home placement may be necessary. Protecting the child from further injuries requires a multidisciplinary approach including day-care facilities for the child, home visits by social workers and nurses, child rearing and homemaking assistance for the parents and individual, parental, and family psychotherapy aimed at breaking the abusive cycle and strengthening the family unit.

Bibliography

American Psychiatric Association, Diagnostic and Statistical Manual of Mental Disorders, 3rd ed. Washington, DC, American Psychiatric Association, 1980

Bemporad JR: Child Development in Normality and Psychopathology. New York, Brunner/Mazel, 1980

Erikson E: Symposium on the Healthy Personality, Supp II In Senn JE (ed). New York, Josiah May Jr. Foundation, 1950

Freedman AM, Sadock BJ, Kaplan HI: Comprehensive Textbook of Psychiatry, 2nd ed. Vol 2, pp 2032–2284. Baltimore, Williams & Wilkins, 1975

Group for the Advancement of Psychiatry, Committee on Child Psychiatry. Psychopathological Disorders in Childhood: Theoretical Considerations and a Proposed Classification, Vol 6, Report 62. New York, Group for the Advancement of Psychiatry, 1966

Harrison SI, McDermott JF: New Directions in Childhood Psychopathology, Vol II. New York, International Universities Press, 1982

Kessler J: Psychopathology of Childhood. Englewood Cliffs, New Jersey, Prentice–Hall, 1966

Noshpitz JD (ed): Basic Handbook of Child Psychiatry, Vol 2. New York, Basic Books, 1979

Piaget J: The stages of the intellectual development of the child. Bull Menninger Clin 26:120, 1962

Sarnoff CA: Latency. New York, Aronson, 1976

Richard D. Marciniak

17 Other Psychiatric Disorders

Writing a chapter about "other psychiatric disorders" poses some interesting problems due to the diversity of the subject matter to be discussed. Some topics are included here because although they constitute distinct clinical entities, they are not easily subsumed under other categories of major mental illnesses. Others are found here because our present level of understanding concerning etiology, phenomenology, treatment, prognosis, and family history prevents us from rendering more precise syndromal classifications. We must therefore be content with labeling such disorders as "unusual" or "atypical." Indeed, those persons so classified will no doubt prove in time to be a very heterogeneous group.

With this disclaimer as a preface, I hope to provide the reader with useful information about a variety of interesting and often perplexing disorders that fall within the purview of psychiatry, and are often encountered by other medical specialists.

Adjustment Disorders

In the course of daily living, every individual is confronted with a variety of emotional challenges to which he or she must respond. These situations range in degree from the mundane, and therefore easily handled, to the catastrophic, which are likely to produce a strong emotional reaction in nearly everyone.

In addition to encountering different stressors, people differ with respect to the meanings they attribute to a particular event, as well as in their ability to respond to emotional stresses in ways that are adaptive rather than symptomatic. Here I am alluding to the concepts of personality and ego-defense mechanisms. Likewise, a person's genetic predisposition toward particular affective or other reactions to stress must be considered in any discussion of adaptability.

The topics of personality and ego defense, as well as genetic aspects of affective illness and psychosis, are discussed in detail in other portions of this text. Our purpose in this section is rather to examine the issues of the diagnosis and treatment of maladaptive responses to stress, paying specific attention to the variety of possible symptomatic presentations. It is essential to remember that in regard to the presently accepted definition of adjustment disorders, the prior existence of a personality disorder, organic mental disorder, or other functional psychiatric disorder may significantly impact on someone's ability to respond adaptively to stress. Conversely, stress can greatly influence the symptomatic course of other psychiatric disorders.

As currently defined in the Diagnostic and Statistical Manual of Mental Disorders, 3rd ed (DSM-III), an adjustment disorder consists of a "maladaptive reaction to an identifiable psychosocial stressor." The reaction, be it affective, behavioral, or a mixture of the two, should begin within 3 months of the occurrence of the stress. A response to stress is considered maladaptive when the resultant affective symptoms exceed a level that can be expected as a "reasonable" reaction to such an event, or when there is significant deterioration in occupational functioning or social relations. Also implicit in the diagnosis of an adjustment disorder is the concept that the symptoms should abate with disappearance of the stressor, or when the individual discovers a means of substituting for a loss or learns more effective strategies for coping with the stress.

The term *stress* is itself rather vague and can consist of isolated events or chronic ongoing situations, or it may be the additive result of several minor stressors, which if present singly would not pose a significant problem of adaptation. A person's response to stress cannot be predicted by an assessment of the stressor alone, because people are unique in their adaptive capabilities, the meanings they apply to a given situation, and the degree to which other social and family support is available.

DSM-III defines eight different adjustment disorders based on which affective or behavioral symptoms predominate. These types are as follows:

Adjustment disorder with depressed mood
Adjustment disorder with anxious mood
Adjustment disorder with mixed emotional features
Adjustment disorder with conduct disturbance
Adjustment disorder with mixed disturbance of emotion and conduct
Adjustment disorder with work or academic inhibition
Adjustment disorder with social withdrawal
Adjustment disorder with atypical features

□ CL was an 18-year-old women enrolled as a freshman at a prestigious college. High school had not been particularly easy, but with hard work she was able to achieve very good grades, which was always a source of great pride for her.

CL found college to be even more difficult and despite long hours of study and limited socializing she was able to achieve only average marks. She began dating a young man at this time but felt torn between the need to study and her desire to see her boyfriend, who eventually broke off the relationship in favor of another women who was willing to spend more time with him.

CL was brought to the emergency room by her roommate about 2 weeks later. She reportedly had grown increasingly withdrawn and irritable, often being tearful or angry. Her schoolwork was also declining in quality despite a nearly obsessive preoccupation with studying.

After a brief hospitalization CL entered into a course of brief, goal-limited psychotherapy, during which she grew to understand the degree to which she used academic success as a predominant source of self-esteem. She decided to reduce her courseload to a more manageable level so she could both attain good grades and enjoy her social life.

The case of CL outlines the development of depressive symptoms, social withdrawal, irritability, and academic inhibition in a young woman subjected to the cumulative effects of several stressors, including a recent move away from her family, previously unexperienced academic difficulty, and the break-up with her boyfriend. The case also illustrates how previously successful coping mechanisms, in this case sublimation through academics, may in certain circumstances become maladaptive. The approach to treatment used here, that is, a brief hospitalization followed by goal-limited psychotherapy, is both a typical and highly successful approach to such patients. Occasionally, it may be desirable to use a benzodiazepine for a brief period if anxiety symptoms are severe and incapacitating.

When assessing a patient who is suspected of suffering from an adjustment disorder, several differential diagnostic points should be considered. If the affective symptomatology is very prominent and seems to have attained a state of autonomy separate from the psychosocial stressor, then a diagnosis of major depressive episode or generalized anxiety disorder must be entertained. Also, it should be kept in mind that stress often aggravates the affective and behavioral symptoms associated with a personality disorder. Therefore, it is only when new clinical features appear in such a patient in conjunction with a stressor that the additional diagnosis of adjustment disorder is made. Finally, an uncomplicated mourning or bereavement is characterized by the presence of affective symptoms and perhaps even some degree of social and occupational dysfunction. These symptoms, however, can be expected to follow a predictable course of development and resolution and remain within a degree of severity considered normal.

Brief Reactive Psychoses

The term *psychosis* refers not to a specific psychiatric disorder but rather to a syndrome, or symptom complex. This consists of a disorganization of the processes of rational thought, loss of reality testing (often manifest as delusional beliefs), hallucinations in one or more sensory modalities, affective lability or blunting, and behavior that can be bizarre and grossly disorganized. The various psychiatric disorders in which psychotic symptoms can be present are distinguished therefore not on the basis of psychosis itself, but rather by such factors as family history, duration of symptoms, course of the illness over time, response to various treatment modalities, and the presence or absence of precipitant psychosocial stressors.

DSM-III defines brief reactive psychosis as a disorder characterized by the symptoms of psychosis as outlined above, appearing closely following a recognizable psychosocial stressor that would provoke significant distress in almost anyone. In addition, these symptoms must persist for more than a few hours but no more than 2 weeks, and cannot be secondary to an organic mental disorder, psychoactive drug use, or another functional psychiatric disorder such as acute mania.

Although not classified as such, a brief reactive psychosis might be considered to be a type of adjustment disorder because it is preceded by stressful life events to which the person has a strongly dysphoric emotional reaction. People with histrionic, narcissistic, schizotypal, and especially borderline personality organizations are particularly vulnerable to the development of reactive psychoses. In contrast to the schizophrenic patient who typically shows a blunting of affective responsiveness, these patients generally demonstrate significant emotional lability and often explosiveness. Suicidal and aggressive behavior are also frequently present.

> ☐ KR was a married 35-year-old woman hospitalized for 2 days after an incomplete, spontaneous abortion of a 3-month pregnancy, which was her first. When her husband was late in arriving to pick her up on her scheduled day of discharge, Mrs. R grew quite anxious and began calling home repeatedly in an effort to locate her husband. She became increasingly hostile, began accusing her husband of infidelity, and eventually accused a nurse of being her husband's mistress and of being pregnant with his child.
>
> When Mr. R arrived approximately 6 hours later, Mrs. R had begun throwing furniture in an attempt to get away from the staff in order to "save the dying babies" whose screams she claimed to hear coming from outside her window. She was transferred to the psychiatric service at this point and treated with supportive care and antipsychotic medications.
>
> Within 2 days Mrs. R had essentially fully reconstituted, and neuroleptic medication was no longer needed. It was learned that she had often expressed extreme jealousy toward her husband during their 7-year marriage, often used benzodiazepines to "calm her nerves," and had taken excessive amounts of them as suicidal gestures on several occasions after arguing with her husband. It became apparent that while she viewed her pregnancy as a means of securing her marriage, she was very anxious about the responsibilities that motherhood would bring. Arrangements were made with Mr. and Mrs. R to continue in couple's therapy after her discharge.

The case of KR illustrates several important characteristics of a brief reactive psychosis. First, reactive psychotic symptoms, by definition, resolve within 2 weeks, and the patient returns to his premorbid level of functioning. If symptoms persist longer, the diagnosis of schizophreniform disorder should be considered. Second, in contrast to schizophrenic patients who often demonstrate a blunted affect, those with reactive psychoses present with very intense affective responses. Premorbid history, family history, and the longitudinal course of the illness also help distinguish reactive psychoses from schizophrenia. Third, a particularly meaningful psychosocial stressor was clearly present in KR's case. If such a stressor is not identifiable, the more appropriate diagnosis would be atypical psychosis.

Although the symptoms of a brief reactive psychosis are acute in onset, self-limited, and occur in response to a specific stressor, this in no way precludes the use of antipsychotic medications and a structured, supportive hospital environment to control the florid psychotic symptoms and behavioral disorganization. Finally, it should be remembered that it is often extremely difficult to distinguish a reactive psychosis from an acute drug intoxication, particularly with central nervous system (CNS) stimulants. Therefore, toxicologic screens of urine and blood should be a routine part of the assessment of patients presenting with acute psychoses.

Atypical Psychoses

As is the case with other psychiatric diagnostic categories containing the word "atypical," the diagnosis of atypical psychosis subsumes several clinical entities that for various reasons do not easily fit into more clearly defined categories. These illnesses' being grouped together should not be taken as evidence for a common etiology or for a similar response to treatment or prognosis.

The diagnosis of atypical psychotic disorder is made in cases where the symptoms of psychosis are present (as described in Brief Reactive Psychoses) that do not meet criteria for other more specific psychotic disorders. Examples of such cases cited in DSM-III include:

- Psychoses with unusual features such as monosymptomatic delusions or isolated, persistent auditory hallucinations
- *Postpartum psychoses* that do not meet the criteria for organic mental disorder or affective disorder
- Brief psychoses without specific precipitant stressors
- Psychoses about which there is inadequate information to make a more specific diagnosis
- Psychoses with confusing clinical features that make a more specific diagnosis impossible

As is true with other atypical psychiatric disorders, periodic reevaluation of patients with an atypical psychosis may eventually allow a more specific diagnosis to be made as more information becomes available. As with all psychotic illnesses, treatment should be multidimensional and should include appropriate pharmacotherapy with antipsychotic medication, a structured and supportive environment, and mobilization of family and social supports and appropriate remedial education and training resources. All treatment efforts are directed toward the ultimate goal of maximizing the patient's function while reducing the risk of recurrent psychotic episodes.

Dissociative Disorders

Like the adjustment disorders and brief reactive psychoses, dissociative disorders occur in a setting of extreme anxiety, usually in association with an emotionally

psychiatric conditions to be considered in the differential diagnosis include catatonic stupor and depressive stupor. The acuteness of onset, however, and other associated historical and clinical features help differentiate psychogenic amnesia from chronic psychotic and affective disorders.

Psychogenic Fugue

Like patients with psychogenic amnesia, those with psychogenic fugue suffer from circumscribed periods of amnesia. The difference, however, is that during the fugue state the person assumes a new identity, with complete loss of memory of their previous identity. When the fugue state ends, recall for events occurring during the period of fugue is generally lacking.

Patients with psychogenic fugue often come to the attention of physicians when they "come to" in an unfamiliar place after a period of fugue. Although they are unaware of events that occurred during that time, evidence obtained from other sources indicates that the person did indeed assume a new identity, often radically different from their own.

Other conditions that involve circumscribed periods of total amnesia must be distinguished from psychogenic fugue. Partial-complex epilepsy, though often accompanied by seemingly purposeful motor behavior, does not involve the assumption of a new identity, nor is the person responsive to his environment. Patients with psychogenic amnesia, as mentioned, do not demonstrate purposeful travel or the taking of a new identity. This is also true of people suffering episodes of confusion and memory loss associated with various organic mental disorders. On the other hand, malingering, or feigned inability to recall one's identity or past behavior, may be very difficult to distinguish from psychogenic fugue. Such malingering, however, usually occurs in the setting of potentially adverse legal consequences for the patient due to his past behavior.

Treatment of psychogenic fugue is primarily psychotherapeutic in nature, with the focus on identifying and eliminating precipitating psychosocial stressors.

Multiple Personality

Multiple personality is a complex and fascinating disorder that has received much attention since the publication of such popular books as *Sybil* and *The Three Faces of Eve*. Also, several widely publicized cases in forensic psychiatry in which a diagnosis of multiple personality was used in support of an insanity defense have served to draw the public's attention.

This condition is characterized by the coexistence of two or more relatively distinct personalities within the same person. The transition from one personality to another often occurs suddenly and in times of stress. Generally, the original or primary personality is unaware of the existence of the other personalities, although one or more of the secondary personalities will often have some degree of knowledge of the other personalities, including the primary one.

The apparent similarities to psychogenic fugue make the classification of multiple personality disorder as a dissociative disorder seem appropriate. It should be mentioned, however, that some authors also cite similarities between multiple personality and severe borderline personality disorders. Also, preliminary research with the functional neuroimaging technique of positron emission tomography (PET) has revealed some fascinating regional differences in brain metabolic activity associated with the expression of the different personalities, raising interesting questions about the underlying neurologic substrate of multiple personality.

Depersonalization Disorder

Depersonalization disorder, unlike the other dissociative disorders, does not produce periods of memory loss for the patient. Rather, the person experiences a temporary change in his quality of self-awareness, which often takes the form of feelings of unreality, changes in body image, feelings of detachment from the environment, or a sense of observing oneself from outside one's body.

There is considerable debate as to whether depersonalization experiences should be considered a disorder since such phenomena occur in a variety of psychiatric illnesses such as schizophrenia, depression, anxiety states, and organic mental disorders including drug intoxications. Indeed, it is estimated that up to 50% of "healthy" adults experience transient episodes of depersonalization.

Once organic or functional mental disorders have been excluded as causes of depersonalization experiences, the vast majority will be found to occur in the setting of significant stress and anxiety. Treatment in these cases should be directed toward stress reduction, elucidation and resolution of anxiety-provoking conflicts, and in cases of severe anxiety, the conservative use of benzodiazepine anxiolytics.

Factitious Disorders

Factitious is defined as "not genuine nor authentic." When applied to psychiatric illness, however, the definition should be extended to include "unnatural," because in many cases of factitious disorder real physical illness or injury is present, but is self-inflicted and therefore not of "natural" origin.

DSM-III defines two distinct types of factitious disorders; those occurring with physical symptoms, those with psychological symptoms, and those with mixed or atypical symptoms. Factitious disorders are diagnosed when:

Physical or psychological symptoms exist that are under the voluntary control of the patient

The only apparent motivation for the patient's behavior is the assumption of the patient role, and the behavior is not otherwise understandable in light of his environmental circumstances.

The presentation is plausible enough to have resulted in several hospitalizations (in the case of factitious disorders with physical symptoms).

The issue of the voluntary production of symptomatology is fundamental to the concept of factitious illness. It implies the conscious feigning of symptoms and possible self-infliction of injury. This process, however, is perpetuated by unconscious needs and is, therefore, out of the realm of the patient's volition to stop. The presentation of physical complaints in those people with a factitious disorder may be a total fabrication, may involve interference with diagnostic tests, or be the result of self-inflicted illnesses and injuries. Factitious psychological symptoms are extreme, often psychotic in nature, and frequently quite bizarre.

The most difficult task for the physician is to distinguish factitious illness from genuine physical and psychiatric disorders. Although it can be a difficult task, certain characteristics help to distinguish these patients. These include the following:

- A history of multiple hospitalizations, especially when occurring in a variety of different locations
- Habitual, uncontrollable, and exaggerated lying about many areas of their lives, which is often referred to as pseudologia fantastica.
- Medical knowledge that is unusually sophisticated
- A notable lessening of symptoms in situations in which the patient is unaware of being observed
- A tendency toward drug abuse and demandingness for medications, especially narcotic analgesics
- The sudden emergence of new complaints as suspected disorders are ruled out
- Evidence of extensive prior medical and surgical interventions
- Nonchalance about submitting to noxious diagnostic and treatment procedures
- Poor interpersonal relationships, as evidenced by the patient's receiving few or no visitors, and his hostility to the medical staff
- A history of hospital discharges, against medical advice

When present, the above features not only assist the clinician in identifying patients with a high likelihood of factitious complaints, but also help distinguish these patients from those with somatization disorders, hypochondriasis, or conversion disorders.

Specific causes of factitious disorders are unknown; however, it is generally accepted that the presence of such disorders implies the coexistence of a severe personality disturbance. Factitious disorders have their symptomatic onset in early adulthood, but the physician usually obtains a history of the patient's hospitalization in childhood for genuine physical illnesses. The disorders appear to be equally prevalent in men and women.

Much has been written about various approaches to psychiatric intervention with these patients, including techniques for confrontation of patients with the factitious nature of their illness, and speculations about the usefulness of long-term psychiatric hospitalization. Even with extensive treatment however, the prognosis is generally regarded as very poor.

☐ MH was a divorced 47-year-old woman hospitalized for complaints of generalized weakness and easy fatigability. Physical examination found her to be lethargic, with poor concentration and short-term recall, and revealed generalized hyporeflexia. Laboratory evaluation showed an elevated serum calcium level of 13 mEq/L, and an electrocardiogram (ECG) revealed prolongation of the P-R and Q-T intervals.

An exhaustive medical work-up did not determine the etiology of the patient's hypercalcemia, which persisted despite conservative treatment. Treatment with the antiosteoclastic medication mithramycin was being considered, when a member of the nursing staff found a large number of calcium carbonate tablets in the patient's suitcase. When confronted with this discovery the patient requested immediate discharge and declined any follow-up.

Sleep Disorders

According to surveys, 95% of American adults have experienced some sort of trouble sleeping. It is estimated that 30 million people suffer from chronic insomnia and that millions more encounter temporary disruptions of sleep resulting from such problems as emotional upset, environmental distractions, jet lag, and changing work schedules.

Patients in a variety of clinical and home settings report similar symptoms of disrupted sleep, and many physicians perceive and treat insomnia as a one-dimensional disorder. In reality, patients present a wide variety of symptoms that stem from vastly differing causes and that require differential diagnosis and treatment. An analogy can easily be drawn between the patient's complaint of "I can't sleep" and the complaint of "I have pain in my abdomen." It is readily acknowledged that the latter complaint can be symptomatic of a wide variety of possible problems, some potentially serious, and that each case must be treated individually. Clinicians should also be aware that with insomnia, as with acute abdominal pain, misdiagnosis and inappropriate treatment can lead to heightened morbidity for the patient.

Traditionally, treatment for both chronic and transient insomnia has involved recognition of the symptom and a prescription for sleep medication. Recent clinical research on the nature of sleep has revealed that insomnia is symptomatic of a wide variety of physiologic and psychological disorders with vastly different causes. Patients relating the same symptoms may suffer from disorders as diverse as sleep apnea, major depression, or drug-related insomnia. Rather than describe in detail the pathophysiology of the many illnesses in which insomnia may be a feature, it is our purpose here to provide an overview of the differential diagnostic process involved in the evaluation of sleep disorders.

When presented with the complaint "I can't sleep," the physician must elicit information vital to the differential diagnosis of insomnia. Questions should explore the issues of transient vs chronic insomnia, insomnia due to physical illnesses, delayed sleep-phase syndrome, insomnia secondary to functional psychiatric or psychophysiologic disorders, nocturnal myoclonus, and sleep apnea. As each major type of insomnia is considered and its symptomatology elucidated, it becomes clear that the complaint "I can't sleep" can be symptomatic of a wide variety of conditions, despite similarities in the initial presentations.

The most important question by far in the differential diagnosis of insomnia is whether it is transient (duration of less than 3 weeks) or chronic (duration of more than 3 weeks). The major causes of transient insomnia include the following:

Situational reactions such as temporary, stressful, emotionally upsetting experiences

Environmental disturbances, such as ambient noise
Sleep schedule changes, such as work-shift changes or jet lag

The daytime consequences of disordered sleep are clear-cut in patients with transient insomnia. Patients report exhaustion, somnolence, and poor concentration. Transient insomnia is that category of sleep disturbance for which the drugs of choice are the sedative–hypnotic benzodiazepines. It is becoming increasingly accepted in clinical practice to use those benzodiazepines that have a relatively short half-life in order to avoid excessive daytime drowsiness, cognitive and motor deficits, and long-term drug accumulation.

Insomnia that persists more than 3 weeks is classified as *chronic,* and must be differently diagnosed for both cause and appropriate treatment. Frequent causes of chronic insomnia are as follows:

Psychophysiologic disorders, such as psychogenic pain
Functional psychiatric disorders, such as major affective disorders and anxiety disorders
Drug- or alcohol-induced insomnia, such as tolerance to and withdrawal from CNS depressants or sustained use of CNS stimulants
Sleep-induced respiratory impairment, such as sleep apnea
Sleep-related myoclonus and "restless legs" syndrome
Delayed sleep-phase syndrome
Other medical conditions, such as paroxysmal nocturnal dyspnea associated with congestive heart failure

Although referral to a sleep disorders center and subsequent polysomnography may be necessary in some cases to obtain a definitive diagnosis, the clinician can, by using a systematic approach, make a presumptive diagnosis and institute appropriate treatment in most cases that present with a sleep disturbance.

Paranoid Disorders

Guardedness, secretiveness, doubting others' loyalty, and overconcern with the hidden motives of others is a universally experienced emotional state, if only for brief periods of time. Such feelings, like euphoria or sadness, constitute a psychiatric disorder only when they become extreme, prolonged, and rigidly fixed. Strong paranoid feelings can occur in several psychopathologic conditions, including organic mental disorders such as delirium, dementia, and drug intoxication. Schizophrenic disorders, affective disorders, and paranoid personalities can also present with prominent symptoms of paranoia.

DSM-III defines the essential features of paranoid disorders as follows:

Persistent persecutory delusions or delusional jealousy
Emotion and behavior appropriate to the content of the delusional system
Persistent symptoms for at least 1 week
Symptoms of paranoia not due to schizophrenic, affective, or organic mental disorders

Three distinct paranoid disorders are currently recognized:

Paranoia, distinguished by a duration of at least 6 months

Acute paranoid disorder, with symptoms of less than 6 months' duration

Shared paranoid disorder, in which a paranoid state develops in a person having a close relationship with an individual already suffering from paranoia. This has been previously referred to as *folie a deux*.

The delusional beliefs experienced by the person with a paranoid disorder are generally well defined and usually encompass a limited number of other people and situations. This distinction helps differentiate these disorders from other psychotic illnesses and organic brain disorders in which paranoia, if present, is usually generalized and less well organized. Also lacking in paranoid disorders is the deterioration of coherent, logical thinking (*i.e.*, the *formal thought disorder*, which characterizes schizophrenic, affective, and organic psychoses.)

☐ SB was a single 37-year-old man employed as a laboratory research assistant when he became engaged to be married. SB gradually developed the belief that a previous boyfriend of his fiancée was plotting to kill him. He began purchasing and accumulating weapons and ammunition, began secretly observing the other man's activities, and even attempted to have the man arrested. SB continued to work, and from all available information showed no significant decline in job performance.

SB presented in an acutely agitated state shortly after his marriage, when he became convinced that a "contract" had been issued to have him killed. Initial treatment in the hospital with antipsychotic medication resulted in quieting of his acute agitation, but had no impact on his delusional beliefs. He soon became hostile toward the staff, accusing them of being "coconspirators," and left the hospital against medical advice. Over the next 3 years SB was hospitalized several times, all during periods of severe agitation in which he feared for his life. Eventually he moved to a different city, abandoning his wife, and was lost to follow-up.

The case of SB illustrates several salient features of paranoia, including well-circumscribed delusions, poor treatment compliance, and the poor response of such delusions to antipsychotic medications. Like SB, most paranoiacs experience the onset of their illness in middle or late adult life, and many can remain functional at work and in other areas of their lives, even while engaging in other behaviors that are based on delusional beliefs. Premorbid risk factors for paranoid disorders include paranoid and schizoid personality disorders, and although precise statistics are not available, anecdotal reports indicate that these disorders occur most commonly in men.

The prognosis of patients with paranoid disorders is believed to be very poor. As mentioned, neuroleptics are most useful in controlling agitation, but are not particularly effective against the delusions of paranoid disorders. Psychotherapeutic intervention, although difficult, should begin with an unwavering effort to establish a reliable and trusting relationship with the patient. Treatment should focus on maintaining satisfactory social and occupational adjustment, whether or not the patient's delusions abate. With this in mind it has been estimated that as many as two thirds of all patients with paranoid disorders can benefit from a combination of medication and psychotherapy.

Bibliography

Aguilera DC, Messick JM: Crisis Intervention: Theory and Methodology. St Louis, CV Mosby, 1978

American Psychiatric Association: Diagnostic and Statistical Manual of Mental Disorders, 3rd ed. Washington, DC, American Psychiatric Association, 1980

Hauri P: The Sleep Disorders. Kalamazoo, Michigan, Upjohn, 1977

Kaplan HI, Freedman AM, Sadock BJ (eds): Comprehensive Textbook of Psychiatry, 3rd ed. Baltimore, Williams & Wilkins, 1980

Kolb LC, Brodie HKH: Modern Clinical Psychiatry, 10th ed. Philadelphia, WB Saunders, 1982

Walker, JI: Psychiatric Emergencies. Philadelphia, JB Lippincott, 1983

Part III
The Therapies

David S. Werman

18 Supportive Psychotherapy

Although the majority of patients seen in psychiatric clinics and mental health centers require some form of supportive psychotherapy, this modality of treatment has received much less attention than it deserves. It tends to be regarded as inferior and unchallenging in comparison with insight-oriented psychotherapy. Most psychiatry programs devote little or no time to teaching supportive psychotherapy. There is even a tendency to devalue the patients who receive such therapy.

Although the distinction between insight-oriented psychotherapy and supportive psychotherapy has been challenged,[1] and regardless of the awkwardness of these or other synonyms, the two forms of treatment, as concepts of therapy, represent critically different entities. While they rarely exist in their "pure" forms, the specific premises of each form of treatment must be understood, lest a confusion of technique and goals ensue that can only weaken the therapeutic process.

Comparison of Supportive Psychotherapy and Insight-Oriented Psychotherapy

Although the theoretical differences between insight-oriented psychotherapy and supportive psychotherapy have been well described,[2] observations of clinical practice reveal that these differences are insufficiently clear. More strikingly, the technical differences are unclear, particularly in respect to the practice of supportive psychotherapy in which one regularly sees a stereotyped adherence to procedures appropriate to psychoanalysis or insight-oriented psychotherapy. This is especially unfortunate because psychoanalytic theory remains the most useful conceptualization of both these psychotherapies. The following comments, which attempt to clarify selected technical features in supportive psychotherapy, stem from a psychoanalytic perspective.

Insight-oriented psychotherapy seeks to alleviate painful affective states (especially of anxiety and depression), modulate ego-alien or destructive behavior, diminish neurotic symptoms and guilt-provoking behavior, and enhance previously nongratifying interpersonal relationships. It also addresses problems primarily relating to the patient's self-concept. Insight-oriented psychotherapy attempts to increase the patient's awareness of the psychodynamic and psychogenetic framework within which these undesired psychological phenomena operate. The anachronistic and self-destructive nature of such behavior is elucidated by systematically diminishing the resistances that keep critical affects and ideas from consciousness. Through interpretations of transference phenomena, fantasies, dreams, symptomatic acts, parapraxia, and patterns of behavior, the patient progressively tends to become aware of his unconscious propensity to deal with current life in ways that are heavily influenced by earlier modes of dealing with stress. As a result, the most poorly adaptive defense mechanisms—denial, projection, and splitting—are diminished, and healthier mechanisms, such as repression and sublimation, are enhanced. Inhibitions standing in the way of adult gratifications are explored, so that the patient can better gratify his wishes. Similarly, neurotic symptoms arising from intrapsychic conflicts are examined with the expectation that he can integrate this insight into his mental life so that his life in the world can be enriched.

Insight-oriented psychotherapy is an effective modality of treatment for the appropriate patient, when treated by a knowledgeable psychotherapist. When it fails, it is usually because it is inappropriate for a given patient. The resulting stalemate disenchants the patient with his therapy, and the therapist loses confidence in the potential efficacy of the treatment; he may angrily perceive the stalemate to be due to a lack of cooperativeness by the patient. The therapist's narcissistic mortification can easily obscure the realities of the situation. In other cases, both patient and therapist may continue meeting for an inordinately long period of time under the illusion that explorative psychotherapy is actually taking place.

Difficulties such as these may stem from the patient's unrealistic goals that are shared with or may originate with the psychotherapist. The therapist's fantasy is that he is able to bring about substantial modifications in psychological "structures"; that is, enduring patterns of behavior, affective responses, defense organizations, self-representations and object representations, symptom and conflict formations, superego functions, interpersonal relationships, and self-concept. However, and this point is never sufficiently stressed, these structures may be so significantly distorted or defective that they can be only minimally modified, if at all. Instead of an endless, idle pursuit of a fundamental psychological change, the psychotherapist is more successful if he helps the patient in the same manner physicians manage diabetes mellitus—not by attempting to cure the disease, but by minimizing its effects with medication, diet, and counseling. It would be absurd to regard such substitutive (supportive) treatment as less worthy of the physician's skill than when he cures pneumonia. Analogously, supportive psychotherapy is an important form of treatment for which a solid background in psychodynamic psychiatry is necessary.

Supportive psychotherapy primarily, but not exclusively, refers to a form of treatment whose principal focus is, in fact, to support—in the sense of shoring up—mental structures that are acutely or chronically deficient. The acute deficiency, or the "crisis," applies to patients whose lives have been in a state of reasonable equilibrium, but which have suddenly been disturbed by an external event that is real, symbolic, or fantasied, and which precipitates a condition of psychological insufficiency.

The Crisis As a Model

The work in supportive psychotherapy can be illustrated by an example of crisis intervention: A student who has functioned well throughout his life is overwhelmed when jilted by his fiancée. He is overwhelmed because the pain—sadness, anger, and narcissistic mortification—is so great that he cannot adequately exercise his cognitive functions. He feels that he will never find anyone else to love, he perceives himself to be empty and worthless without his fiancée, and he believes the pain will continue indefinitely; he feels unable to either think rationally about his situation or to do anything about it. He feels so worthless that he not only feels he is incapable of benefiting from help, but also that no one would want to help him. The hopelessness of his situation may lead to suicidal thoughts or acts. Self-destructive trends may reflect a punitive turning of his anger with his fiancée against himself. The world seems to reflect his feelings of emptiness and he withdraws from it into feelings of despair. His distorted view of his situation does not permit him to appreciate that the pain will ever abate; he cannot imagine that another woman can replace his fiancée in his affections because the world seems empty without her.

In such a situation, the therapist can perform a number of useful tasks. By merely interviewing the patient he implicitly suggests that something can be done to alleviate the pain, that he does not find the patient loathsome, and that he can accept him as he is. The therapist verbally and nonverbally communicates to the patient that he appreciates the extent of his pain. If some rapport is then established, the therapist will attempt to do with the patient what the patient himself might well have been able to do for a friend only a few weeks earlier: He will carefully explore the realities of the situation and help the patient find realistic solutions, and if the patient is unable to do the latter, the therapist may suggest them. He will tactfully challenge unrealistic notions and examine the possible consequences of one path or another. Thus he nurtures, suggests, guides, and helps distinguish reality from fantasy. In short, he acts as an accepting, benevolent, levelheaded parent.

In many crises the impact of the blow begins to lighten in a matter of days or weeks, and the patient's own ego resources take over. Most psychological crises are surmounted without formal or even informal psychotherapy; mourning reactions are typical of this sort of crisis. Perhaps those individuals who are unable to deal with the usual life crises by themselves or with the help of people in their environment demonstrate some significant degree of ego weakness.

The patient who is seen in longer-term supportive psychotherapy is similar to someone in a crisis except that his inadequate coping has usually been chronic and may be expected to continue for some time; also, the symptoms present are not necessarily precipitated by external events. My focus here, then, is on the longer-term supportive therapy that is conceptualized as a substitutive form of treatment, supplying the patient with those psychological elements that he either lacks or possesses insufficiently.

Evaluation

The issues involved in evaluating patients for insight-oriented psychotherapy or supportive psychotherapy depend on the quality of psychic function; in the first place this addresses the question of ego strength. A recognized paradox is that the best-integrated people derive the most benefit from insight psychotherapy or psychoanalysis. This is not surprising since it merely recalls the universal observation that what is only minimally disrupted can most readily be improved, whether it be the human body, social institutions, or the ego. The ego functions considered in evaluation of patients include reality testing, intelligence, verbal skills, evidence of object relations, a good work or school history, and psychological-mindedness. In addition, a good candidate for insight-oriented psychotherapy should be aware of his feelings, be able to tolerate the painful ones, and be able to describe them. He should have at least enough basic trust to enter a therapeutic relationship. Patients who somatize extensively are not usually helped very much from insight-oriented therapy unless they are eventually able to recognize the psychological nature of their difficulties. The patient who tends to act rather than talk presents specific problems because rash and destructive behavior may represent either a primary impulse disorder or acting out of conflict, the latter being much more amenable to influence than the former. Patients with severe impulse disorders are usually unable to tolerate insight-oriented psychotherapy.

The foregoing are generally accepted as the main criteria in selecting patients for insight-oriented psychotherapy. Other factors of critical importance, however, may be obscured by the psychiatric diagnosis. There is often an assumption that schizophrenics in remission and patients described as "borderline personalities" are at one end of the supportive therapy/insight-oriented psychotherapy continuum, while patients with neurosis are on the opposite end. Character disorders, alcohol and drug abuse, and depressive syndromes are placed somewhere in between, depending on severity, chronicity, and disability. Although such a schema has some merit, it does not account for many exceptions across diagnostic entities. For example, patients whose schizophrenic symptoms are in remission, and formerly psychotically depressed patients, may be able to derive more benefit from insight-oriented psychotherapy than are certain obsessive–compulsive neurotics.

Additional criteria for "workability" in insight-oriented psychotherapy are difficult to delineate with high precision, but relate to the following:

1. A high degree of motivation. The patient is intensely uncomfortable with painful feelings of guilt, shame, sadness, anxiety, or with the psychological problem for which he is seeking help. Furthermore, the problem must be one that can actually be alleviated to some extent—either it can be diminished, or the patient can be expected to find a more comfortable way of living with the condition. Birth defects, one's sex, homosexuality, and so forth, are typical of the latter conditions.
2. An autoplastic conviction: The patient realizes that despite any stresses that arise from the people and the world around him, his psychological liberation primarily depends on changes that will occur in himself, and will come about only if he tries strenuously to effect those changes. He is curious about his behavior and his emotions. Related to this is a sense that his life is more influenced by knowable factors than occult forces.
3. A reasonable degree of physical and psychic energy. This factor is difficult to describe, but concerns lifelong patterns of passivity or activity. If such patterns are strongly passive in nature, the patient may not be able to summon up the effort to change. It is often reflected in his physical behavior, in which he demonstrates that he would rather do without something desired than expend energy to obtain it.
4. The patient must not only have the ability to talk, but he must actually do so, with relative ease, about his feelings, ideas, dreams, fantasies, and physical sensations. (Phrases such as "verbal ability" or "ability to communicate" do not adequately convey the sense of this criterion.) The inability to talk freely usually represents resistance, but could indicate other factors, such as a lack of trust, an immediate transference reaction, or some reality factor. If this resistance is not diminished early in treatment it may stalemate the entire therapeutic endeavor. The most destructive resistance to treatment is when the patient literally does not come to the interview. Initial and continual silence may be modified by confrontations, clarifications, and perhaps interpretations, but if it does not diminish after various attempts, it may indicate an incorrect evaluation.

Goals of Treatment

A major pitfall in supportive psychotherapy concerns goals of treatment and the time for termination. It is reasonable, in a form of treatment defined as *substitutive*, to contemplate that the patient may need to maintain, to some degree, life-long contact with his therapist. One of the therapist's tasks is to determine, as early in treatment as possible, whether reasonable goals can be set and achieved, and treatment terminated, or if the patient will indefinitely need external "supplies." A decision once made can be reversed, but unless the therapist has a sense of direction in this matter, supportive psychotherapy can go on indefinitely and unnecessarily;

it may also be terminated prematurely. At times, the prolongation of therapy proves to be a greater problem in supportive psychotherapy than the danger, often alluded to, of inadvertently stripping a patient of his defenses and thereby precipitating a psychotic episode.

The attachment that the patient develops toward the therapist is a double-edged sword; on the one hand it leads to the rapport without which no psychotherapy can take place. In supportive psychotherapy it is the cement that holds the therapeutic relationship together, not only in the early phase of treatment, but at any point afterwards, and particularly in those cases for which the treatment must go on for many years. On the other hand, however, this very attachment that makes the therapist an important and useful figure in the patient's life can also become a barrier to his achieving a maximum degree of autonomy, by creating a relationship of excessive dependency. There are no simple remedies for this matter, but one can best deal with it by being aware of it.

A clear goal in treatment does not necessarily correspond to what the patient desires but to what an either overzealous or nihilistic therapist thinks is appropriate. It is essential to determine what the *patient* wants from therapy. Sometimes he only wants medication, referral to a medical specialist, or a letter for legal purposes. Patients sometimes agree to psychotherapy—for a variety of reasons—even though it is not what they want. Alternatively, therapists occasionally begin treatment and agree to goals that are highly unrealistic, allowing themselves to be swayed by the patient's yearning for help, his mental anguish, or his ability to charm. In the not-very-long run, the inappropriate use of these goals becomes apparent, and this realization can be injurious to the patient because he has had his hopes raised, only to have them crushed. This "killing with kindness" should suggest that countertransference issues do exist; accordingly, the therapist should carefully examine his own thoughts and feelings.

The Therapist's Work

Supportive psychotherapy, no less and perhaps more than other forms of psychotherapy, provides a *holding environment* for the patient.[3,4] Such an environment provides the patient with an illusion of safety and protection, an "illusion that depends upon the bond of affective communication between the caretaker and the child."[3] Protection here serves both against external dangers as well as the patient's impulses. In supportive psychotherapy, the therapist can point out these external dangers when the patient is unable to recognize them, and can serve as a benevolent, limit-setting parent when the patient's impulses threaten to erupt. In contrast to insight-oriented psychotherapy, in supportive psychotherapy the therapist must be explicit and direct, when the occasion demands it, about his attitude toward the patient's destructive impulses. He should identify them as harmful and let the patient know that he is personally concerned about such behavior. If necessary, the patient should be told that uncontrolled behavior during the therapy hour cannot be permitted. In a similar vein, the therapist may inform the patient that he cannot treat him unless the patient cooperates in some activity such as taking essential medication, attending AA meetings, desisting from antisocial behavior, etc.

These interventions raise the question of how much and what kind of talking the therapist should do in supportive psychotherapy. A simple yardstick is that the therapist's comments should either support the therapeutic process or at least do nothing to disrupt it. In insight-oriented psychotherapy and psychoanalysis, minimal intervention permits the free flow of the patient's thoughts, feelings and fantasies without the pressure to orient himself to something external. This process fosters a desirable, controlled regression, which is obviously inappropriate in supportive psychotherapy. Silence also tends to preserve the relative anonymity of the therapist and thereby permits the development of transference, which is to be avoided in supportive psychotherapy. What seems to be most useful in supportive psychotherapy is a form of discourse that resembles social conversation, yet differs from it in that the therapist specifically directs his comments toward certain goals. This procedure is not without its own pitfalls: The therapeutic relationship can become one that not only has the form of social discourse, but its content as well, leaving therapeutic goals behind. The friendly relationship, which permits the therapist to function as an agent of support, is transformed into a relationship of friendship in which the auxiliary role of the therapist is lost.

Schafer, doing brief psychoanalytic psychotherapy with college students, speaks of a "pedagogical and personal" approach, which is especially appropriate in supportive psychotherapy.[5] By "pedagogic" he means the appropriate sharing of the therapist's knowledge about the patient or about psychological processes with the patient. Talking to patients "personally" relates to the therapist's attempt to couch his comments in language that not only does not set him apart from the patient's concerns, but empathically relates him to those concerns. While this personal approach is appropriate in all forms of therapy, it is indispensable in supportive psychotherapy, where the patient is not expected to be able to tolerate significant levels of frustration.

A common misunderstanding of supportive psychotherapy is that it concerns "reassurance." This ill-defined concept usually means one of three things: first, that the therapist attempts to make the patient feel happier by glossing over or denying unpleasant realities and by offering pleasing untruths. This brings the therapist into collusion with the patient's misperceptions of reality. In specific circumstances, of course, it may be useful to reinforce a patient's denial of a frightening reality—impending death, for example—by introducing a justifiable element of hope. A second meaning of reassurance relates to the therapist's empathic attitude, and this should be present in every form of treatment. Finally, the reassurance that is characteristic of supportive psychotherapy occurs when the patient is unable to exercise a realistic appraisal of a given situation: The cognitive ego functions he should be using, are operating inadequately, either because of longstanding ego defects or because the function is overwhelmed by massive affect. In this situation, the therapist works with the patient to help him become aware of real possibilities, contingencies, and so forth, and to help him make valid choices. This last concept of reassurance is used in counseling techniques, which, in fact, make up some of the techniques used in supportive psychotherapy, and are more central to this strategy of treatment than they are to insight-oriented psychotherapy.

A patient may be an appropriate candidate for insight-oriented psychotherapy, but live in so tumultuous an environment that any gains he makes are immediately negated by the surrounding stress. Although one may begin individual treatment with such a patient, the therapy should be complemented by work with other family members. The family, or spouse, should then be seen in evaluative interviews to determine how one can best intervene. Subsequent contacts with the family may be necessary when critical situations arise. Whenever possible, the patient should be present when family members are being seen, in order to maintain his trust in the therapist.

Resistance

The handling of resistance and transference in supportive psychotherapy has been dealt with by other authors; only a brief recapitulation of general principles follows. In supportive psychotherapy, contrary to insight-oriented psychotherapy, one should not attempt to weaken resistances and defenses, but should try to strengthen those that are adaptive. Although this is an appropriate strategy, it requires some qualification. For example, a patient who comes progressively late to therapy, or frequently misses his hours, is communicating his need to avoid contact with the therapist for some reason. Not to confront this behavior is to give it tacit approval; moreover, not confronting this behavior implicitly encourages doing rather than reflecting. (But here again, the entire situation must be considered; it is possible that in a passive, obsessional patient, one might encourage such behavior as a progressive step away from excessive rumination.) The therapist should ascertain whether the reasons for the patient's avoidance of therapy are conscious, and if they are, the patient should be encouraged to discuss them with the therapist as candidly as he can. Appropriate measures can perhaps be taken to mitigate the problem; this might entail, for example, spacing visits farther apart or shortening each interview. If the patient is unaware of the feelings or thoughts that prompted his behavior, the therapist may be able to grasp the sense of these acts from the general flow of the therapeutic material, and be able to discuss his conjectures with the patient.

Other manifestations of resistance, which weaken the rapport between the patient and therapist, should also be dealt with. Such situations might involve the setting of limits within the interview. Similarly, severely maladaptive defenses, such as projection and denial, should be dealt with. It is especially important, when the patient incorrectly claims that the therapist dislikes him or has hostile intentions towards him, that the therapist correct such defective reality testing in order to safeguard the therapeutic relationship. In this connection, it is most useful for the patient to learn to recognize and identify his feelings so that he can understand why he experiences certain events in distorted ways. For example, he may begin to recognize, and avow, his own hostility to the therapist.

Pseudo–Insight-Oriented Psychotherapy

Some psychotherapy that is intended by the therapist to be insight-oriented is, in fact, supportive psychotherapy. This notion is borne out through evaluations or treatment of patients who have previously undergone "insight-oriented psychotherapy." One learns that from the earliest hours the therapist has made "interpretations" of a psychogenetic and psychodynamic nature—in fact, it often appears that most of the former therapist's work consisted of making such "interpretations." To a large extent, regardless of their validity, these "interpretations" remain sequestered, intellectual ideas, not integrated into the patient's life. This failure of integration may occur because the interpretations have not been built up from a careful exploration of the patient's associations, dreams, and fantasies, made rich by a decrease in resistance, and perhaps more significantly, they are not made in the affectively charged situation of the transference. At times, therapists themselves tend to intellectualize and rationalize, and pass these defenses on to the patient. The enhancement of intellectualization may also exist in forms of therapy in which patients are assigned specific roles, are given rational explanations of their behavior, and are subject to considerable pedagogic pressure from the therapist or other patients in a group psychotherapy setting. In all of these situations, insight into conscious and unconscious processes is peripheral to the overall strategy of the treatment. If the foregoing processes, however, do not constitute insight-oriented psychotherapy, they do represent an excellent model of supportive psychotherapy, and for the properly selected patient this use of intellectualization and rationalization is most appropriate. Dreams can be used in a similar way.[6] Certain individuals can probably obtain benefit from self-help books, also serving to enhance intellectualization and rationalization.

Once a specific intellectualized formulation has been accepted by the patient, he should be encouraged to bring this idea to mind when he is in a perplexing, frightening, or depressing situation; this practice can help him gain control of his feelings and provide him with time to plan a useful response. It is also helpful to have the patient rehearse such characteristic, frequently-occurring situations in the therapist's presence. In such a rehearsal, the patient can learn to intellectually situate the problem and then to recall formerly useful techniques for dealing with it. This kind of work is clearly derived from the techniques of behavior modification, which should be considered in supportive psychotherapy when deemed appropriate.

Identification With the Therapist

In addition to using the therapist's interventions to shore up defenses, the patient can benefit by identifying with various perceived aspects of the therapist's personality. Such identification may range from genuine introjects to superficial imitation. The more the identification becomes an enduring aspect of the patient's mental function, the more reliable it will be; however, even imitation can be useful if it works. Identification occurs in all forms of therapy, as well as in human relationships in general, but it can be a significant therapeutic factor in supportive psychotherapy and should be fostered.

Among the therapist's traits with which the patient may identify for his own benefit are consistency, empathy, trustworthiness and trust, self-observation, compassion, and control of impulses. The therapist's capacity to tolerate the patient's considerate and affectionate feelings along with his hostile and vengeful attitudes encourages the patient to develop a more empathic attitude toward the people around him as well as toward himself. This process tends to diminish the propensity of many patients with severe chronic ego disturbances to view objects and themselves as totally good or totally bad—the "splitting" described by some authors.[7] Such patients often project their worst feelings onto the therapist, who may react angrily when he feels himself attacked or degraded: This validates the patient's perceptions. To the contrary, if the therapist maintains his empathic attitude, it can have a beneficial effect on the patient, whose worst expectations of the therapist fail to materialize; he can then move toward perceiving him as a fundamentally benevolent individual with whom identification becomes desirable. Such a process can only take place through repeated experiences and much testing of the therapist; reassurances of benevolence are of little if any value.

Values

The therapist's role in being an "auxilliary superego" is important, but is complicated by the question of values. One can say, in broad terms, that disturbances in superego functioning become appropriate issues in psychotherapy when they are conflictual for the patient, destructive or constrictive for the patient or for others, or are apt to become social or legal problems. In these situations, the therapist can direct his efforts toward counterbalancing the effects of an overly strict or insufficiently effective superego. The traditional task of "giving permission" is often useful in helping the patient overcome inhibitions related to sexual behavior and assertiveness. The patient who gives evidence of superego weakness should be clearly told that he is poorly served by his behavior and that it is potentially destructive; more benign, substitutive behaviors that can provide gratification without danger to himself or others should be explored.

Transference

The problem of transference is similar to that of resistance. Only a brief mention of the principles need be made. Interviews should be no more frequent than necessary to do the work of supportive therapy; if necessary, because of evidence of a developing transference, the length of each interview can be shortened. Instead of the therapist attempting to be a "blank screen," he should be sufficiently a "real person" to inhibit the free play of fantasy. Specific transference material can be "interpreted upward" by deliberately avoiding unconscious and archaic content and describing this material as a response to overt events occurring in therapy. A rapidly developing transference should be dealt with energetically by limiting contact with the patient and by a firm, reality-based explanation of the patient's feelings. Transference psychoses are rare; should it be evident that such a development is occurring, the use of psychotropic medication, if not already prescribed, is indicated, and hospitalization may be necessary.

Use of Dreams

Exploration and interpretation of dreams is usually not advisable in supportive psychotherapy, especially in patients with a history of severe regression. When establishing the therapeutic agreement, I do not request that these patients report their dreams. If they do so nevertheless, it is helpful to simply ask their general thoughts about the dream. Such an approach acknowledges the patient's desire to be cooperative; additionally, the manifest content of the dream may provide the therapist with material that can be helpful in understanding the patient's current behavior; here again the "upward interpretation," relating the dream to matters in the patient's current life, can be useful.

Problems of Self-Concept

Patients who present with significantly lowered self-esteem, or grandiosity, may or may not be able to be helped in insight-oriented psychotherapy. The criteria outlined earlier for this form of treatment apply here also. When patients with these problems are seen in supportive psychotherapy, they usually have other psychological problems that deserve attention. The patient can benefit by using the therapist to "mirror" his grandiosity or as an idealized parent who he experiences as part of himself for the enhancement of his self-concept. Such developments often lead to a diminution of anxiety, depression, and self-destructive behavior, and permit the patient to enjoy gratification in his personal life and work. Since such a therapeutic relationship cannot be continued indefinitely, the therapist must decide on goals early in treatment. Attempts to move toward an insight-oriented mode of treatment should be made with those patients who demonstrate sufficient ego strength. For those who are more apt to regress, therapy can be interrupted when the patient's psychological life is in a state of relative equilibrium, with the explicit understanding that the patient may return for further (supportive) therapy if this equilibrium is upset.

Chronically Dysphoric Patients

The chronically depressed, oral-dependent, "needy" patient can be considerably helped in supportive psychotherapy when the therapist renounces the unreachable goal of transforming this patient into a mature, independent individual. Once significant improvement in this direction seems unlikely, supportive psychotherapy can provide these patients with many desired "supplies." The conscientiousness of the therapist, his taking the patient and his distress seriously, and his treating the patient with a respect that is often unique in the patient's life will lead to a reasonable degree of rapport. Some demands for medicines and infantilizing favors will subside when the patient realizes that no matter how meager he may find the relationship, it is more than he has had; it is also a reasonable gratification because it is regular, dignified, and above all, dependable. Even strongly dependent adults hardly ever totally lose the wish to be independent, and the therapist should ally himself with the patient's ideal self. Once rapport with this patient is established, and the patient's life is in equilibrium, "weaning" attempts should be made to reduce the frequency and duration of visits. Again, as with most patients in supportive psychotherapy, and perhaps to some extent in all therapies, at termination it must clearly be established that there is the possibility of returning to therapy if it becomes necessary.

Changing From Supportive to Insight-Oriented Psychotherapy

The foregoing view is regarded by some therapists as therapeutic nihilism. I contend that this model of psychotherapy is not negativistic; it simply tries to take account of realities. Nothing should prevent the therapist who practices supportive psychotherapy from attempting to move toward a more insight-directed therapy once the patient is in equilibrium and his defenses are reasonably strong. It then becomes a matter of delicately testing the possibilities; if this is done with attention paid to progressive developments, it can be done safely. The critical point is to avoid subjecting the patient to an experience that will waste his time, energy and money, and make him feel that he is a failure. The most skilled therapist cannot be effective treating a patient in a mode of psychotherapy that is inappropriate. Moreover, such enterprises often lead to harmful countertransferences: The therapist who pushes his patient toward unrealizable goals will feel defeated by the patient's inability or unwillingness to progress, and will react with feelings of impotence and rage. It is unusual, however, for therapy to continue without the patient gaining some insight into his illness. Attempts can and should be made, at this point, to affect the roots of the patient's difficulties. Progress may lead to further attempts, and lack of progress suggests that this approach is not useful. One failure does not mean that one should abandon all chances of success at insight therapy; the conditions for change may not be auspicious at a given time. Repeated failures will of course lead a therapist to confine his work to a more purely supportive mode.

Adjunctive Measures

Supportive psychotherapy need not be an exclusive treatment. On the contrary, many of the patients for whom it is indicated benefit from adjunctive treatments and experiences such as medication, behavior modification, Alcoholics Anonymous (AA), group therapy (especially for those with difficulties in socialization), hospitalization, and a variety of community support services ranging from halfway houses to sheltered workshops. As previously mentioned, it may be useful, and at times necessary, to see other members of the patient's family. With especially disturbed patients, it is appropriate to plan on support modalities according to shifts in the patient's current problems. Whenever possible, the patient should be given the opportunity of being on his own; the more confident he becomes that the therapist's door is open, if he needs help, the more he will try to be on his own.

Conclusion

The diversity of the disturbances of these patients makes it impossible to do more than give broad guidelines. The central issue here, is that supportive psychotherapy is more than a mere exercise in ambulatory custodial care. A psychoanalytically-informed profile of the patient's psychological strengths and weaknesses, of his home situation and his wider social environment, can lead to a rational and fruitful plan of treatment that is as gratifying for the therapist as it can be for the patient.[8] Much of medicine is devoted to treating patients whose illnesses remain with them throughout life; psychotherapy can do no less.

References

1. Schlesinger HJ: Diagnosis and prescription for psychotherapy. Bull Menninger Clin 33:269–279, 1969
2. Dewald P: Psychotherapy. New York, Basic Books, 1964
3. Modell AH: The holding environment and the therapeutic action of psychoanalysis. J Am Psychoanal Assoc 24:285–307, 1976
4. Winnicott D: Psychiatric disorders in terms of infantile maturational processes. In: The Naturational Process and the Facilitating Environment. New York, International Universities Press, 1965
5. Schafer, R: Talking to patients in psychotherapy. Bull Menninger Clin 38:503–515, 1974
6. Werman DS: The use of dreams in psychotherapy: Practical guidelines. Can Psychiatr Assoc J 23:153–158, 1978
7. Racker H: The meanings and uses of countertransference. Psychoanal Q 26:303–357, 1957
8. Werman D: The Practice of Supportive Psychotherapy. New York, Brunner/Mazel, 1984

Tracey Potts Carson

19 The Behavioral Approach

Like any other vital and developing approach to disorders of living, the behavioral approach defies exact and invariant definition when considered over time. Indeed, as in the case of other approaches, its contemporary proponents would doubtless be found severely wanting at least in good sense, if not intellectual integrity, compared with any "second coming" of the founders of the behavioral tradition in psychology. Nevertheless, it is possible to identify a certain common core of fundamental assumptions that probably characterize most behavioral practitioners today, and that distinguish them in greater or lesser degree from their colleagues who use other approaches. And, as will be seen, this core belief system guiding modern practice bears a readily discernible relationship to the earliest formulations of the behaviorist position.

The central tenets of the behavioral approach are these:

1. For the most part, disorders of behavior (including certain kinds of "internal," physiologic behavior) are acquired or *learned* in the course of the individual's attempts to adapt to the circumstances and contingencies uniquely characteristic of that person's environment.
2. Since maladaptive behavior is the product of having learned poor methods of coping, or of having failed to learn more adequate and successful ones, appropriate therapeutic intervention consists of the planning and deployment of *new learning experiences* specifically tailored to the correction of behavioral deficiencies.

3. Inasmuch as patterns of dysfunctional behavior for given persons are both complex and highly individualistic, their detailed assessment must be accomplished prior to planning a treatment (*i.e.,* what is to be newly learned) program; complete assessment includes specification of those aspects of the environment or other behaviors of the individual *currently* associated with variation in the occurrence or intensity of the problematic behavior, an assessment process termed *behavioral analysis.*
4. Etiologic hypotheses bearing only a distal or remote relationship to the observable problematic behavior are to be eschewed; the proximal cognitive operations thought to underlie and support maladaptive behavior, however, are a suitable target of corrective therapeutic intervention in what has come to be called *cognitive behavior therapy.*

This last, in its legitimization of attributed mental events as having causal significance, represents a considerable liberalization of the original behaviorist "program."

History

The potent behavioral movement that has dominated much of American academic psychology since the 1920s owes its origins primarily to one man, John Broadus Watson, who was then a professor at Johns Hopkins University. Until Watson, psychology had largely concerned itself with mapping the domain of subjective experience. Watson's basic contribution was to point out the central scientific flaw in this enterprise; namely, since such experience must forever remain private within the individual, there can be no such thing as an intersubjectively reliable observation concerning it. Watson therefore championed, and very effectively, the abandonment of all merely "mental" phenomena as the proper domain of a truly scientific psychology and proclaimed that, henceforth, psychology should concern itself only with *behavior,* behavior that could be directly and objectively (*i.e.,* intersubjectively and reliably) observed.

Watson was decidedly not an "ivory tower" academician. On the contrary, girded with the new information coming out of the Soviet Union on the conditioned reflex, he embarked on a campaign to convince his colleagues and a curious public of what he felt would be the enormous practical benefits behaviorism could bestow. He boasted, for example, that he could take any healthy child and turn him into whatever kind of adult one might wish the child to become. With his colleague Rosalie Rayna, he also published the first demonstration of a deliberately conditioned phobia in a human being—the celebrated case of "Little Albert." By the end of the 1930s, Watson had been joined in his cause by Thorndike and Skinner, who added the idea of the potential power of operant or instrumental conditioning to the Pavlovian or classical conditioning Watson had emphasized.

Despite the auspicious beginning, however, behaviorism did not take hold in a mental health field largely dominated by psychodynamic thinking, and the few clinicians who openly espoused the viewpoint were for many years considered eccentric, at best. This general rejection began to abate in about 1950, with the publication by John Dollard and Neal Miller, then both at Yale, of *Personality and Psychotherapy*. This milestone book, written by authors who had been psychoanalyzed themselves, reinterpreted psychodynamics into the language and concepts of behavioral psychology. From that point, it was only a matter of time until clinicians in large numbers would become attracted to the possibilities inherent in a behavioral approach and seek training in its methods.

That promise in fact materialized during the 1960s with an explosion of publications describing the invention of new behavioral treatment methods, the reports typically containing unusually rigorous assessments of treatment outcomes. The 1970s, in turn, marked a period of rapid development for behavioral psychology. Impressive initial gains were consolidated, new inroads were made in assessment methodology, and behavioral techniques were successfully applied to alter both cognitive and physiologic processes. In fact, the behavioral approach underwent considerable revision during the 1970s, at which time the effectiveness of cognitive therapies allied with Albert Ellis (1962) and Aaron Beck (1967) encouraged behaviorists to incorporate cognitive events within the behavioral framework. As a consequence, behavioral theory now recognizes cognitions as treatable responses that—similar to observable behavior—develop and change as a function of learning experience. Also during the 1970s, applications of behavioral procedures to the treatment of disorders previously regarded as purely medical or organic in origin spurred development of a new and burgeoning field called *behavioral medicine*. Behavioral scientists now collaborate with physicians in treating a number of medical problems, such as cardiovascular disease, hypertension, diabetes, gastrointestinal and dermatological disorders, anorexia nervosa, stuttering, pain, enuresis, asthma, seizures, and obesity.

Basic Principles of Classical and Instrumental Conditioning

While the requirements for a clinical approach to be designated *behavioral* have undergone considerable relaxation in recent times, it is probably fair to say that the principles of classical (also termed *Pavlovian* or *respondent*) and instrumental (also termed *Skinnerian* or *operant*) conditioning still form the backbone of most behavioral therapeutic interventions. We turn now to a very brief overview of these processes.

In classical conditioning, a reinforcing stimulus—one that on presentation reliably evokes a given response—is paired with a previously neutral stimulus, with the result that the latter also acquires the property of eliciting the response in question. Maladaptive anxiety responses are readily conceptualized within this learning paradigm. Thus, for example, behavioral clinicians are likely to interpret phobias as fear responses that, although originally elicited on an innate basis by genuinely dangerous circumstances, have become conditioned, often through accidental pairing, to stimuli that are trivial from a survival standpoint. In the aforementioned case of "Little Albert," a normal child's innate fearful response to loud noises was conditioned to a previously neutral stimulus—a white rat—by repeatedly pairing presentations of a loud noise with presentations of the rat. As a consequence of this deliberate exercise of classical conditioning principles, Albert became phobic of white rats, and his anxiety response subsequently generalized to rabbits, fur, cotton, and other similar stimuli.

Whereas the clinically important aspects of classical conditioning are thought to relate chiefly to autonomic responding, the instrumental conditioning paradigm (with the possible exception of certain types of biofeedback training) is useful chiefly in the understanding and planned modification of behaviors mediated by the somatic nervous system. A crucial tenet of the behavioral clinician is that most if not all such behavior is acquired and maintained by the consequences it produces—*reinforcing* consequences; hence, by altering these consequences it should be possible to effect an alteration in the pertinent behavioral output. While the definition of "reinforcement" in instrumental or operant conditioning often comes dangerously close to circular reasoning, there exist certain ingenious theoretical solutions to this problem, the details of which need not concern us here.

Even with this sketchy overview of simple conditioning processes, the reader may anticipate an important and very general technique in the behaviorist repertoire of therapeutic interventions, namely the technique of *extinction* of problematic and presumably conditioned behaviors. Extinction, in either the classical or the instrumental paradigm, is accomplished simply by arranging for the "reinforcement" *not* to occur. In the extinction of classically conditioned responses (*e.g.*, anxiety), the therapist arranges for the patient to be exposed repeatedly to the originally neutral but now anxiety-producing stimulus, while preventing in one way or another the occurrence of the originally (and sometimes objectively) fearful stimulus, technically referred to as the *unconditioned* stimulus. Because the patient will usually have learned, instrumentally, various ways of avoiding such exposure, the therapist will often need to employ special techniques to minimize such avoidant responding, which unless effectively combatted would render extinction impossible. The extinction of *instrumentally* learned behaviors is normally a straightforward matter once the maintaining (reinforcing) stimuli have been identified; one simply endeavors to prevent their occurrence or to limit their provision contingent on the emitting of more desirable behavior.

The planned use of extinction processes by no means exhausts available behavioral techniques based on classical and instrumental conditioning paradigms. In practice, classically conditioned responses often prove quite resistant to the singular application of extinction procedures and respond more favorably to *counterconditioning* or *aversive conditioning* techniques. Counterconditioning theoretically weakens or eliminates the learned connection between specific stimuli and some type of maladaptive behavior by conditioning an alternative, more adaptive response to the stimuli involved, thereby replacing the madaladaptive response (usually anxiety) with a preferable alternative. The most effective derivative of counterconditioning, *desensitization,* exposes the patient to a carefully defined hierarchy of anxiety-evoking stimuli and juxtaposes each exposure with a trained state of deep relaxation, such that a relaxation response eventually becomes conditioned to the relevant stimuli. With *systematic* desensitization, the patient is exposed to the anxiety-producing stimuli in imagery; another variant of desensitization, *in vivo,* instead requires a real-life exposure to those situations eliciting anxiety.

The commonly used but sometimes controversial technique known as *aversive conditioning* is essentially the reverse of the procedure employed in extinquishing conditioned anxiety. Here, the therapist attempts to *create* a (classically) conditioned anxiety response to stimuli associated with some unwanted or problematic behavior pattern by pairing these stimuli repeatedly with noxious stimulation of one sort or another, either real (in vivo) or imagined (in vitro). Applications of aversive conditioning have been effective in treating deviant sexual arousal patterns, alchoholism, cigarette smoking, overeating, and enuresis. With one variant of aversive conditioning, *convert sensitization,* both performance of the undesirable behavior and presentation of the noxious stimulus (*e.g.,* vomit) occur in vitro.

Behavioral techniques derived from the instrumental conditioning paradigm, too numerous to comprehensively summarize in the present context, basically subdivide into those that facilitate acquisition or increase of desirable behaviors and those that facilitate a decrease or elimination of undesirable behaviors. Most importantly, all such techniques change behavior through systematic regulation of its consequences. Those behavioral techniques used to develop or increase behavior primarily involve applications of *positive reinforcement*—the presentation of positively reinforcing stimuli contingent on (following) emission of the targeted behavior. Positively reinforcing stimuli not only include material and verbal rewards, but also the avoidance of aversive stimuli, such as discomfort or pain. By definition, a positive reinforcer includes any object, behavior, or event whose contingent presentation increases the frequency of a response. Thus, positive reinforcers need not be pleasant and, in fact, may be idiosyncratic and seemingly unpleasant (consider, for example, the positive reinforcement for an autistic child's head-banging behavior).

Although *negative reinforcement* also generates an increase in behavior, its incorporation into therapeutic procedures occurs much less frequently. Aversive conditioning techniques, however, may include an application of negative reinforcement, when, as a part of a two-stage aversive conditioning program, emission of a desirable behavior predictably terminates an ongoing aversive stimulus. Technically, a negative reinforcer can be any stimulus (object, behavior, or event) whose contingent withdrawal yields an increase in the frequency of a response. Those stimuli that function as negative reinforcers are usually unpleasant or aversive in nature.

With some patients, the clinician will find it difficult to identify a functional incentive or positive reinforcer for behavior change. The "Premack Principle" can fortunately remedy this dilemma in most cases. As the Premack Principle specifies, a relatively high-frequency behavior will function as a positive reinforcer for behaviors that occur at a lower frequency. When applying this principle, the clinician simply identifies a high-frequency behavior for the individual patient (*e.g.,* housework, napping, reading, depressive speech) and then instructs the patient that such behavior is only to occur following a period of engagement in a previously-defined adaptive activity that has been targeted for increase.

One form of positive reinforcement used to develop a new response, called *shaping,* initially reinforces the patient for an existing behavior that has some similarity to the desired new response, and then proceeds to reinforce the emission of successively closer approximations to the desired response. Shaping facilitates the eventual learning of a new behavior that is initially too complex for the patient, by breaking that behavior down into its simpler components or approximations. While clinical applications of this technique are unlimited, shaping has been quite essential in the teaching of self-care, language, and prosocial skills to institutionalized patients. As an example, nonverbal, psychotic children have learned to speak through a program using techniques of shaping, modeling, and imitation (see Lovaas). These children were initially rewarded for merely looking at a trainer's mouth, then were reinforced for emitting any vocalization, and eventually received all reinforcement contingent on their imitating increasingly complex sounds and words modeled by the trainer.

Extinction and *punishment* underlie most instrumental conditioning techniques used to eliminate or suppress undesirable behavior. Extinction procedures eliminate a behavior by discontinuing reinforcement relevant to its occurrence; maladaptive behavior that is sustained by the attention it draws from other people, for example, should extinguish when consistently ignored. Punishment, in contrast, involves the delivery of an aversive stimulus contingent on a response targeted for suppression. Thus, the punished individual is confronted with an aversive consequence or "cost" after emitting the undesirable response in question. Not surprisingly, punishment techniques employ a variety of unpleasant stimuli, ranging from electric shock (usually limited for behaviors injurious to self or others), to verbal reprimands, to the forfeiture of positive reinforcers. For instance, the *response cost* technique involves forfeiture of a salient positive reinforcer (*e.g.*, money, television viewing, therapy time) after emission of a problematic behavior. *Time-out,* a punishment procedure commonly used to accomplish suppression of disruptive classroom behavior, alternatively requires that the individual be physically separated from all major reinforcers for a temporary period of time following misbehavior. Punishment has at best a time-limited effect in the suppression of undesirable behavior; nevertheless, such suppression may make possible the substitution of desirable behavior that can be positively reinforced.

The use of treatment techniques based on the principles of classical and instrumental conditioning is limited only by the therapist's imaginativeness in conceptualizing the patient's problems, by certain species-specific constraints on what is (and is not) likely to be conditionable, and, of course, by important ethical and professional considerations. Judicious application of any technique or combination of techniques ultimately depends on the clinician's skill in identifying those antecedent or consequent stimuli that regulate the occurrence of an individual's behavioral deficiencies. It should also be noted that the effectiveness of any technique to suppress or extinguish undesirable behavior is augmented when treatment also provides positive reinforcement for alternative, appropriate behavior.

Other Frequently Employed Techniques

Much learning at the human level is accomplished by modeling, imitating, and rehearsing the behavior of an accomplished model; yet *modeling* as an important principle of learning was slow to gain acceptance in behavioral academia, in large part because it proved difficult to cast within a strict conditioning mold. Over time, however, thanks mostly to the persistence of a small but very active group of investigators, notably among them Albert Bandura, modeling processes gradually came to be accepted as potentially important to a comprehensive psychology of learning, particularly in relation to the acquisition of complex skills. The implications for clinical work were fairly obvious from the beginning, in part because much of the background research on modeling involved behaviors having more-or-less direct clinical relevance, such as children being instigated to aggression by an aggressive model. Also, many clinically important behaviors seemed so complex in organization as to be beyond the ken of a simple, single-response conditioning approach. For example, how does one teach appropriate heterosocial dating behavior to a man in his 30s having no previous experience in that area?

Modeling and associated techniques of role playing and the like have in all probability an exciting future in behavioral treatment technology relating to complex social behaviors. Somewhat surprisingly, they may prove to be as potent as the conditioning-based techniques, even with respect to more circumscribed behavior dysfunctions. For example, there is sufficient evidence that snake phobias may be effectively treated by having the phobic person observe, and subsequently imitate, a fearless person approach and handle a large but nonvenomous reptile.

We have already had occasion to refer to the infusion of cognitive thinking into the behavioral understanding and treatment of disorder. While we often regard this as a relatively new development, its roots do go back at least into the 1950s with the development by Albert Ellis of what he called *Rational-Emotive Therapy* (RET). According to this view, cognitions assume primacy in the organization of affect and behavior; hence, instances of dysfunction in affect or behavior are always traceable to dysfunctional *beliefs,* of which, according to Ellis, there are certain more-or-less routine and predictable types. A common example offered by Ellis is the belief that "it would be an utter catastrophe unless everyone who knew me loved me." Ellis's technique involves a forceful verbal unearthing of such "irrationalities" and their equally forceful refutation in direct confrontive debate with the patient. He and his colleagues have persuasively presented RET as an effective program, particularly for the modification of maladaptive emotional responses; however, the highly confrontive therapeutic style demonstrated by Ellis and seemingly requisite to successful execution of RET is not comfortable for all clinicians.

Probably the best known of the cognitive-behavior therapies currently is that developed by Aaron Beck for the treatment of depression, chiefly unipolar depression. This therapy, for which specialized training is recommended, has compiled a very respectable, even superior outcome record in direct competitive trials with antidepressant medication, tending to support Beck's contention that dysfunctional cognitive processes are at the root of many depressive behavioral phenomena, including some grave and severe ones. Essentially, Beck's cognitive therapy for depression uses a variable combination of cognitive and behavioral techniques to alter those idiosyncratic, self-defeating cognitions that lead to or sustain a person's depression. Therapist and patient work together as "scientific collaborators" to find the depressed person's relevant alternatives to depressogenic thought patterns. (See Beck, et al, 1979, for an excellent introduction to this therapy.)

In very recent years, the proliferation of proposed cognitively based therapies has been so great that no serious attempt can be made to catalog them here. The interested reader is referred to Kendall and Hollon (1979) for a reasonably current review of the field.

Case Application

The following case of gender identity disorder (Barlow and Abel, 1976; Barlow, Reynolds, and Agras, 1973), a disorder generally considered highly refractory to treatment of any sort, is offered as an example of a comprehensive and exclusively behavioral approach to the treatment of this difficult problem. In it, as will be seen, several different behavioral techniques were deployed in a thoughtfully sequenced manner in order to achieve what appears to be an excellent result.

☐ A 17-year-old transsexual man who wanted to change his sex agreed to try therapy designed to alter his gender identity. He had wanted to be female for as long as he could remember and had spontaneously begun cross-dressing before the age of five. At the time of initial assessment, his behavior in general was markedly effeminate. Additionally, he was depressed and withdrawn, in part because people ridiculed his effeminate appearance and behavior.

The first step of treatment, directed toward altering this man's gender role behavior, taught the client masculine styles of sitting, standing, and walking. Appropriate behaviors were modeled by a male therapist, than imitated and rehearsed by the client. Therapists provided both instructive feedback to improve the client's imitation attempts and effusive praise to reinforce successful reproductions of the modeled responses. As these newly acquired behaviors generalized outside of therapy, their emission was reinforced by the client's social environment (in terms of decreased ridicule and staring), and the client began to enjoy his new "masculine" style.

The next step of treatment involved social skills training, with an emphasis on teaching appropriate heterosocial behaviors. Using once again the techniques of modeling, behavioral rehearsal, and immediate feedback, therapists succeeded in modifying the client's social presentation to the extent that he was feeling more confident and effective in his interactions with peers. Interestingly, the social skills program included voice retraining, which effectively altered the client's high-pitched, effeminate manner of speaking.

Following this therapeutic emphasis on appropriate gender behavior and social skill acquisition, the client was introduced to a fantasy-retraining procedure. More specifically, he was taught to envision himself enacting a masculine role in his sexual and other fantasies. At the conclusion of this treatment phase, however, a repeat assessment of his psychophysiologic response to erotic stimuli indicated that he was still unaroused by heterosexual material and was still responsive to homosexually oriented material.

Therapy then began to focus directly on a modification of this man's sexual arousal pattern. First, his arousal to heterosexual stimuli was enhanced through a classical conditioning procedure that systematically paired orgasm with heterosexual stimuli. The procedure was effective in establishing heterosexual arousal, and at this stage of treatment, continuing assessment showed

> that the client was erotically responsive to both heterosexual and homosexual material. Suppression of the homosexual arousal was then indicated.
>
> The last stage of treatment used classical conditioning procedures (a combination of covert sensitization and aversive conditioning with electric shock) to successfully suppress the client's homosexual arousal. Follow-up assessment 2 years later indicated that this man was effectively functioning as a heterosexual man, dating regularly, and attending college.

This example was selected in part to highlight the multifaceted nature of behavioral intervention. Treatment of this transsexual man addressed many problems relevant to the maintenance of his variant gender identity: inappropriate gender behavior, lack of social skills, inappropriate gender fantasy, homosexual arousal, and lack of heterosexual arousal. Therapy not only suppressed unwanted behavior but also taught the client new and appropriate alternatives. Finally, this case illustrates the behavioral emphasis on continuing assessment both during and after treatment intervention.

Summary

Although behavioral psychology is commonly mistaken for a school of psychotherapy or a mere collection of diverse treatment techniques, it actually represents a distinctive orientation to psychopathology. Central to this approach is a commitment to empirical validation of any presumed influence over behavior, both in research and clinical practice. The foundation of the behavioral approach thus consists of empirically derived principles of psychology and related disciplines, relevant to the prediction and control of human behavior. Having demonstrated that abnormal behavior can be produced, altered, and eliminated through manipulation of stimulus conditions (*i.e.*, new learning experience), behaviorists can effectively argue that most psychopathologic responses need not be conceptualized as symptoms of unconcious conflicts or anomalous somatic functioning. From a behavioral perspective, the appropriate target for clinical intervention is the maladaptive behavior itself, not some hypothesized "underlying" mental disorder that proves to be both untestable and unessential for accomplishing successful behavior change.

Behavioral theorists recognize a multiplicity of causes for problematic response patterns but emphasize that treatment-relevant assessment must determine what aspects of the person's environment and which of his other responses are *currently* associated with a fluctuation in the expression of problematic behavior. This process of identifying currently operative determinants or modulators of maladaptive responding, referred to as *behavioral analysis,* addresses early influences on the targeted problem behavior only insofar as they continue to play a role in the regulation of this behavior. Observation and measurement of the problem behavior as well as those events that are contiguous with its fluctuation provide the data needed to generate objective hypotheses about what sustains the learned maladaptive responding. Treatment then modifies those environmental stimuli or responses of the individual thought to sustain a pattern of dysfunctional behavior, and in the process, provides the conditions necessary for more adaptive functioning.

Although the behavioral approach is still relatively new in comparison with other approaches to psychopathology, it has developed significantly within a short time period and has proven itself capable of addressing even the most complex of clinical presentations. With continued success in applications of this approach, the behavioral community has acquired a certain self-assurance, with consequent reduction in what had once been somewhat shrill attacks on nonbelievers. Today, many behavioral clinicians are seeking integration and rapprochement with other approaches, and are for the most part being warmly received in this collaborative venture.

Bibliography

Barlow DH, Abel GG: Sexual deviation. In Craighead WE, Kazdin AE, Mahoney MJ (eds): Behavior Modification: Principles, Issues, and Applications. Boston, Houghton Mifflin, 1976

Barlow DH, Reynolds EJ, Agras WS: Gender identity change in a transsexual. Arch Gen Psychiatry 28 (4): 569–76, 1973

Beck AT: Depression: Causes and Treatment. Philadelphia, University of Pennsylvania Press, 1967

Beck AT, Rush AJ, Shaw BF, et al: Cognitive Therapy of Depression. New York, Guilford Press, 1979

Dollard J, Miller NE: Personality and Psychotherapy. New York, McGraw-Hill, 1950

Ellis A: Reason and Emotion in Psychotherapy. New York, Lyle Stuart, 1962

Kendall PC, Hollon SD: (eds): Cognitive Behavioral Intervention: Theory, Research and Procedures. New York, Academic Press, 1979

Lovaas OI: Reinforcement Therapy (film). Philadelphia, Smith, Kline, and French Laboratories, 1966

Premack D: Toward empirical behavioral laws: I. Positive reinforcement. Psychol Rev 66: 219–233, 1959

E. Michael Kahn

20 Group Psychotherapy

Group psychotherapy is an effective, economical mode of treatment for a variety of psychiatric problems. In the group, the insights and the caring of all members are brought to bear as each member struggles with his problems. Problems may be less difficult to discern than in the dyadic (one-on-one) setting, for they are seen in each individual's transactions with other group members. In addition, one or two well-trained group leaders will be able to provide "state-of-the-art" care for up to ten patients simultaneously. In these ways, group psychotherapy gains both efficacy and economy.

This chapter will (1) delineate the major schools of group psychotherapy, (2) present the theoretical rationale for group treatment, (3) review the ways in which a therapeutic group climate is developed and maintained, and (4) define the means by which appropriate group interventions may be chosen for individual patients.

Schools of Group Psychotherapy

Theories of group psychotherapy have grown from each of the major therapeutic traditions. Over the years, these concepts have been shaped to emphasize the unique aspects of the group experience. At present, there are four major schools: (1) psychoanalytic and object relations, (2) interpersonal and interactive, (3) Gestalt, and (4) Bionian/Tavistock.

Psychoanalytic and Object-Relations Theory

In psychoanalytic and object-relations theory, the patient's reactions to situations, relationships, and transferences developing in the group are believed to provide clues to the nature of the patient's unconscious psychological conflicts and characteristic defense mechanisms. Through interpretation, these intrapsychic experiences are brought into awareness. Continued confrontation of these maladaptive patterns leads to more mature behavior. Immature ego defenses and fragmented personality structures are supplanted by a mature, well-integrated self.

Interpersonal and Interactive Modes

Interpersonal and interactive modes of therapy focus on the individual patient's characteristic modes of relating to others in the group setting. Their transactions betray habitual patterns of behavior that bar intimacy and sabotage the development of satisfying commitments. With the help of the group members, the leaders challenge each person to reflect on his behavior, and to understand the reasons why these actions do not bring them happiness. Through feedback from other members, and an opportunity to practice in a controlled situation, each patient develops more successful modes of interaction.

Gestalt Therapy

The focus of gestalt therapy is the individual's awareness, both cognitively and emotionally, of his ongoing experience in the group setting. Through describing these experiences as they occur, often in "experiments," the individual comes to understand the "hidden" parts of himself, and to feel more comfortable with them. For example, the therapist may say to the patient, "You smile as you talk of your boss, but your hands are clenched. Focus on your hands now; clench them more tightly. How do they feel?" Simultaneously, the patient is challenged to take responsibility for acting to meet his needs, resolving conflict and internal confusion. Replay of past traumatic events through psychodrama may be used to facilitate recovery of lost aspects of the self. Each member, in turn, works with the therapist, while the other members serve as a "Greek chorus," supporting that person's work.

The Bionian/Tavistock Method

The focus in Bionian/Tavistock groups is the dynamics of the group as a whole. The leaders wait for issues to emerge in the group's interactions, then offer global interpretations. This method is excellent for training people about group dynamics. Research has shown, however, that this method is not useful to people seeking conventional therapeutic change.

Curative Factors

There is general agreement on the curative factors active in a group setting. The relative importance of any one factor will vary from patient and from group to group. These factors are as follows:

Cohesion: a feeling of closeness and belonging engendered by the group, which provides the supportive backdrop for confrontation and risk-taking

Catharsis: expression of feelings about the past or current situations, which provides release of emotional tension

Self-understanding: insight into motivation and patterns of interaction

Interpersonal feedback: an opportunity to find out how one "comes across" to people, a chance to practice new ways of relating, and a way to share impressions of others

Universality: finding out that other people have similar problems, that one is not alone

Instillation of hope: developing positive expectations through one's own success experiences, and through sharing others' success experiences

Altruism: gaining satisfaction from giving to others, and feeling competent from having been of help to them

Family Reenactment: the group's providing an opportunity, with its "parents" (leaders) and "siblings" (members), to work through issues that stemmed the family of origin

Guidance: provision of helpful advice by therapists and other members

Existential: developing awareness that one must take responsibility for one's own actions and accept the limitations of the human condition (see Yalom)

The Change Process

The processes by which change occurs through psychotherapy are at once both self-evident and obscure. Each of the schools uses its own metaphor to describe the process, and the techniques by which the process is facilitated. A general framework for understanding this process will be presented below, with examples taken from the group therapy setting.

Ongoing Experience

The raw substance of psychotherapy is the inner experience of the patient as he reacts to the present, recalls the past, or anticipates the future. The therapist will help stimulate this reflection, and will assist the patient in finding clues to the nature of his problems, and to the solutions for these problems.

☐ A male graduate student came to group psychotherapy because conflict with his dissertation advisor blocked completion of his degree. He stated that he felt "helpless" in his interactions with this "domineering" faculty member. The therapist prompted the member to watch for situations in the group in which he felt "helpless" or "domineered."

Tension

As situations arise in the group that resemble the problematic situations causing the patient to come for therapy, the patient will become increasingly tense. In many

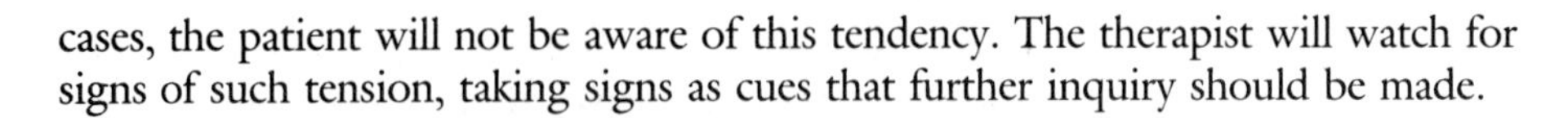

cases, the patient will not be aware of this tendency. The therapist will watch for signs of such tension, taking signs as cues that further inquiry should be made.

☐ During the student's third group meeting, one woman sought advice and reassurance concerning her impending divorce. One of the older group members offered superficial advice, and this was rejected quickly. The older member reacted angrily, stating that he felt no one respected him. At this point, one of the leaders noted that the graduate student appeared stiff and frightened. The leader asked, "How are you feeling right now? Are these feelings similar to those you have in other situations?"

Awareness

The patient gradually gains awareness of his characteristic patterns of reaction. At this point, the therapist strives to help him understand what's going on "behind the scenes" emotionally.

☐ The student answered, "I felt really sad for Mary, like I'm not sure anyone can help her." The therapist asked, "How so?" "I was starting to think that John was angry at her for having any problems," replied the student. "Is that something you saw happen in your home when you were growing up?" the therapist queried.

Levels of Change

The change process occurs on three levels, the cognitive, emotional, and behavioral. Cognitive change requires insight into the thought process that has maintained a particular pattern of behavior, a decision to alter that pattern, and the development of a strategy to accomplish this alteration. Emotional change requires emotional arousal (catharsis) and a setting in which the patient is safely supported, so that emotional healing can occur. Behavioral change requires the opportunity to practice new ways of doing things, as well as the means by which successful experiences are reinforced and may be generalized.

☐ In the sixth group session, a similar situation arose, and the student again became frightened. The therapist said, "Talk about your fear." The student stammered. The therapist offered, "Something makes it hard for you to talk about your fear." "People will think I'm weak if I tell them," the student replied. "Is that so?" asked the therapist. At that point, the student began to sob, and he was comforted by several other group members. With their support and reassurance, he talked about his relationship with his demanding, insensitive father. With guidance by the therapist, he asked the other members for continued support. They said that they saw his willingness to talk about problems and to ask for support as signs of strength rather than weakness.

Reflection

Once the change process has begun, the individual will be more aware of problematic interactions, both inside and outside the group, and will begin to study these

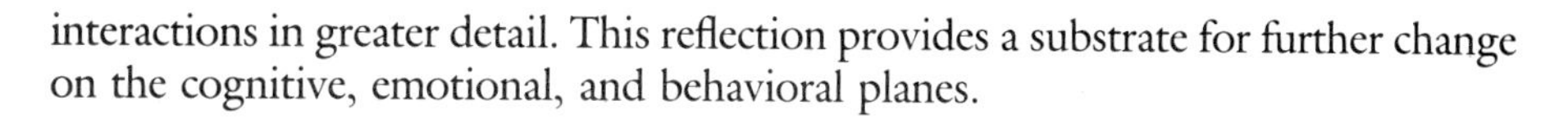

interactions in greater detail. This reflection provides a substrate for further change on the cognitive, emotional, and behavioral planes.

> ☐ In the following week, the student reported, he noticed that he became fearful whenever he spoke with his graduate advisor. After much thought, he concluded that he dreaded rejection by this man. He related this to his wish for acceptance by his father, which he felt had never been granted.

Integration

With time, the patient will generalize the changes made in the group to other life situations. More effective strategies dealing with problems will be elaborated, and the emotional burden of unresolved conflict will be reduced. Support, guidance, and confrontation may be needed at times to keep this process active.

> ☐ Gradually, the student became more willing to express his own ideas to his advisor. He was able to critique papers he had written with this older man without feeling "like I was just a little kid." His productivity increased. Rejection of a manuscript submitted to a journal later triggered a return of the work block. After confrontation with his advisor and support from the group, he worked through this episode.

The Patient, the Therapist, and the Group

Format and Contract

Therapy groups usually consist of six to ten people, led by one or two therapists. Groups of smaller size are often unsuccessful because the development of cohesion is stymied by competition for leader attention. Larger groups, for the most part, are unmanageable; members may be ignored or excluded. Because of the complexity of the events that can occur in a group, it is helpful to have two leaders. They work synergistically to accomplish leader tasks, and provide support for each other. Still, the tasks of the leader are difficult; careful training and skillful collaboration are needed. Most groups meet on a regularly scheduled basis. In the outpatient setting, the interval is usually once a week; in the inpatient setting, groups may meet from two to five times a week, depending on the patients average length of stay and the goals of treatment. For patients with short attention spans (children and adolescents), or those who become agitated or anxious easily (schizophrenics), the usual meeting length is 1 hour. For individuals with greater capacity to withstand the strains of a group, meetings of 90 to 120 minutes are more fruitful. Fees are usually less than one half those of individual therapy, and most insurance companies reimburse for group psychotherapy.

Norms and Leader Tasks

It is the responsibility of the therapist to make and enforce a contract with the patients regarding the format of the group. Tardiness, absence, contact with other members outside the group setting, and breach of confidentiality are strongly discouraged. Establishment of these rules seems to be a precondition for development of a cohesive, "safe" atmosphere within the group. The leaders will also facilitate the development of group norms that promote closeness, activate the change process, encourage disclosure and risk-taking, and establish a supportive atmosphere. The leaders will block the development of antitherapeutic norms, such as "People can't talk about sex in here," or "It's not OK to be angry." They are responsible for bringing each patient's emotional resources, however great or small, to bear on the problems at hand.

Patient Selection

Group treatment is well-suited both to patients who have trouble establishing good relationships with other people and to patients who will benefit from peer support. Group therapy may be especially helpful in the treatment of patients who are skillful at hiding their problems or defenses in one-on-one therapy, or patients who are prone to develop strong transference to their individual therapists. On a pragmatic level, group treatment is a likely choice in agencies short of personnel or funds.

Therapists usually screen patients to assure that all members of a group maintain similar levels of adaptive function (ego strength). Otherwise, the disparity of resources will interfere with development of a consistent pace. In most cases, therapists strive to avoid patients whose problems are all alike, unless they are forming a special-purpose group. Homogeneity may lead to defensive stalemates.

The therapist must ask whether a particular patient, with his or her psychological resources, can work with the group as it already exists to obtain his or her goals. Patients whose level of function is inconsistent with other group members and patients whose defensive styles will place them at odds with the group are likely to become "drop-outs" who have obtained little benefit from treatment. With time and support, however, patients with very modest resources can achieve considerable benefit from treatment.

Patient Preparation

Many patients find group therapy particularly threatening because "Everyone's looking at me." Patient education regarding the group contract, the types of activities that are undertaken in the group, and the role of the therapist in "protecting" patients will help minimize the negative impact of these fears. For many patients, a brief course of individual therapy is a useful prologue to the group, for it helps them gain confidence in the therapeutic process and to feel more confortable talking about their problems. Outpatient therapists often suggest that the patient attend three to twelve group sessions before reaching a decision to discontinue group therapy; most patients who stay beyond this introductory period will stay with the group until the natural conclusion of the therapeutic process.

Stages of Group Development

Therapy groups pass through four developmental stages in their natural course. Each state is marked by a particular issue, which is shared by all the members, and often by the leaders as well. Traumatic events in the life of the group may trigger a regression to earlier issues. Awareness of these stages helps the therapist to understand the events within the group, and to shape them therapeutically; each stage provides unique opportunities for therapeutic work. These stages are:

Inclusion. Questions such as "Do I belong here?" and "What role am I to play in this group?" characterize this early stage of development. This is a good time to observe the ways that members approach others and seek their acceptance. Deficits in self-esteem or identity confusion may be readily apparent.

Testing. Having gained a sense of belonging, the members begin to seek ways to assert their individuality. They will begin to reveal their more guarded feelings and impulses, and will watch the responses of the other members and the leaders quite closely. Conflicts about the expression of feelings (sad or angry) and about dominance and independence may be apparent.

Cohesion and Working. Having developed a sense of belonging and established a feeling of personal safety, each member will feel free to pursue his or her therapeutic goals. The group matrix will function as a source of advice, interpretation, and support in the course of this work.

Termination. Departure of a member from the group or dissolution of the group itself will activate feelings of grief and loss. Gains made during the earlier stages will be reworked and integrated. The members may find new ways to deal with the inevitable hurts and losses that are part of life's course.

Special-Purpose Groups

Originally, group therapists strove to work primarily with higher-functioning (neurotic) patients on a long-term basis in the outpatient setting. A body of theory and technique, the core of the material presented above, was developed in this setting. In recent years, however, theory and technique have been modified to encompass a wide variety of patients and settings. These include the following:

- Medication maintenance for schizophrenics
- Social-skill development for schizophrenics
- Treatment of post-traumatic stress disorder in Viet Nam veterans
- Treatment of inpatients on short-term units
- Support for people in stressful vocational positions such as physicians-in-training or business managers
- Crisis intervention for people facing difficult life changes such as retirement, divorce, or physical illness
- Treatment of adolescents with behavioral disturbances, such as anorexia nervosa

A number of factors may complicate the leadership of such groups. The members may have few emotional resources; they may be brought to treatment by adverse circumstance or others' dictates; their outlook may be so narrow as to preclude peer confrontation. On the other hand, each group is unified by a common feature, an experience, a goal, and a diagnosis, which may serve as a nidus for cohesion. The leaders in such groups will work to overcome the aforementioned hindrances by (1) infusing energy, (2) providing direction and support, and (3) using special technical maneuvers, such as role playing or psychodrama. The leaders will supplement the assets of the members with the energy and knowledge that make it possible to reach their joint goals. The leaders will also help the members define practical, meaningful objectives.

Bibliography

Bion WR: Experience in Groups. London, Tavistock Pubications, 1961
Fagan J, Shepherd IL: Gestalt Therapy Now. New York, Harper and Row, 1970
Ganzarain R: General systems theory and object relations theories: Their usefulness in group psychotherapy. Int Group Psychother. 27: 441–456, 1977
Polster E, Polster M: Gestalt Therapy Integrated. New York, Brunner/Mazel, 1973
Rioch MJ, The Work of Wilfred Bion on Groups. Psychiatry 33:55–66, 1970
Wolf A, Schwartz EK: Psychoanalysis in Groups. New York, Grune and Stratton, 1962
Yalom ID: The Theory and Practice of Group Psychotherapy. New York, Basic Books, 1975

Gail McLeod

21 Marital and Family Therapy

In the past few decades, treatment of marital and family problems has become a common psychotherapeutic modality. Sager and associates (1968) report that as many as 50% of people undergoing psychotherapy express concerns regarding their marital relationships. Forty percent of marriages end with divorce, while increasing numbers of dysfunctional families seek psychotherapy. Marital and family therapy based on the research and treatment efforts of Clifford Sager, James Framo, Ira Glick, David Kessler, Nathan Ackerman, Murray Bowen, Virginia Satir, Jay Haley, and Salvador Minuchin will be discussed in this chapter.

Marital Therapy

Couples generally approach matrimony with minimal preparation and extremely unrealistic expectations. Courtship is often brief and intensely romantic; there is a magical promise that intimacy, affection, and passion will continue and that needs will be met. The relationship is rarely examined closely, and the potential mate is often idealized. When the honeymoon is over, however, most marriages quickly evolve into a long succession of days that are routine and familiar. Many couples can face and accept the disappointments of romanticized love, build a satisfying relationship based on what each partner has to offer, and find beauty and comfort in the ordinary. Others cannot, and feelings of dissatisfaction and resentment surface quickly and escalate as the marriage continues.

Factors Influencing Marital Adjustment

Mate Selection

Mate selection is complex and multidetermined (see Framo). For example, a shy, passive man may choose a dominant, outspoken wife—the "opposite attract" or "need complementarity" concept. Another person may choose a mate whose needs and level of emotional maturity are similar to his or her own. Here, an anxious, dependent woman might select a husband who is withdrawn and chronically dysphoric. Mates may select one another unconsciously as a result of early childhood experiences within the family of origin, possibly as a parental substitute, as an attempt to reestablish the original family constellation, or to heal previous unresolved conflicts there. The patterns described here are not inherently pathologic and can lead to marriages that are satisfying and positive.

Marital Contracts

Sager (1976) has used the term *marital contracts* to describe largely unspoken expectations, agreements, and fantasies of marital life that are held by most couples. There are three basic types of marital contracts. The conscious, verbalized marital contract generally occurs in some cursory fashion prior to the wedding ceremony or in the early months of marriage. Here the obvious and superficial arrangements dealing with the basic aspects of living together—housekeeping, vacations, and money management—are discussed.

The conscious, nonverbal marital contract, Sager's second category, contains the wishes and expectations of each spouse regarding the marriage and mate that are not discussed, but kept hidden usually out of shame or apprehension, or to avoid conflict during courtship. These surface fairly quickly in the marriage and can be the source of much strife. Often, a spouse will seemingly agree with his mate's expectations prior to the wedding, but quickly begin to try to change the agreement or transform the spouse soon after the ceremony. A wife might verbalize agreement with her husband's frugality during courtship and engagement, for example, but attempt after the wedding to make him into the generous, carefree "big spender" that she had secretly envisioned and desired.

The unconscious marital contract, Sager's third category, contains those expectations and fantasies rooted in the individual's family of origin, childhood experiences, and intrapsychic processes. Such expectations are often complex and contraindicatory and nearly always outside the individual's level of awareness. Issues of power, control, and closeness or distance are contained here. For example, a husband might state that he wants his spouse to share decision making equally. In reality, he has deep-seated fears regarding submission and control, and feels dominated and angry when the wife makes a decision without consulting him. She, in turn, senses his anger, is confused and irritated by it, and conflict ensues.

All marriages have such contractual arrangements or "understandings." Mates routinely expect that their spouse accepts and agrees with their conceptualization of what the relationship will be. The contractual expectations of some couples are complementary and can lead to interaction that is gratifying and reciprocal. Reflection and discussion with one's potential spouse regarding needs, expectations, and possible sources of conflict can aid in the development of a stable marriage. Conflict occurs when needs and expectations clash or when the basic marital "arrangement" must be renegotiated to encompass the birth of a child, major illness of a spouse, or departure of children from the home.

Environmental and Personality Factors

The opportunity to grow up in a family where parents have a stable, well-functioning marriage is the best preparation one can have for later marital life. Emotional maturity and a well-differentiated sense of self are also important.

McGoldrick identifies the following factors that may negatively affect marital adjustment:

- Entering a serious relationship or marrying quickly after a major loss
- Significantly different family backgrounds
- Alienation of either spouse from his or her parents or siblings
- Excessive emotional or financial dependence on either family of origin
- Unstable parental marital models
- Marriage prior to 20 years of age or after 30
- Pregnancy before or during the first year of marriage

The Marital Life Cycle

Berman and Lief have described a marital life cycle that delineates the stages of marriage with the associated tasks and potential conflicts of each stage. The marital tasks associated with young adulthood (ages 22–28) involve differentiation from families of origin, establishing a firm commitment to the spouse, and coping with the responsibilities and demands of parenthood. Conflict develops when youthful mates fail to separate from parents and build a workable marital alliance or are unable to maintain the marriage and adapt to the pressures of childrearing and parental roles.

The transitional 30s (ages 29–39) coincide with the pivotal 10-year marital impasse that Warkentin and Whitaker have described. During this interval, the final dissolution of the intense, romanticized love of courtship occurs as the demands of childrearing steadily increase. Mates are often restless, bored, and questioning regarding their choice of a spouse. Their rates of personal growth and development have varied and they seek therapy usually as a result of gradual estrangement and mounting conflict, frequently wondering if they have "fallen out of love."

Middle adulthood (ages 43–59) and older age (60 years and over) are also critical marital years, with conflicts often intensifying after children leave the home or serious illness necessitates a major change in marital roles. Knowledge of these stages and their associated potential stressors and conflicts is vital and can be a valuable aid to the therapist in assessing troubled marital relationships.

Indications for Marital Therapy

Couples seek treatment for a variety of complaints or concerns. In an exhaustive survey of over 700 couples seeking marital therapy, Green listed, in order of frequency, the most common reasons couples seek marital therapy: communication problems, frequent disagreements or arguments, unmet emotional needs, sexual dysfunction, monetary problems, extended-family difficulties, infidelity, and dissension regarding childrearing. *Conjoint* marital therapy, in which the couple is seen together by an individual therapist or cotherapists, is the indicated treatment for such problems or for other issues that are primarily based in the marital relationship. Marital therapy may also be the treatment of choice or an adjunctive treatment modality when one spouse is symptomatic, experiencing anxiety, depression, or psychosomatic illness, for example.

When the presenting problem involves a child or children, the preferred form of treatment (marital vs family) is less clear and necessitates careful evaluation by the therapist to determine whether the major focus of difficulty rests in the marital relationship or the family relationship. Often, in these situations, a combination of marital and family sessions is necessary.

Marital Assessment—The Initial Interview

Couples, arriving for therapy after a period of mounting conflict and estrangement, often feel frightened, demoralized, and ashamed. It is important that the therapist be attuned to the couple's distress and assist them to feel as comfortable as possible. Initial contacts are focused on building a therapeutic alliance, taking a detailed history regarding the marital relationship and the couple's presenting problem(s), and developing a tentative plan for treatment.

Areas of Conflict

In performing a marital evaluation, certain basic areas are routinely addressed. The couple's anxiety and defensiveness are lowered by first gathering nonthreatening, basic identifying data, such as age, employment, length of marriage, ages of children, and information regarding previous marriages and previous therapies. Each spouse is asked to discuss briefly the most significant areas of marital conflict and their duration. It is helpful to ascertain the couple's reasons for seeking therapy at this particular time and their perceptions as to when the marriage was last gratifying and not excessively conflictual. Is the decision to seek therapy a joint one made early in a period of strife or alienation by a couple whose relationship has basically been a satisfying one? Such couples are likely to engage actively in treatment and respond well. Has one spouse coerced the other to come as a prelude to divorce after many years of marital distress? These couples frequently benefit less because their maladaptive interactional patterns are rigid and entrenched; they are less hopeful, have more lingering bitterness and anger, and are afraid to take risks.

Therapy Expectation

An experienced therapist will elicit the couple's understanding and expectations of the marital therapy process. Some couples expect a sudden and magical transformation. Many, as Framo notes, enter therapy believing that their spouse is really the "sick" one who must change and that the therapist, of course, will direct this process. In these situations, the focus is redirected immediately from that of changing the mate to identifying and altering one's own behaviors that are fostering the marital dysfunction. The therapist must remind the couple that improvement in the marital relationship will take time and that the process will, likely, be painful.

Family History

A history is obtained from each spouse regarding his or her family of origin. Descriptions of early childhood experiences, parental marital relationships and personality styles, birth order and sibling constellation, and unusual events or significant stresses within the family, such as the death or illness of a parent or sibling or extreme financial hardship, reveal potential factors significantly shaping one's views of marriage and possible sources of conflict.

As Framo indicates, couples are often extremely reluctant to discuss this information and almost never volunteer it unless it is solicited by the therapist. One husband, for example, revealed only in response to very close questioning by the author that his parents were deaf-mutes. He mentioned this unusual family circumstance only briefly and made no connection between it and his wife's complaints that he was distant and did not seem to know how to talk to her.

Exploring the Marital Contract

Most spouses will eagerly explore and discuss their courtship and initial marital adjustment. What qualities or factors attracted each mate to the other? Was the decision to marry reciprocal or desired more strongly by one? Did unusual circumstances or events (the strong desire by one spouse to leave the family of origin, an out-of-wedlock pregnancy) affect the couple's decision to wed? Sager's marital contract notion is particularly applicable here. It is helpful to clarify whether hopes, needs, and expectations were discussed in detail and to determine if these were complementary or conflictual. What changes have occurred in the original marital contracts as the marriage has developed, and have these alterations been sought and accepted by both mates, or have they occurred only because one spouse has decided to change the basic marital arrangement?

Sexual History

Exploration of the sexual relationship is significant also. Framo observes that a satisfying sexual adjustment can lead to greater tolerance and acceptance in other areas of the relationship, while such difficulties are often amplified if the sexual relationship is poor or nonexistent. Is either partner involved in an extramarital relationship?

Communication Skills

In addition to providing helpful historical information, discussion of the aforementioned areas offers opportunities for the therapist to assess the couple's basic communication patterns and skills. Do mates speak simultaneously, making global "we" statements rather than giving the spouse the opportunity to directly express his or her own feelings and opinions? What is the most frequent source of arguments, and what is the general tenor of the relationship? What joint interests and recreational activities do the couple share?

Treatment Techniques and Strategies

The therapist uses information obtained during assessment as a framework for addressing the couple's particular problems or conflictual areas. Certainly, no particular therapeutic technique or techniques are appropriate for use with all couples, and it is the therapist's task to identify major problem areas and the best strategies to approach them.

Nearly all couples seeking therapy require assistance with basic communication skills as well as interventions to alter faulty communication patterns. The marital contracts of most couples also need examination, with particular emphasis given to aspects that are conflictual or need renegotiation. Many need help with conflict management. Some have never learned to disagree and must be taught to express differences. Others differ at every turn, fight in destructive ways, and need assistance in developing negotiation strategies and learning to fight more constructively. Mates attempting to reestablish the family of origin or master old conflicts there will hopefully gain greater understanding of the effects of this process on the marriage and are helped to see and relate to their spouse in new and different ways. For some couples, attention to sexual dysfunction is required.

Throughout the marital therapy process, it is necessary that the therapist build on the strengths of the marriage. Healthy personality traits must be accentuated and the positive regard each partner has for the other must be underscored.

Measuring Progress in Therapy

Duration of therapy is determined by the nature and severity of the marital distress, the couple's basic commitment and motivation, and the theoretical perspective and individual style of the therapist. Measurement of the couple's progress is usually evidenced by the following:

- Improvement in or resolution of the presenting problem
- Decreased tension and conflict
- Improved problem solving, negotiation, and communication skills
- An increased sense of separate identity
- Greater intimacy and enjoyment of the mate and the marriage in general

Family Therapy

Family therapy is defined as the treatment of the family group for the purposes of improving general family functioning, altering troubled relationships, and lessening distress. Many valid schools of family therapy exist, and the following basic ideas are common to all these schools.

The Family As a System

The family is the most unique and important group to which we as individuals belong. In it, we develop physically and emotionally; it teaches us about life and colors our perceptions in ways that we cannot fully imagine or even accept. Consensus exists throughout the family therapy field that the family can be viewed as a system. Members are constantly interacting, and the effects of these interactions are felt by all. As with other systems, the family attempts to maintain equilibrium when confronted with stress from within or without. For example, the family system may accommodate itself to the serious illness and hospitalization of a parent, one of the most significant stresses it may face, by assigning parental tasks or roles to other family members until such time that the parent returns home and some sense of harmony or order is restored.

Like other systems, the family has rules that delineate interactional patterns among members and govern other aspects of their life together. Some rules are clearly stated, such as, "Children must knock to enter the parents' bedroom if the door is closed." Others are often unspoken but clearly understood; for example, "Always discuss problems first with Mom and let her pave the way with Dad." Such covert rules often restrict expression of feeling and differences between family members, and can frequently be pathologic by promoting the view that all members must think and feel the same.

The Family Life Cycle

As with marriage, the family is significantly affected by the developmental stages through which it passes (see Carter and McGoldrick). This developmental process begins, of course, with marriage, enters a new phase with the birth of children, is often severely tested with the onset of adolescence and the departure of children from the home, and continues with the retirement and eventual deaths of the parents. The family therapist must give attention to the developmental stage of the family that he is evaluating or treating. Problems of young families with small children frequently are rooted in the marital relationship and require different treatment techniques from those utilized with families of rebellious teenagers struggling with issues of independence and responsibility.

Sometimes developmental events occur out of turn or unpredictably such as the death of a parent or child, the midlife birth of a child, or serious illness. Such events are extremely stressful to a family and many seek therapy to resolve these crises.

Functional and Dysfunctional Families

Which factors promote health and satisfactory functioning in families and which lead to possible pathology and distress? Although no absolute criteria exist to delineate "normal" or "abnormal" family adjustment, considerable agreement exists as to characteristics of family life that are *functional,* fostering health and stability, and those that are *dysfunctional,* often leading to impaired family functioning and conflict.

Lewis and associates have discussed the following traits characteristic of functional families:

- Families with a stable marital union
- Families with parents who exercise firm, consistent childrearing practices
- Families who have rules that are clearly stated and understood
- Families with members who are encouraged to differ, express feelings openly, and to be independent

These families care, cooperate, and are flexible in their dealings with one another. Conflict is handled openly and is resolved; there is no lingering anger or estrangement. Developmental stages and their associated potential problems are met and mastered; the family, by using its own resources, can adapt to the stresses and strains of life.

Dysfunctional families, as Lewis and his associates report, are characterized by relationships that are excessively close or distant. In those with an excessive sense of togetherness, independent thought and action, or direct expression of feeling is discouraged. In families where emotional distance predominates, family members are estranged, with little awareness or concern demonstrated for the needs of others or for the general welfare of the family system. Inconsistency in childrearing is common. A parent will often form an inappropriate alliance with a child against the other spouse, and the marital relationship is fragile. In both categories of dysfunctional families, communication patterns are faulty and direct expression of feeling is discouraged. Problem-solving skills are often impaired.

Indications for Family Therapy

Family therapy is indicated in those families in which the family interaction exacerbates the illness of an individual family member, or for families experiencing relationship difficulties; for example, persistent conflict between children or strife between parent and child. Family therapy is also indicated in families that are struggling with a severe situational crisis such as illness, death, or divorce.

Family Assessment

A variety of approaches to family evaluation are described in the literature. None have improved on the recommendations regarding family assessment made separately by Haley and Minuchin, two of the leading family therapists today. If possible, all members of the family are seen together during the assessment period. Haley views the evaluation interview as composed of structured, easy-to-follow stages.

Social Stage

The first, or social stage, is designed to lessen the family's anxiety and discomfort related to beginning treatment. Consisting of an informal period where therapist and family members are introduced and basic identifying information is obtained, its purpose is to facilitate the family's adjustment to the office and therapy setting. Despite its benign nature, the social stage can be an extremely enlightening introduction to the basic affective tone of the family and to the structure of the family system. The seating arrangement chosen by members is important: Does the identified child sit between the parents or do some members absent themselves from the main family group by sitting across the room? Similarly, significant communication patterns are often demonstrated here. Does one member speak for all? Are members reluctant to speak independently?

Information-Gathering Stage

After a reasonable period of introduction, the therapist shifts the focus by outlining his purposes for the session, usually mentioning how the meeting was arranged, stating in general terms his interest in getting to know the family as a group, and learning more about the particular problem that has brought them. Family members are asked to describe the presenting problem(s) in their own words. It is best, as Haley and Minuchin note, not to begin with the referred patient, who often feels attacked and frightened. Rather, they recommend that the therapist first contact the adult family member who appears most peripheral, and proceed then to address other family members, ending with the identified patient. It is helpful, as well, to seek information regarding possible steps the family has taken to solve the problem. During this interval, the therapist discreetly surveys the family's mood, verbal and nonverbal communication, and general patterns of interaction.

Interaction Stage

After each member has individually described and discussed his thoughts and feelings about the presenting problem, members are encouraged to discuss the problem among themselves. This part of the assessment interview, the interaction stage, can even include a brief reenactment of the problem in the therapy session. It can be revealing in terms of sequences and patterns of behavior, and in uncovering alliances or coalitions between family members.

Reviewing and Summarizing Stage

After completion of the interaction stage, the therapist moves to the final part of the assessment interview. Here, he reviews the problem as presented by various family members and briefly summarizes his own assessment of it in terms the family can easily understand. He aids the family in listing problems in order of priority. All cannot be addressed at once and the family can usually identify those needing immediate attention. Here the therapist is careful to change the focus from an individual—the identified patient—to a family system where all are involved. Plans for future treatment are tentatively discussed and arrangements made for subsequent appointments.

Decathecting Stage

The final phase of the interview should be spent allowing the family members to express their thoughts and feelings about the evaluation session. An attempt is made to make all family members feel less threatened, isolated, or detached. This building of a therapeutic alliance is one of the most important tasks the therapist has if he is to effect change and alter dysfunctional family patterns as treatment progresses. The use of metaphors or style of language that are similar to the family's, playfulness and attention to the children, and gentle, nonsarcastic use of humor are other techniques that assist in establishing such a relationship.

After the first interview the therapist will be able, as Minuchin has discussed, to formulate a "family map" or conceptualization of the general structure of the group. The family's developmental stage is noted and the functioning of the various subsystems of the family is assessed. Is the marriage basically sound and free from overinvolvement by children or in-laws? How well do the spouses serve as parents and make decisions regarding their children? What is the nature of the relationship among siblings? Communication styles and patterns are identified as are alliances between different family members. The therapist carefully monitors and evaluates the degree of rigidity or flexibility in the family and its predominant affect or mood. General functioning, conflictual areas, interactional patterns, and the function of the referred patient and his behaviors or symptoms in the broader family context are identified.

Treatment Techniques and Strategies

Strategies employed as therapy progresses are determined by the particular needs and problem areas of the family and the goals that they and the therapist have identified. Treatment initially focuses on the presenting problem that has led the family to therapy. When the primary problem is stabilized, improved, or resolved, attention is given to other areas of family functioning that need improvement or change. As Glick and Kessler indicate, a variety of interventions are used by the therapist throughout the treatment process. Change occurs slowly and by degree, and such interventions are often interwoven and frequently repeated. Strategies cannot be employed mechanistically and the therapist's experience and intuitive ability often determine the manner in which they are adapted or employed to meet a family's particular needs. Glick and Kessler have described three broad categories of treatment strategies, which are discussed below.

Improving Communication

Therapeutic techniques can be used to improve communication and to support direct expression of thoughts and feelings. The therapist demonstrates straightforward and clear communication and good listening, and interacts with sensitivity and empathy as he deals with various family members. He guides the family's exploration of very painful, potentially volatile material by helping them discuss and interact with less anger and defensiveness regarding their problem. At these times, long-repressed feelings and major areas of conflict that can be significant factors in the family's current problems are addressed. Nonproductive family communication patterns (interrupting, topic-switching, overgeneralization, blaming) are identified and altered as the therapist repeatedly coaches the family to attempt alternative ways of talking and interacting.

Altering Family Alliances

The second category of interventions and strategies focuses on the family's inappropriate alliances and inflexible coalitions. Functional family systems have marital, parental, and sibling subsystems that are separated by clear but flexible boundaries. In many families seeking therapy, however, the family's subsystems are poorly functioning, boundaries are weakened, and dysfunctional alliances or coalitions develop. Generally, this occurs when the marital relationship is poor and one spouse develops an inappropriate alliance with a child against a mate. The father may become very closely aligned with an adolescent daughter, for example, and repeatedly ally himself with her against the mother.

A variation of this type of cross-generational coalition is also frequently seen when parents become focused on the particular psychosomatic illness or behavioral problems of a child, which serves to direct attention from their outwardly harmonious, but fragile marriage (see Minuchin). The child and his behaviors or illness are their sole focus; they describe at great length the problems they have encountered because of the designated problem. The child's behavioral disturbance or illness serves, in effect, to keep the spouses together and to conceal or diffuse their marital difficulties.

Special care must be taken in implementing therapeutic strategies to alter these dysfunctional alliances. The therapist must not be seen as condemning or moving with haste. A gradual restructuring of family relationships is necessary, with particular attention paid to strengthening and improving the marital relationship, removing the child from his place between the parents, and returning him to his proper position among the siblings. Often, such efforts dictate that hidden, longstanding conflict between the parents or family be addressed and resolved. The therapist monitors the family's ability to deal with emotionally charged material and is supportive of their pain as he helps them to discuss issues that they had previously avoided.

Minuchin and Haley recommend active interventions (such as reenactment of conflict) within the session to provide direct opportunities for alternative problem solving. The use of family assignments gives members the opportunity to practice new behaviors and interactional patterns. Alteration of seating arrangements during the session is an outwardly small but powerful tool to increase distance or closeness symbolically. For example, the therapist could ask a child sitting between the parents to sit with the other children as the therapist talks with the husband and wife regarding their marital relationship.

Educational Strategies

Glick and Kessler's third category of interventions could best be described as *educational*. The therapist provides information about family life while also serving as a role model. Many families benefit, for example, from discussions regarding age-appropriate behaviors of children and basic child-management skills. Similarly, their identification with the therapist's appropriate behavior can lead to more mature attitudes and actions. For example, controlling parents locked in bitter, nonproductive struggles with an adolescent may gradually begin to emulate the therapist's more relaxed and flexible attitude, and thus allow the adolescent increased independence and age-appropriate responsibility.

Measuring Progress in Therapy

As with treatment of couples, the duration of family therapy is variable and depends on the family's particular problems and desired goals. Treatment focusing specifically on amelioration of the presenting problem or behavior is usually brief (10–15 sessions). Resolution of complex family issues or implementation of broader change in the general family system indicates longer, more in-depth therapy. Of course, no family leaves therapy with all their problems solved. Generally, termination occurs when the family and therapist agree that (1) the presenting problem has improved or resolved; (2) communication patterns have been altered and replaced with clearer, more positive interaction and reduction in the level of tension and conflict; (3) problem-solving skills have been strengthened, with the family now able to negotiate differences and resolve conflicts outside of therapy sessions; and (4) greater flexibility, empathy, and increased enjoyment of family life are present.

Conclusion

Marital and family therapy is a common and respected form of treatment used in a variety of clinical settings. Basic theoretical concepts related to marriage and the family have been reviewed with assessment and treatment strategies outlined. The techniques presented here offer a basic framework for assessment and treatment of marital and family dysfunction.

Bibliography

Berman EM, Lief HI: Marital therapy from a psychiatric perspective. Am J Psychiatry 132:583–592, 1975

Carter, EA, McGoldrick M: The Family Life Cycle. New York, Gardner Press, 1980

Framo JL: Marriage and Marital Therapy. In Andolfi M, Zwerling I (eds): Dimensions of Family Therapy. New York, The Guilford Press, 1980

Glick ID, Kessler DR: Marital and Family Therapy, 2nd ed. New York, Grune and Stratton, 1980

Green BL: A Clinical Approach to Marital Problems: Evaluation and Management. Springfield, Charles C Thomas, 1970

Haley J: Problem-Solving Therapy. San Francisco, Josey–Bass, 1976

Lewis JM, Beavers WR, Gossett JT et al: No Single-Thread Psychological Health in Family Systems. New York, Brunner/Mazel, 1976

Minuchin S: Families and Family Therapy. Cambridge, Harvard University Press, 1974

Sager CJ: Marriage Contracts and Couple Therapy. New York, Brunner/Mazel, 1976

Sager CJ, Gundlach R, Kremer M et al: The married in treatment. Arch Gen Psychiatry 19:205–217, 1968

Warkentin J, Whitaker C: Serial Impasses in Marriage. In Cohen JM (ed): Family Structure, Dynamics, and Therapy. Washington, DC, American Psychiatric Association, 1966

Floyd C. Wiseman

22 Other Psychotherapies

Psychotherapy has been shown to be beneficial in over 70 well-designed studies. Eighty-one percent of just over 1,000 patients treated with intensive psychotherapy had no exacerbation of their illness during a 5-year follow-up period. Not only did these patients demonstrate subjective improvement, relief of symptoms, and favorable personality changes, but medical and psychiatric hospitalizations were also markedly reduced from a pretreatment average rate of 5.3 days each year to a post-treatment rate of 0.78 days per year. A Blue Cross study involving 136 patients revealed that the average monthly medical and surgical cost decreased from $16.47 per patient before psychotherapy to $7.06 per patient after psychotherapy. Preceding chapters have discussed the more traditional forms of psychotherapy: supportive psychotherapy, group psychotherapy, cognitive therapy, and family and marital therapy. This chapter will discuss some of the other, less commonly used psychotherapies.

Curative Factors

Psychotherapy, regardless of type, has three goals: (1) to reduce suffering, (2) to improve work performance, and (3) to improve social functioning. Similarly, almost every type of psychotherapy has eight factors that produce emotional change. They are as follows:

The physician–patient relationship
Tension release
Cognitive understanding or insight
Reward and reinforcement
Modeling
Persuasion
Practice of new techniques
Emotional support

The trusting relationship between therapist and patient encourages behavioral change. The so-called "therapeutic triad" of empathy, nonpossessive warmth, and genuineness of the therapist correlates with a favorable outcome in psychotherapy. Ventilation of guilts, hidden shames, and anxieties allow relief from emotional tension. Insight–an understanding of the causes of the emotional conflict—contributes to improved behavior, while the therapist's approval of socially appropriate behavior acts as a reinforcement to change. Patients tend to model themselves after their therapist. In addition, therapists can persuade the patient to practice new techniques while providing them with consistent emotional support.

Hypnosis

Hypnosis, artificially induced alterations of consciousness of one person by another, if used properly, increases the effectiveness of psychotherapeutic interventions by intensifying the influence of the therapist. Hypnotizability has been shown by the Spiegel eye-roll technique to be a quantifiable, stable trait. The subject is asked to face forward, look upward as far as possible as if he were trying to look at the top of his head, and then close his eyelids slowly. The maximum amount of white of the eye visible to the observer is scored on a scale of 0 to 4, with 4 (all white) being present in the most hypnotizable subject. Roughly 20% of the population have a score of 4 and are easily hypnotizable, 20% of the population score 0 and cannot be hypnotized, and 60% fall somewhere in between with scores of 1 to 3, in whom a moderate trance can be induced. Patients with disturbances in affect and thought, or with a variety of neurologic problems, are less susceptible to the trance state.

Hypnosis is most commonly used in pain control, relaxation therapy, control of phobic reaction, and elimination of habits such as overeating and cigarette smoking. The hypnotherapist instills in his patients a sense of self-mastery, an effect that is continued through the use of self-hypnotism. In addition, hypnosis effectively provides a fresh outlook on a patient's particular concern; for example, in smoking control the patient is urged to appreciate the importance of his healed body and to see himself as the "protector of his body" rather than dwell on the damage due to cigarette smoking. The patient is also encouraged to use self-hypnosis whenever he feels an urge to smoke, as well as at scheduled intervals throughout the day. Hypnosis can be used as an adjunct in chronic pain treatment by increasing relaxation and changing pain perception; in a hypnotized subject, pain sensation can be turned into a tingling, buzzing, or cold sensation.

As with most other forms of therapy, success in the clinical use of hypnosis depends on patient selection. Hypnosis is contraindicated in organic brain syndrome, psychotic depression, schizophrenia, and paranoid disorders, because intact reality testing must be present for a trance to be induced, and attempted trance induction in a patient who is out of touch with reality may increase psychotic symptoms. Hypnosis may be useful as an adjunct for treating certain symptom complexes such as weight and smoking control, conversion disorders, phobias, and chronic pain.

Directive Therapy

Often associated with the techniques of Milton Erickson, and used in conjunction with hypnosis, directive therapy focuses on specific symptoms that are causing the patient distress and attempts to alter them by introducing a "paradoxical" framework. The therapist attempts to take complete charge of the patient's symptoms and devises paradoxes that make symptom use more difficult. The patient is told to commence a specific activity that appears on the surface to be the opposite of the intended goal. He may be asked to become more symptomatic, to practice his symptoms until he becomes better at them, or to perform the symptom at the command of the therapist. The patient may be ordered to follow each occurrence of his symptom with an act that he believes he should accomplish but does not enjoy, such as housecleaning.

The main difficulty with directive therapy is that the techniques are difficult to teach systematically. Although skilled directive therapists understand the power of suggestion to unlock unconscious conflicts, unskilled therapists can easily misapply directive therapy and use it as a sadistic weapon.

Client-Centered (Rogerian) Therapy

Client-centered or Rogerian therapy rejects the medical model of psychological distress; instead, the patient becomes a client, and the therapist becomes a nondirective helper who aids in self-actualization. Problems are believed to arise from developmental disturbances that block the natural "actualizing tendency." Self-understanding leads to emotional growth, healthy relationships, and self-fulfillment.

The nondirective therapist provides an environment that encourages the client to gain a fuller understanding of the self; and with understanding comes change. The therapist accepts the client completely, an attitude known as *unconditional positive regard,* which allows the client to express feelings, thoughts, and attitudes. As the client begins to more fully experience and live the emotions, feelings, and self-concepts of which he was previously unaware, change and self-actualization occur.

According to its proponents, Rogerian therapy is not a form of "treatment," but instead a model for all human interactions. Because of this universality, and its humanistic view of the underlying positive core of mankind, Carl Rogers' work has been used in counseling, education, transcultural relations, corporate organization, and in working with individuals suffering from illnesses as diverse as schizophrenia and mild anxiety. A typical therapeutic relationship may last for a year, with weekly sessions.

Rogerian therapy apparently has much to offer those who live in our alienated world, where the experience of being with someone who understands us may be an infrequent occurrence. The feeling of acceptance by another, which leads to self-acceptance, can be a powerful force, especially when the client's distress focuses on feelings of alienation and aloneness. Positive regard has limits to its usefulness, however, because it views humans as basically positive, and only acknowledges those experiences within our awareness; client-centered therapy ignores any unconscious motivations as well as the hostile side of human nature. The Rogerian therapist believes that positive reinforcement is more important than an objective understanding of the client's personality or the real-life elements of his existence. Although Rogerian therapy is often thought to be most applicable either to those who benefit most from a supportive environment, such as chronic schizophrenics, or to mildly neurotic patients who do not require extensive therapy, client-centered therapy has shown success in a diverse assortment of psychological problems and has provided a useful model for education and race relations.

Reality Therapy

Proposed by William Glasser to help delinquent children learn socially appropriate behavior, reality therapy asserts that healthy adjustment depends on our ability to assume responsibility for our actions. To teach responsibility the therapist (or parent) must demonstrate that he cares for the patient (or child). A set of rules and regulations are then established. For reality therapy to be effective, the patient (child) must have a say in making the rules, must understand the rules clearly, must agree with the rules, and must know the punishment for breaking the rules. Finally, the punishment should fit the crime. For example, if the teenager does not wash the car, he cannot use it for a Saturday night date. A warm, genuinely concerned therapist who demonstrates firm and consistent enforcement of the rules will gradually help the patient learn responsibility.

Reality therapy is useful in helping parents and teachers teach responsibility to children, can effectively encourage adolescent delinquents to learn more socially appropriate behavior, and may be useful in teaching prisoners socially acceptable behavior as well. Changing longstanding antisocial behavior is a lengthy process and almost always requires initial confinement to provide the criminal enough structure to effect change. Reality therapy is ineffective in treating psychosis, because psychotics do not understand cause and effect. It is not effective for neurotics, either, because they have an overly rigid sense of responsibility; they benefit from loosening up, not from learning more responsibility.

Rational–Emotive Therapy

One form of cognitive therapy, rational–emotive therapy (RET), developed by Albert Ellis, is based on the belief that psychological distress results from irrational thinking promoted by society. The RET therapist attempts to help the patient "analyze" these false social assumptions ("I must be loved by everyone . . . any failure of mine must be all my fault."). To effect change, the therapist uses an extremely active, confrontative manner that emphasizes intellect over emotion. The RET method can be used for individual therapy or presented in a lecture format in a group setting. Treatment is short-term and goal-directed.

As with many of the more cognitively oriented therapies, RET demands a certain level of intellectual sophistication in the patient. The underlying theory, with no concept of the unconscious, presumes that insight promoted in an educational, authoritarian approach will lead to change. This presumption may be true in those high-functioning individuals who can understand that their problems are based on false assumptions.

Transactional Analysis

With its catchwords of "strokes," "warm fuzzies," and "I'm OK, you're OK," transactional analysis (TA) took the psychotherapy-seeking public by storm in the late 1960s and early 1970s. Originated by Eric Berne and elaborated by Thomas A. Harris, the proponents of TA have suggested that it is an effective method of treating interpersonal difficulties, managerial problems, and societal ills. TA postulates its own tripartite view of human personality, consisting of three ego states: *adult,* the synthesizer and evaluator of information from the environment and from the other ego states; *parent,* the external lessons and values of the parents; and *child,* the source of internal urges and feelings. The information of all three ego states is assumed to be gathered in direct "recordings" that are encoded as memories in the brain during the first 5 years of life, unencumbered by fantasies or interpretations.

Although TA can be used for individual therapy, it is more commonly employed in a group setting. The leader first presents the TA formulation as a lecture. An attempt is then made to understand the reciprocal interaction between patient and therapist or between patient and patient in terms of which ego state is being expressed. These interactions may be seen as "games," or "scripts," repeating patterns of behavior that are outgrowths of childhood memories and experiences. Rewards or "strokes" are given by the therapist if the patient resolves conflicts by using the *adult* ego state instead of the harsh *parent* or the impetuous *child* ego states.

The strength of transactional analysis lies in its ability to describe a model of human interactions that is easily understood by the public while providing a framework for possible change that depends on insights and rewards supplied by the therapist. Transactional analysis therapists have proposed a mechanistic, reductionistic theory of personality that views acceptance of the *adult*—or socially encouraged role—as the means to psychological health. Transactional analysis, however, fails to allow a view of personality that extends beyond immediate social interactions. For patients who are able to observe their own social interactions in an objective manner, and use this insight to alter their outward behavior, transactional analysis may offer considerable benefit.

Gestalt Therapy

Gestalt therapy is one of the original "body therapies" that attempts to treat psychic distress by active expression of emotions in a supportive group environment. Originated by Fritz Perls, a therapist trained in psychoanalysis, and borrowing its name from the branch of psychology that attempts to understand the perception of the "whole," gestalt therapy postulates that anxiety and neurosis are the result of an unnatural splitting of emotional needs from consciousness, thus making their gratification impossible. Perls and his followers believe that intellectual reasoning is not adequate to heal this split; the individual must be made aware of his needs in order to be free of neurosis. A combination of sensorimotor and psychological exercises helps the individual better understand his emotional needs. For example, in a two-chair technique the therapist asks a patient who has been unable to grieve the death of his mother to imagine that his dead mother sits in a chair placed in front of him. "Talking" to his mother allows hurt, loss, anger, and other repressed emotions to pour out.

A frequent criticism of gestalt therapy has been the unclear goals and unsystematized approach to therapy. Any of the "body therapies," which emphasize intense expression of affect, tend to place significant responsibility on the group leader; often transference issues are ignored. Aside from the simple cathartic effect of expressed emotion, certain forms of gestalt therapy may be beneficial for the restricted, mildly obsessional individual who has difficulty identifying and communicating feelings.

Neurolinguistic Programming

Originating in the mid 1970s as an amalgam of gestalt therapy and linguistics, neurolinguistic programming (NLP) professes to be useful in training psychotherapists, businessmen, and salesmen, while at the same time being effective in treating emotional disturbances. Neurolinguistic programming attempts to formulate methods on how to observe and alter the way the brain organizes and uses sensory experience. People have a "preferred" mode of sensory input, whether visual, auditory, or kinetic. Proponents of NLP believe that the preferred mode is expressed in language: "I can see that," "I hear you," "I'll go along with that." Neurolinguistic programming therapists are trained to become adept at observing subtle body motions such as finger twitching, nasal flaring, and especially eye movement. Eye movement is believed to be directly associated with sensory processing: When a right-handed person looks up and to the observer's left, he is trying to envision an event never seen, whereas eyes up and to the observer's right indicates that the patient is picturing an event that he has already seen. Detecting input information allows the therapist to understand the mental organization of the patient and to induce rapport and facilitate change through suggestion.

The elements of sensory input and relevance of eye movement are without scientific proof so far. Proponents' claims have been anecdotal and often extreme, with 10-minute cures of phobias and one-session cures of depression cited. No formal studies or follow-up reports are available. Corporate America appears to have confidence in NLP, since seminars for salesmen and executives are available. Whether NLP proves to have true therapeutic efficacy or is able to further our understanding of human behavior remains to be seen.

Psychodrama

Psychodrama has its origins in primitive tribal rituals that reenacted aspects of human behavior in a group setting. Contributions from the early Greek and Roman civilizations formalized the dramatic concept in terms of an "audience," and often attempted to understand human behavior as a result of inner and outer conflicts. Modern psychodrama has its origins in the 20th century under the guidance of Joseph Moreno (1891–1974), a Rumanian-born psychiatrist who began developing his therapeutic methods in Vienna in the 1920s. He used the robust experimental theater movement as a basis for the special techniques associated with psychodrama. He continued his work in the United States from the 1930s onward.

Psychodrama employs the familiar triad of director, actor, and audience to gain insight into the conflicting roles that the patient is often asked to assume in society. The protagonist (patient) selects a scene that has strong emotional meaning. The scene may be an occurrence from the past or present, or even the patient's fantasy of the future. The director (therapist) adds to the scene other members of the group who serve either as the other characters with whom the protagonist is interacting or as the protagonist's *auxiliary egos*. These egos portray some aspect of the protagonist's psychic structure, whether it be a memory of a lover, a fantasy, a parent, or a conflicting aspect of the patient's inner drives. Often a group member is chosen to portray a particular auxiliary ego in the hope that the participant will, in the process, gain some insight into his own, often similar problem. The scene is reenacted with input from the players while the director attempts to guide the action, promoting the emergence of spontaneous feelings and insight. Psychodrama can be used, not only to discover previously unconscious material, but to prepare the individual for an upcoming anxiety-laden situation.

The supportive environment of the group encourages the patient to accept and ultimately resolve his conflicts. As with many other forms of therapy, there have been no formal outcome studies. For the well-selected patient, psychodrama has the potential to help the individual master difficult situations and, at the same time, gain insight into his emotional problems.

Primal Therapy

Originated by Arthur Janov, primal therapy postulates that neurotic behavior results from unmet needs of the infant. At an early age the infant realizes that the parents are not going to satisfy all of his demands for food, affection, warmth, or love. This realization causes such psychic pain that he represses his "true" self and begins to express a "neurotic" self that is more acceptable to the parents. Primal therapists believe that the individual must reexperience the primal scene and reintegrate it without the neurotic elements.

Candidates for therapy are selected after an extensive interviewing process from a large pool of applicants. The chosen participants sequester themselves in hotel rooms for 48 hours to lower their defenses and then begin individual, daily, open-ended therapy sessions. After approximately 3 weeks of active confrontation by the therapist, with the goal of expressing and experiencing childhood memories, the patient undergoes a spontaneous *full primal*—a reenactment of the primal scene accompanied by repressed memories and affects. The patient cries, lies in a fetal position, and may engage in sucking motions, baby talk or other infantile behavior. Following the full primal stage, the patient spends several months reenacting the primal scene with a group of others who have also experienced this event. The neurotic patterns reportedly cease with the emergence of the true person after 6 to 8 months of therapy.

Primal therapy is one of the many body therapy outgrowths of the human potential movement that depend on the process of abreaction and catharsis to facilitate change. The effectiveness of primal therapy is unsubstantiated.

est

In the late 1960s and early 1970s, est, or as it is also known, Erhard Seminar Training, carried the iconoclastic human potential movement to an authoritarian peak. The product of Werner Erhard (née Jack Rosenberg), est achieved wide media attention due to the extreme nature of the seminars. Training involves gathering approximately 250 to 300 people in a hotel convention room, where they spend 15 to 18 hours per day on Saturday and Sunday of two consecutive weekends. The trainees must stay in the room for the entire session, with only 2 or 3 short breaks during the day for eating or bathroom necessities. The seminar begins with a lecture presentation of est philosophy followed by "processes," which include group relaxation exercises, sense memory, meditation, and psychodrama. The group leader uses ridicule and double-blind messages to encourage self-disclosure and intense emotional experiences in the trainees.

With its forced physical discomfort, ridiculing approach of the leader, and the cultlike adoration of Erhard, est may be of no harm to people with stable personalities and mature defense mechanisms, but it is contraindicated in psychologically vulnerable individuals with any history of emotional distress, no matter how slight.

Summary

The importance of the primary care physicians' understanding psychotherapy is underscored by the fact that of the 15% of the population that suffers from a major mental disorder, only 15% of these are treated by psychiatrists or mental health professionals. A full 60% are treated by family physicians, with 22% receiving no treatment at all. An informed physician, who can either treat the illness himself or make the appropriate referral, will have an enormous influence on the emotional and physical health of his patients.

Bibliography

Ellis A, Grieger R: Handbook of Rational–Emotive Therapy. New York, Springer, 1977
Glasser W: Reality Therapy. New York, Harper and Row, 1965
Haley J: Strategies of Psychotherapy. New York, Grune and Stratton, 1963
Harris TA: I'm OK, You're OK: A Practical Guide to Transactional Analysis. New York, Harper and Row, 1969
Janov A: The Primal Scream: Primal Therapy, the Cure for Neurosis. New York, GP Putnam & Sons, 1970
Kaplan H, Friedman AM, Sadock BJ: Comprehensive Textbook of Psychiatry, 3rd ed, Baltimore, Williams & Wilkins, 1980
Kirsch MA, Glass LL: Psychiatric disturbances associated with Erhard Training Seminars: II. Additional cases and theoretical considerations. Am J Psychiatry 134:1254, 1977
Kovel J: A Complete Guide to Therapy. New York, Pantheon Books, 1976
Lankton SR: Practical Magic: A Translation of Basic Neurolinguistic Programming into Clinical Psychotherapy, Cupertino, California, Meta Publications, 1980
Marmor J: The Physician as Psychotherapist. In Usdin G, Lewis JM (eds): Psychiatry in General Medical Practice. New York, McGraw-Hill, 1979
Rogers CR: Client-Centered Therapy. Boston, Houghton Mifflin, 1951
Walker JI: Psychiatry in Primary Care. Menlo Park, California, Addison-Wesley, 1981

Steven Lipper

23 Clinical Psychopharmacology

The era of modern clinical psychopharmacology is generally considered to have begun either in 1949 with Cade's report of the antimanic effects of lithium, or in 1952 with the first reports of the antipsychotic efficacy of chlorpromazine (Thorazine). A few years later, two classes of antidepressant medications, the tricyclic agents and the monoamine oxidase (MAO) inhibitors, were introduced into clinical practice. The tricyclic antidepressants are chemical analogues of the phenothiazine antipsychotic agents, while the MAO-inhibiting antidepressants were developed as the result of an observation that tuberculosis patients treated with isoniazid (INH) and similar agents became less depressed. The first benzodiazepine antianxiety agent, chlordiazepoxide (Librium), was synthesized in 1957 and became available for clinical use in 1960.

The availability of antipsychotic, antimanic, antidepressant, and antianxiety agents has enormously enhanced the ability of psychiatrists to treat severely impaired patients, and attempts to understand the mechanisms of action of these medications have led to the development of important new hypotheses concerning the possible neurochemical bases of several major psychiatric disorders. For example, the dopamine hypothesis of schizophrenia and the catecholamine or biogenic amine hypothesis of affective disorders, although now regarded as simplistic, initiated what has become a sustained inquiry into the biology of these illnesses.

The proper use of psychopharmacologic agents requires more than knowledge of the actions, kinetics, and side effects of the individual medications. If the physician has not developed skill at diagnosing psychiatric disorders, or has not mastered the art of forming psychotherapeutic relationships with patients, it is unlikely that optimal benefit will be achieved from the prescription of psychopharmacologic agents. Under such circumstances, the prescribed medication might be inappropriate for the patient's disorder or, alternatively, treatment might founder because of the patient's noncompliance in taking the medication. Among many possible transference and countertransference issues, those involving trust and dependence, in particular, commonly arise in the context of medication-taking and compliance.

The most frequently prescribed psychopharmacologic agents can be subsumed within five major categories: (1) antipsychotic agents, (2) antidepressant agents, (3) lithium, (4) antianxiety agents, and (5) hypnotic agents. These categories, however, are not rigidly distinct with respect to the clinical utility of the agents. For example, both imipramine (Tofranil) and phenelzine (Nardil), which are routinely classified as antidepressant medications, are effective in the treatment of panic disorder, a diagnostic entity subsumed under the rubric of the anxiety disorders.

Antipsychotic Medications

Antipsychotic medications are useful in the treatment of schizophrenia, acute and chronic organic brain syndromes, psychotic depression, the acute phase of manic episodes, and Gilles de la Tourette's syndrome.

Five major classes of antipsychotic agents are currently available for clinical use: the phenothiazines, the thioxanthenes, the butyrophenones, the dibenzoxazepines, and the dihydroindolones (Table 23-1). In general, the agents are equally effective when equipotent doses are employed. Their antipsychotic efficacy is considered to result from their shared activity in blocking brain dopamine receptors. The selection of an antipsychotic agent may be made on the basis of the difference in incidence of side effects associated with a particular medication, in relation to both the profile of psychiatric symptoms and the medical history of an individual patient. For example, one may select an antipsychotic agent with a high incidence of sedation to treat a very agitated patient and a less sedating agent to treat a withdrawn patient with psychomotor retardation. Similarly, it would be desirable to avoid antipsychotic agents with a high incidence of orthostatic hypotension for use in patients whose medical conditions might be jeopardized by lowered blood pressure.

The first major class of antipsychotic medications, the phenothiazines, contain three types of compounds: the aliphatic type as exemplified by chlorpromazine (Thorazine), the piperidine type as exemplified by thioridazine (Mellaril), and the piperazine type as exemplified by trifluoperazine (Stelazine). Representative of the thioxanthene class is thiothixene (Navane). Each of the three remaining classes of antipsychotic agents contains only one compound approved for clinical use.

The maximum daily dosage of chlorpromazine is about 2000 mg/day. Dosage

Table 23-1
Prototypic Antipsychotic Agents

Generic Name	Trade Name	Relative Potency*
Phenothiazines		
Aliphatic; chlorpromazine	Thorazine	100
Piperidine; thioridazine	Mellaril	100
Piperazine; trifluoperazine	Stelazine	5
Thioxanthene		
Thiothixene	Navane	5
Butyrophenone		
Haloperidol	Haldol	2
Dibenzoxazepine		
Loxapine	Loxitane	10
Dihydroindolone		
Molindone	Moban	10

* The approximate number of milligrams of each agent equivalent to 100 milligrams of chlorpromazine. In practice, dosages must be individualized for each patient

greater than 800 mg/day of thioridazine should not be used because of its potential of producing a toxic retinopathy. The maximum daily dosage of trifluoperazine, thiothixene, and haloperidol is about 60 mg/day. The maximum daily dosage of loxapine or molindone is about 225 mg/day. While these "maximum" doses may be exceeded for a good clinical reason, the use of megadosages of antipsychotic medications, such as 1200 mg/day of fluphenazine or haloperidol, is not recommended, because the number of patients benefited has not been found to be substantial. While no patient should be considered a drug failure without an intensive course of therapy, extremely high doses are not routinely required for most patients. An adequate trial of an antipsychotic agent at or slightly above standard therapeutic doses is generally considered to be of 3 or 4 weeks' duration, provided severe or intolerable side effects do not occur.

If a patient does not respond to adequate doses of an antipsychotic agent given for an adequate length of time, that agent should be discontinued and replaced by an agent in a different chemical class. Patients who do not respond to one medication may respond to another. In general, one should not change antipsychotic medications every few days unless intolerable side effects supervene. When switching from one antipsychotic medication to another, one should start the substitute medication at a dose that is less potent than that achieved with the first agent in order to diminish the possibility of adverse reactions from the second drug. Patients may be more sensitive to the side effects of a particular medication, even when used at doses equipotent to those of a previously used agent.

The failure of a patient to respond to adequate trials of two oral antipsychotic agents may be followed by use of a long-acting intramuscular agent such as fluphenazine (Prolixin) decanoate in order to bypass extensive first-pass gut and liver metabolism that may preclude adequate delivery of the drug to the central nervous system (CNS) in some patients. Long-acting injectable medication may be useful also in the treatment of patients who are noncompliant about taking oral medication, but who are willing to attend an outpatient clinic on a regular basis, usually every other week, in order to receive an intramuscular injection. At the present time, further investigation is required before the measurement of erythrocyte or plasma levels of antipsychotic medications can be usefully applied to clinical practice.

Among the prototypic phenothiazines, chlorpromazine (Thorazine) has the advantage of having a relatively low incidence of extrapyramidal side effects (EPS) compared to piperazine agents. On the other hand, chlorpromazine has a higher incidence of sedation, orthostatic hypotension, dermatitis, and possibly convulsions, than that associated with agents in the other two phenothiazine classes. An advantage of thioridazine (Mellaril) is that it has the lowest incidence of EPS of any currently available antipsychotic agent. The major disadvantage of thioridazine is that it has the greatest anticholinergic activity of all the antipsychotic agents. Consequently, thioridazine is associated with a higher incidence of such symptoms as constipation and difficulty urinating. Additionally, patients receiving thioridazine not uncommonly complain of absent or retrograde ejaculation, even on standard doses of thioridazine; this side effect may limit the usefulness of thioridazine in men. Trifluoperazine (Stelazine), the prototypic piperazine phenothiazine, has a higher incidence of EPS than chlorpromazine or thioridazine, but is less sedating and produces significant orthostatic hypotension less frequently. Fluphenazine (Prolixin), another piperazine phenothiazine, is available in two forms, as a hydrochloride for oral administration and as a long-acting injectable decanoate (or enanthate) compound. Fluphenazine decanoate is an ester that is slowly hydrolyzed in muscle and released to achieve therapeutic activity over approximately 2 weeks. Some patients may prefer, or be more compliant with, receiving biweekly injections averaging 25 mg intramuscularly (IM), to having to take daily oral medication. The long-acting injectable form of fluphenazine should be distinguished from the intramuscular forms of many other antipsychotic agents available for use in emergency situations in which oral dosage forms cannot be administered or are unacceptable. Additionally, many antipsychotic medications are available as liquid concentrates that may be useful at times for enhancing medication compliance or drug absorption.

The routine use of *rapid neuroleptization,* the intramuscular administration of small doses of an antipsychotic agent, usually haloperidol (Haldol) or thiothixene (Navane), at 30-minute intervals for several hours, is not recommended because treatment goals can usually be accomplished with adequate oral doses of the agents.

Thiothixene (Navane), molindone (Moban), and loxapine (Loxitane) may be considered to have side effects of an intensity in between those of chlorpromazine and trifluoperazine. An advantage of molindone is that weight gain has not been reported when the agent is used for chronic treatment, in contrast to the other antipsychotic agents, particularly the phenothiazines, which may be associated with a considerable weight gain over extended periods of time. No one of the agents has been found to be superior over another for use in a particular subgroup or subtype of schizophrenic disorder.

Haloperidol (Haldol) has a high incidence of extrapyramidal side effects associated with its use. Haloperidol, however, is relatively nonsedating, rarely produces allergic reactions, and has a low incidence of ocular damage, liver dysfunction, severe orthostatic hypotension, hematologic abnormalities, or photosensitivity associated with its use. This profile of side effects may make haloperidol a useful agent in the treatment of psychotic patients with certain concomitant medical illnesses.

For most patients, the maintenance dose of antipsychotic medication is less than that initially employed to control an acute psychotic episode. For maintenance therapy, one should minimize the amount of antipsychotic medication required to control psychotic symptomatology in order to minimize side effects and diminish the potential for tardive dyskinesia. Some patients who have had a psychotic episode may not relapse, despite discontinuation of antipsychotic medication. Every patient, therefore, is entitled to a drug-free period at some time, with frequent follow-up evaluations, to determine the necessity for continued maintenance medication with antipsychotic agents. At the same time, the most common factor in the relapse of chronically psychotic patients is the discontinuation of antipsychotic medication. The rate of relapse is exponential; approximately 5% to 10% of schizophrenic patients relapse per month after discontinuation of antipsychotic medication.

In attempting to discontinue an antipsychotic agent in a patient with a history of chronic illness, one should gradually taper the dose of medication, probably over months, in order to minimize the risk of reemergence of psychosis. One should also assess the risk–benefit ratio of discontinuing a medication in a patient with a prior history of repeated psychotic episodes that have involved job loss, intolerable family disruption, suicide attempts, or homicidal behavior. If it is clinically indicated to stop an antipsychotic medication within a few days, and the patient has required an antiparkinsonian agent, it is advisable to maintain the patient on the antiparkinsonian medication for several days beyond discontinuation of the antipsychotic medication, because EPS may otherwise emerge at that time.

The long half-life of all the antipsychotic agents makes it possible to administer these agents in a single bedtime dose. Although a single bedtime dose may be most convenient for most patients, some may prefer to take the medication in divided doses. Additionally, one may be reluctant to prescribe large doses of an agent such as chlorpromazine in a single bedtime dose because of the possibility of severe orthostatic hypotension the following morning.

There is no evidence that the use of more than one antipsychotic agent in an individual patient is more efficacious than adequate doses of a single agent. Consequently, combining one antipsychotic agent with another is generally considered to be polypharmacy.

Autonomic Side Effects

Autonomic side effects are the result of the anticholinergic and the α-adrenergic blocking properties of the antipsychotic agents and occur more frequently with the low-potency medications. Anticholinergic side effects include dry mouth, blurred vision, constipation, and confusion (due to a central anticholinergic syndrome). If severe, some of these side effects can become medically significant, for example, if urinary retention or paralytic ileus develop. Orthostatic hypotension is a consequence of α-adrenergic blockade. In general, at least some degree of tolerance to the autonomic side effects frequently develops within the first few weeks of treatment, and some simple measures may alleviate a patient's discomfort. Frequent sips of water or sugar-free gum can make the dry mouth less bothersome, and the use of support stockings, along with advice to change position slowly, may ameliorate the symptoms of orthostatic hypotension.

Extrapyramidal Side Effects

As a result of the dopamine receptor blocking activity of the antipsychotic agents, side effects involving the extrapyramidal system may occur. There are three major categories of extrapyramidal symptoms: drug-induced parkinsonism, akathisia, and acute dystonic reactions. The drug-induced parkinsonism can include tremor at rest, muscular rigidity, akinesia, masklike facies, and shuffling gait. Akathisia, an involuntary motor restlessness that may be misdiagnosed as anxiety or a psychotic symptom, is manifest by constant pacing, fidgeting, and inability to sit still. Common forms of acute dystonic reactions are spasms of the neck muscles, resulting in torticollis or retrocollis, and spasms of the eye muscles, resulting in oculogyric crisis. The high-potency antipsychotic agents such as haloperidol, thiothixene, and the piperazine phenothiazines have a higher incidence of extrapyramidal side effects associated with their use than do the low-potency antipsychotic medications such as the aliphatic and piperidine phenothiazines.

Several antiparkinsonian medications are available for the treatment of drug-induced parkinsonism and akathisia. These include trihexyphenidyl (Artane) 2 mg to 5 mg orally one to three times a day; benztropine mesylate (Cogentin) 2 mg to 4 mg orally one to three times a day; and amantadine (Symmetrel) 100 mg to 200 mg orally one to three times a day. Acute dystonic reactions can usually be resolved rapidly by giving the patient 25 mg to 50 mg of diphenhydramine (Benadryl) orally or by intramuscular injection. If symptom relief is inadequate after half an hour, another dose of Benadryl, an antihistamine with anticholinergic activity, can be administered. Because some patients may never manifest extrapyramidal symptoms, these agents should not be used prophylactically. Additionally, the anticholinergic activity of trihexyphenidyl or benztropine mesylate may be cumulative with that of the antipsychotic medication. Treatment with an antiparkinsonian medication may be required for only 2 or 3 months, after which an attempt to reduce its dosage with a view to discontinuing it should be made, because many patients will no longer manifest extrapyramidal symptoms, despite continued use of an antipsychotic agent.

Tardive Dyskinesia

Tardive dyskinesia is a syndrome of involuntary movements that result from prolonged treatment with antipsychotic medications and that may be irreversible. The classic picture of tardive dyskinesia is a triad of cheek–face–tongue movements, sometimes referred to as the *buccolingual masticatory syndrome,* and can include repetitive bulging of the cheeks, chewing, sucking, lip-smacking, tongue-protruding, and lateral jaw movements. Blinking, grimacing, arching of the eyebrows, and blepharospasm may also occur. In addition to the facial movements, patients with tardive dyskinesia may display choreiform movements of the hands and feet, athetoid movements of the extremities, and truncal movements such as rocking and shoulder shrugging. The involuntary, stereotyped movements that characterize the disorder can be suppressed temporarily by voluntary activity of muscles in the affected area and can be accentuated by movements in distant parts of the body. Fine, wormlike movements of the tongue at rest are considered to be one of the earliest manifestations of tardive dyskinesia.

To assume that previous or current treatment of a patient with an antipsychotic medication is responsible for the development of abnormal movements can be a diagnostic error. Before concluding that a patient has tardive dyskinesia, a thorough medical assessment must be made, since dyskinesias or similar abnormal movements are seen in a variety of conditions other than tardive dyskinesia. Use of medications such as amphetamine, neurologic disorders such as Huntington's chorea, and ill-fitting dentures are some of the conditions that may have manifestations resembling tardive dyskinesia, and that must be considered in the differential diagnosis. Making a differential diagnosis between tardive dyskinesia and the stereotyped movements carried out by some schizophrenic patients may be particularly difficult.

Tardive dyskinesia has been reported to occur with agents in all of the classes of antipsychotic medications. Whether certain types of antipsychotic medications are more likely to produce tardive dyskinesia is, however, unknown. The duration of treatment with antipsychotic medication is believed to be the single most important treatment variable in considering the causes of tardive dyskinesia. Prevalence of the syndrome, which appears to be increasing, is higher in patients who have had long-term treatment with antipsychotic medications than in those who have received short-term treatment. Nevertheless, cases of tardive dyskinesia have been reported to occur within the first 6 months of drug treatment. The prevalence of tardive dyskinesia is considered to be approximately 15% in chronically hospitalized patients.

All of the antipsychotic medications act by blocking dopamine receptor sites in the limbic system and striatum. The major hypothesis for the occurrence of tardive dyskinesia postulates that chronic administration of antipsychotic medications functionally inactivates, in a manner analogous to chemical denervation, striatal dopamine receptors that become supersensitive to ambient dopamine; and that this dopamine receptor supersensitivity is manifested clinically in tardive dyskinesia. Additionally, diminished brain cholinergic activity has been postulated to be associated with tardive dyskinesia; and anticholinergic medications, such as trihexyphenidyl (Artane) and benztropine mesylate (Cogentin), employed to treat the extrapyramidal side effects of antipsychotic medications, have been reported to worsen the symptoms of tardive dyskinesia.

The prolonged and irreversible course of many cases of tardive dyskinesia might be explained if permanent neurotoxic or degenerative effects were anatomically shown to be produced by antipsychotic medications. To date, however, no specific, localized neuroanatomical changes have been demonstrated to be produced by antipsychotic medications in either animals or man.

Tardive dyskinesia usually appears while patients are taking antipsychotic medication, although abnormal movements may appear for the first time or become accentuated after antipsychotic medication has been stopped or after a reduction in dose. In some instances, such dyskinesias last for only a few days and may be considered withdrawal reactions.

Although many therapies have been evaluated, currently there is no satisfactory or uniformly effective treatment for tardive dyskinesia. Discontinuation of antipsychotic medication is, in theory, the ideal treatment, but it is not feasible for many patients. Experimental strategies to treat tardive dyskinesia have used cholinergic agents such as choline, lecithin, and deanol; γ-aminobutyric acid agonists such as benzodiazepines, baclofen, and sodium valproate; amine-depleting agents such as reserpine and tetrabenazine; as well as other compounds postulated to alter neurotransmitter function in the central nervous system (CNS). However, no pharmacologic treatment to date uniformly benefits dyskinesias in all patients.

The decision to stop antipsychotic medication in an attempt to treat tardive dyskinesia must be individualized for each patient, with an assessment made of the relative morbidity of the abnormal movements against the danger of an exacerbation or recrudescence of psychosis. Withdrawal of antipsychotic medication has been reported to result in a reversal of the dyskinesia in about one third of the patients. If an antipsychotic medication must be continued, it may preferably be prescribed in divided daily doses, such as four times a day, rather than in one large daily dose. The dyskinetic symptoms of some patients have been reported to be controlled better by administration of antipsychotic medication in divided doses.

Paradoxically, antipsychotic medications are the most effective and specific agents for suppressing tardive dyskinesia, the improvement being essentially symptomatic with recurrence of dyskinetic movements occurring after later medication withdrawal. Although studies have not shown a worsening of tardive dyskinesia when antipsychotic medications are administered for weeks or months, caution must be exercised in prescribing antipsychotic medications to dyskinetic patients for extended periods of time because longer-term studies have not been performed.

Since tardive dyskinesia is frequently irreversible, prevention assumes great importance. Antipsychotic agents should be used only when indicated, and their use should be avoided in the treatment of nonpsychotic conditions. The lowest doses effective in controlling psychosis should be used, and the continued need of a patient for antiparkinsonian medication should be assessed. Patients should be examined frequently so that tardive dyskinesia can be detected promptly by early signs such as wormlike tongue movements, choreiform finger movements, frequent eye blinks, or facial tics.

Other Side Effects

The antipsychotic agents, particularly the low-potency phenothiazines, may produce sedation to which a tolerance usually develops within the first few weeks of treatment. Use may be made of this side effect if sleep disturbance is part of the clinical picture, particularly because all or most antipsychotic medications can be given in a single bedtime dose.

Antipsychotic medicaitons can lower the seizure threshold.

A variety of skin rashes may occur in association with the use of antipsychotic medication. Additionally, photosensitivity of the skin can occur and result in severe sunburn. Patients should be warned about this possibility and advised to use protective dermatologic preparations and wear appropriate clothes.

Granular deposits in the anterior lens and posterior cornea may occur with chronic use of the antipsychotic medications. These are visible only by slit-lamp examination, and periodic ophthalmologic examinations are recommended for patients on maintenance antipsychotic treatment.

Prolactin levels are increased by antipsychotic medications, and galactorrhea can occur. Glucose tolerance tests may be shifted in a diabetic direction, and false-positive results on pregnancy tests may occur. The weight gain experienced by many patients on antipsychotic medication, with the particular exception of molindone, does not seem to be explicable on an endocrine basis.

Two side effects that are believed to be allergic in nature are uncommon: cholestatic jaundice and agranulocytosis. It is fortunate that agranulocytosis, which usually occurs during the first 6 to 8 weeks of treatment with antipsychotic medication, is so rare, since its onset is abrupt and has an associated mortality rate of approximately 30%. Occasional white blood cell counts are not considered useful in predicting agranulocytosis, a diagnostic possibility that must be considered and quickly evaluated if a patient develops a sudden fever and sore throat within the first few months after antipsychotic medication has been started.

Neuroleptic malignant syndrome, another rare side effect attributed by some but not all investigators to the blockade of central dopamine receptors by antipsychotic agents, is characterized by marked hyperpyrexia, muscular rigidity, and diaphoresis in patients treated with antipsychotic agents. The syndrome develops rapidly over 24 to 72 hours, with hypoactivity developing into akinesia and mutism and eventually stupor or coma. The level of consciousness often fluctuates between alertness and clouding. Up to 20% of reported cases have died. Most patients recover fully within 5 to 10 days after the discontinuation of the antipsychotic agent. The crucial step in treatment is to discontinue the antipsychotic medication immediately. The hyperpyrexia is treated by cooling; fluid imbalance is corrected with intravenous fluids; other complications are managed supportively as they occur. Benzodiazepines or dantrolene sodium (Dantrium) may ameliorate the muscular rigidity.

The risk of severe cardiovascular toxicity is not high with the antipsychotic medications, but they may increase the risk of ventricular arrhythmias by prolonging ventricular repolarization.

In general, the antipsychotic agents have a very high therapeutic index, and patients have survived acute ingestions of many grams of these agents.

Antidepressant Medications

The currently available antidepressant agents can be subdivided into three groups: the tricyclic antidepressants, the more recently introduced or "newer" antidepressants, and the monoamine oxidase (MAO) inhibitors. The term *heterocyclic* encompasses both the newer antidepressants and the tricyclic compounds (Table 23-2).

Table 23-2
Heterocyclic Antidepressant Agents

Generic Name	Trade Name	Dose Range* (mg/day)
Tricyclic:		
Amitriptyline	Elavil	150–300
Desipramine	Norpramin	150–300
Doxepin	Sinequan	150–300
Imipramine	Tofranil	150–300
Nortriptyline	Aventyl	75–150
Protriptyline	Vivactyl	20–60
Trimipramine	Surmontil	150–300
Newer Agents:		
Amoxapine	Asendin	150–600
Maprotiline	Ludiomil	150–300
Trazodone	Desyrel	150–600

* For medically healthy, nongeriatric adults

Tricyclic Agents

Tricyclic antidepressants are primarily used in the treatment of major depression. In combination with lithium, they are useful in treating the depressed phase of bipolar disorder. Other uses include adjunctive roles in the treatment of chronic pain and schizoaffective disorder. Additionally, imipramine (Tofranil), as well as the MAO-inhibitor phenelzine (Nardil) and the benzodiazepine alprazolam (Xanax), have been reported to be effective in the treatment of panic disorder.

Traditionally, the major mechanism of action postulated for the tricyclic antidepressants has been considered to be the block, by way of an amine pump, of the reuptake of biogenic amines (norepinephrine and serotonin) into presynaptic neurons. Such a mechanism is consistent with the catecholamine hypothesis of affective disorders, because it might explain the antidepressant activity of these agents through their reversal of a hypothesized functional deficit of biogenic amines in synaptic clefts between CNS neurons. However, doubt exists whether this is, in fact, the major mechanism of action of the tricyclic antidepressants, in part because the reuptake blocking effect occurs over a few days, while the agents generally do not become effective until after 2 to 3 weeks of administration. Current thinking suggests that the tricyclic agents' antidepressant activity results from a compensatory decrease in the number of β-noradrenergic receptors. It has been hypothesized that this *down-regulation* occurs secondary to the increased concentration of norepinephrine at the synapse, which is the initial effect of antidepressant treatment. The compensatory *down-regulation* represents, therefore, a mechanism for reestablishing a nonpathologic level of noradrenergic activity.

The selection of a heterocyclic antidepressant agent may be made on the basis of the difference in incidence of side effects associated with a particular medication, in relation to both the profile of psychiatric symptoms and the medical history of an individual patient. For example, one would wish to avoid the use of a highly anticholinergic antidepressant medication in a patient with prostatic hypertrophy. Additionally, one might wish to use the sedative effect of some of the medications in treating the insomnia frequently associated with major depression. It is important not to confuse this sedative activity, which occurs immediately, with antidepressant efficacy. At the present time, biological criteria, such as the level of urinary metabolites of norepinephrine, in predicting response to a particular antidepressant or group of antidepressants remains experimental and controversial. If a patient or a relative of his has previously responded to a particular antidepressant, the likelihood of a response to the same agent is increased, and this knowledge may assist in the selection of an antidepressant medication. Additionally, the age of a patient may, in part, determine the choice of an antidepressant. For example, in elderly patients, who may be more sensitive to anticholinergic side effects, orthostatic changes, and their deleterious consequences, one might wish to avoid agents that are highly anticholinergic or that have a high incidence of orthostatic hypotension.

The dose of antidepressant medications is an important consideration because many patients who are ultimately considered to be nonresponders may simply have been receiving inadequate daily doses of medication. For example, in the healthy, nongeriatric adult, amitriptyline (Elavil) may be sedating and may improve sleep at doses of 25 to 75 mg per day without having antidepressant efficacy. The approximate minimum daily doses of the heterocyclic antidepressant agents are listed in Table 23-2 as the doses at the lower end of the dose ranges for each agent. Geriatric patients, however, may have satisfactory antidepressant responses to total daily doses that are considerably less than those presented in Table 23-2, and usual adult doses may be toxic in these patients. The adage "Start low, go slow" certainly applies to the initial daily dose and subsequent dose increments of heterocyclic antidepressants for geriatric patients. Some geriatric patients do require and tolerate standard doses of these agents, but the dose must be individualized for each patient.

For the tricyclic antidepressants, and probably for the newer agents, a 2- to 3-week period at adequate daily doses may elapse before antidepressant activity is observed. Consequently, a therapeutic trail should not be considered adequate before at least 3 weeks of treatment have passed. Patients should be advised of this fact, lest their expectations of immediate relief unnecessarily complicate treatment. For most patients, the entire daily dose of a heterocyclic antidepressant can be administered at bedtime, when it may facilitate sleep. Some patients, however, who find a medication to be "activating" may prefer to take their daily dose at a different time, and medications can also be prescribed in divided doses in order to diminish the occurrence of side effects secondary to a single large daily dose.

Patients who have recovered from a major depressive episode with the help of an antidepressant medication should be maintained on the antidepressant agent for 6 months to a year before discontinuing the medication. The heterocyclic antidepressants should not be abruptly discontinued, because many patients may report symptoms of cholinergic rebound, including anxiety, restlessness, nausea, tremor, diaphoresis, or insomnia. Gradually decreasing the dose of antidepressant medication over 1 or 2 weeks prior to complete medication withdrawal can minimize these symptoms.

Heterocyclic antidepressants can be safely combined with lithium or an antipsychotic agent. The daily dose of a tricyclic may be lower than is usually recommended when used in combination with these medications. Tricyclic antidepressants, when given to bipolar patients not already treated with lithium, may precipitate manic episodes. Similarly, there are reports that tricyclic antidepressants may exacerbate schizophrenic symptoms if the patient is not already taking an antipsychotic medication. Tricyclic administration may increase the plasma levels of antipsychotic agents. If one should choose to add an antidepressant agent to an antipsychotic medication, antiparkinsonian drugs should be discontinued, since the anticholinergic activity of the antidepressant medication can serve the same function. Additionally, the cumulative anticholinergic activity of an antipsychotic agent, an antidepressant agent, and an antiparkinsonian medication may result in toxicity.

Among the more important interactions of the antidepressants with other medications are those with alcohol and the antihypertensive agent guanethidine (Esimil). Patients should be cautioned that antidepressant medications and alcohol are mutually potentiating. Tricyclics, like many of the antipsychotic agents, antagonize the antihypertensive effects of guanethidine, with a resultant, possibly dangerous rise in blood pressure.

Sixty to seventy percent of patients treated with heterocyclic antidepressants can be expected to demonstrate a satisfactory antidepressant response. Patients who do not respond to an adequate therapeutic trial of an antidepressant agent may benefit from a trial of one or more different antidepressant agents. Some clinicians make the controversial suggestion that if a patient has not responded to an antidepressant with high reuptake-blocking activity for norepinephrine, one might switch that patient to an antidepressant with high serotonin reuptake-blocking activity (Table 23-3), and vice versa. Also, the addition of either triiodothyronine (T_3; Cytomel, 25 μg/day), 1-tryptophan, or lithium to an existing antidepressant medication regimen may benefit some patients who have not responded to the antidepressant medication alone. MAO inhibitors may be tried in patients who do not respond to heterocyclic antidepressant agents, and electroconvulsive therapy, if indicated, has been demonstrated to be more effective than either the heterocyclic or MAO-inhibiting antidepressants.

Tricyclic Antidepressant Plasma Levels

Plasma levels of tricyclic antidepressants may be indicated in patients who have not responded to usual doses after an adequate therapeutic trial; patients whose use of alcohol, barbiturates, or other substances may increase antidepressant metabolism; and patients whose health might be at risk from inappropriately high plasma levels of these agents (*e.g.*, geriatric patients). Plasma levels might ensure appropriate doses for such patients. There is a marked variation among patients in their steady-state plasma levels of tricyclic antidepressants, the variability being fivefold to tenfold, and sometimes even as high as thirtyfold.

Several considerations are important in obtaining plasma tricyclic antidepressant levels. First, consistent relationships between plasma level and efficacy for some tricyclic antidepressant agents have been established, to date, only in patients

Table 23-3
Pharmacologic Differences Among Heterocyclic Antidepressant Agents*

Agent	Sedative Effects	Anticholinergic Effects	Block of Amine Pump	
			5HT†	NE‡
Amitriptyline	5	5	3	2
Desipramine	1	1	1	5
Doxepin	5	4	2	2
Imipramine	3	4	3	3
Nortriptyline	2	3	2	4
Protryptyline	0–1	3	1	4
Trimipramine	4	3	3	3
Amoxapine	2	2	2	4
Maprotiline	2	2	1	5
Trazodone	3	0–1	5	1

* Rated on a 0–5 scale (0, absent; 5, very high degree)
† Serotonin
‡ Norepinephrine

with endogenous depressions. Secondly, the number of well-controlled and statistically valid studies of these relationships is limited. Thirdly, the laboratory assay used must be reliable and accurate, which may not be the case for some commercial laboratories.

Consistent relationships between tricyclic plasma levels and antidepressant efficacy have been well established for only two tricyclic antidepressant medications, nortriptyline (Aventyl), and imipramine (Tofranil). The majority of studies with nortriptyline report a "therapeutic window" between 50 ng and 150 ng/ml plasma concentrations. Concentrations below and above these plasma levels are associated with poor clinical responses. Studies with imipramine have demonstrated that maximal antidepressant efficacy occurs at total plasma concentrations (imipramine plus its desmethyl metabolite) greater than or equal to 225 ng to 240 ng/ml. Since total plasma levels of imipramine above 150 ng/ml are linearly related to clinical efficacy, the upper limit for plasma imipramine may be largely determined by the occurrence of side effects. The relationships between clinical efficacy and plasma antidepressant levels for amitriptyline (Elavil), desipramine (Norpramin), doxepin (Sinequan), and protriptyline (Vivactil) are less well established at this time and require further clarification.

Anticholinergic Side Effects

Although some antidepressant agents may be less anticholinergic than others (see Table 23-3), the tricyclic antidepressants, in general, can cause the same anticholinergic side effects as those produced by the antipsychotic agents. These side effects may be more frequent and more pronounced, however, than those resulting from antipsychotic medication. One should be cautious in the use of the heterocyclic antidepressants in treating patients with prostatic hypertrophy, and the agents can precipitate an acute episode in patients with preexisting narrow-angle glaucoma. Some clinicians have found bethanechol (Urecholine) to be useful in ameliorating the peripheral anticholinergic symptoms of the tricyclic agents.

At high doses, and at usual or even low doses in the elderly, the tricyclic antidepressants can produce a central anticholinergic syndrome, a toxic state characterized by disorientation, confusion, severe short-term memory impairment, agitation, and visual or auditory hallucinations. Concomitant peripheral anticholinergic signs, such as dry mouth and skin, flushed face, and tachycardia, may be confirmatory.

Cardiovascular Side Effects

Tachycardia, orthostatic hypotension and, rarely, hypertension can occur with the heterocyclic antidepressants. Imipramine (Tofranil) has a fairly high incidence of orthostatic hypotension, while nortriptyline (Aventyl) has been reported to produce this side effect less frequently.

Electrocardiographic changes secondary to heterocyclic antidepressant agents are generally benign and reversible; they include flattened T waves, prolonged QT intervals, and depressed ST segments. Dangerous arrhythmias, however, can occur in patients with preexisting cardiac disease, and these medications are contraindicated in patients who have sustained a recent miocardial infarction. If used in patients with preexisting cardiac disease, these agents should be initiated at low doses, with only gradual increases in the daily dose and careful cardiac monitoring, for example, by means of serial electrocardiograms (ECGs). Imipramine has quinidine-like effects and may ameliorate some arrhythmias.

Occasionally, at therapeutic doses, atrial fibrillation, first-degree atrioventricular block, or bundle branch block may occur, although these changes occur more frequently at toxic doses.

Other Side Effects

Many of the heterocyclic antidepressants can cause sedation and a lower seizure threshold. Pathologic sweating, an anticholinergic side effect, sometimes occurs. Mild abnormalities in liver function tests may occur.

Overdoses

Unlike the antipsychotic agents, the tricyclic antidepressants have a relatively low therapeutic index, and fatalities can occur following the ingestion of 10 to 30 times the usual daily dose of one of these agents. This fact emphasizes the importance of assessing suicidal ideation and potential in depressed patients for whom one may be prescribing medications that can be lethal in overdose. For patients with increased suicide potential, one should prescribe only limited quantities of antidepressant, perhaps no more than a week's supply at one time.

In tricyclic overdosage, agitation and delirium may proceed, sometimes rapidly, to coma, shock, and respiratory depression. Mydriasis, temperature disturbances (either increased or decreased), seizures, and arrhythmias, including atrial fibrillation, atrioventricular block, intraventricular block, and ventricular flutter or extrasystoles, can occur. Treatment measures must be aggressive because these multiple, serious symptoms are potentially fatal.

The Newer Antidepressants

Three antidepressant medications have recently been introduced into clinical practice: maprotiline (Ludiomil), amoxapine (Asendin), and trazodone (Desyrel). They differ in chemical structure from the tricyclic antidepressants in that they do not have two benzene rings connected by a central seven-atom ring. The claim that these agents have a more rapid onset of action than do the tricyclic antidepressants remains controversial.

Maprotiline

Maprotiline (Ludiomil), a tetracyclic compound, selectively inhibits the reuptake of norepinephrine with little effect on serotonergic systems. It is weakly anticholinergic and may be less cardiotoxic than many of the tricyclic antidepressants, although caution should still be exercised in treating patients with preexisting cardiovascular disease. On the other hand, the incidence of seizures may be higher with maprotiline, at therapeutic doses, than for the other heterocyclic agents.

Amoxapine

Amoxapine (Asendin), a demethylated derivative of loxapine (Loxitane), is prescribed at doses approximately twice those recommended for imipramine. Although amoxapine blocks the presynaptic reuptake primarily of norepinephrine, one metabolite of amoxapine has dopamine-blocking activity that can produce extrapyramidal side effects when amoxapine is used in therapeutic doses. These symptoms respond to standard antiparkinsonian medication. At the present time, there have been several case reports of amoxapine-treated patients who have developed a syndrome closely resembling tardive dyskinesia that has not abated after discontinuation of amoxapine. Consequently, concern is currently being expressed about amoxapine's potential for producing tardive dyskinesia. Additionally, seizures occurring as the result of amoxapine overdose have been reported to be sometimes refractory to usual treatment.

Trazodone

Trazodone (Desyrel) selectively inhibits the reuptake of serotonin into presynaptic neurons, and has been reported to have virtually no effect on muscarinic acetylcholine receptors. Nevertheless, some clinicians have observed what appear to be anticholinergic side effects in some patients. The dose range for trazodone is similar to that for amoxapine. A single daily dose may produce orthostatic hypotension, particularly if trazodone is taken on an empty stomach. For that reason, and also to reduce the possibility of gastric distress, the manufacturer recommends that trazodone be taken with food. While trazodone was initially said to have little tendency to slow intracardiac conduction or to generate arrhythmias, there have been several reports of ventricular arrhythmias, particularly with patients with preexisting cardiac disease. Consequently, trazodone should not be considered to be devoid of cardiac arrhythmogenic effects. The frequency of premature ventricular contractions, specifically, may be substantially increased. More recently, attention has been focused on the fact that trazodone can cause priapism, which, if prolonged and unrelieved, can result in permanent impotence. Some patients with trazodone-induced priapism have required surgery. This suggests that trazodone should probably not be the primary choice in men in the absence of advantages that this agent may have for individual patients.

Monoamine Oxidase Inhibitors

Three MAO inhibitors are currently available for clinical use: phenelzine (Nardil), isocarboxazid (Marplan), and tranylcypromine (Parnate) (Table 23-4). In general, the hydrazine agents have a lower incidence of untoward side effects than the nonhydrazine agent. The major indication for the MAO inhibitors, particularly in patients who may not have responded to one or more heterocyclic antidepressants, is in the treatment of nonendogenous or nonmelancholic atypical depressions characterized by increases, rather than decreases, in appetite, weight, and sleep. Patients experiencing such depressions often report that their mood does respond to environmental changes and they complain of anxiety and phobic or hypochondriacal (somatic) symptoms. Agoraphobia and social phobias are commonly associated anxiety states; headaches and palpitations are representative somatic complaints. Additionally, phenelzine has been reported to be as effective or slightly more effective than imipramine in the treatment of panic disorder.

The MAO inhibitors should not be used in the treatment of major depression with psychotic features, because these medications may exacerbate such depressions and result in an intensification of delusional ideation. A history of cerebrovascular disease is also a contraindication to treatment with MAO inhibitors.

There is evidence that the MAO inhibitors may be of use in the treatment of some patients with depression with concomitant pain and in the treatment of posttraumatic stress disorder. Like the heterocyclic antidepressants, the MAO inhibitors may be combined with lithium in the treatment of the depressive phase of bipolar disorder.

Whether the antidepressant activity of the MAO inhibitors is a direct result of their inhibition of the enzyme MAO is a subject of continued investigation. MAO exists in two forms, or subtypes: MAO type A and MAO type B. The preferred substrates for MAO type A are norepinephrine and serotonin, neurotransmitters that are, according to the biogenic amine hypothesis, considered to be functionally deficient in depressive disorders, while MAO type B preferentially metabolizes phenylethylamine, methylhistamine, and benzylamine. Accordingly, one would

Table 23-4
MAO Inhibitors

Generic Name	Trade Name	Dose Range (mg/day)
Hydrazine:		
Phenelzine	Nardil	45–90
Isocarboxazid	Marplan	30–50
Nonhydrazine:		
Tranylcypromine	Parnate	20–40

expect agents that selectively inhibit MAO type A to have greater antidepressant activity than agents that selectively inhibit MAO type B. Evidence for this hypothesis is provided by the finding that the investigational agent clorgyline, a selective inhibitor of MAO type A, has greater antidepressant efficacy than does pargyline (Eutonyl; marketed as an antihypertensive agent), a selective inhibitor of MAO type B.

The MAO inhibitors currently available for clinical use are mixed inhibitors, that is, they inhibit both the A and B forms of the enzyme. One might speculate that their antidepressant activity results more from their inhibition of MAO type A than of type B, the form of the enzyme present in platelets and commonly assayed to determine the extent of MAO inhibition. Since the clinical antidepressant activity of the MAO inhibitors generally does not occur until after 2 or 3 weeks of drug treatment, and MAO inhibition is usually quite marked after the first few days of drug administration, it is possible that delayed effects on neurotransmitter systems, rather than MAO inhibition or immediate amine concentration changes alone, may be necessary for the therapeutic effects of the MAO inhibitors. One hypothesis is that, in response to MAO inhibitors, subsensitivity gradually develops in central noradrenergic neuronal systems, particularly α_2-noradrenergic receptors, over a period of several weeks.

Phenelzine (Nardil), the MAO inhibitor that has been studied most extensively, has been found to exert its greatest antidepressant effectiveness when at least 80% of platelet MAO (type B) inhibition has been achieved. Generally, this level of inhibition correlates with a dose of phenelzine at or above 60 mg/day. Isocarboxazid, at doses of 30 mg/day, inhibits platelet MAO activity by approximately 80%, a degree of inhibition that can be enhanced at even higher daily doses.

Phenelzine is available in 15-mg tablets; isocarboxazid and tranylcypromine, in 10-mg tablets. In nongeriatric adult patients, the daily dose of an MAO inhibitor should be increased by one tablet a day to achieve a maximum initial dose of 60 mg of phenelzine, 40 mg of isocarboxazid, or 30 mg of tranylcypromine, in order to minimize early side effects. These doses should be maintained for 3 or 4 weeks, the usual lag time for response, unless intolerable side effects occur and necessitate dose reduction, sometimes on a temporary basis. At the end of 3 or 4 weeks, if clinical antidepressant efficacy is inadequate, the daily dose may be gradually increased to the maximum tolerated level of medication. For maintenance MAO inhibitor treatment, usually lasting 6 months to 1 year, daily doses may be considerably lower than those used in the treatment of an acute depressive episode. The MAO inhibitors should be discontinued by tapering the daily dose gradually over 1 or 2 weeks.

Hypertensive Crisis

Hypertensive crisis is one of the most dangerous side effects of the MAO inhibitors and occurs when a patient being treated with an MAO inhibitor ingests foods or medications containing tyramine or other biogenic amines that are normally metabolized and inactivated by the enzyme MAO present in the gut and liver. Since the MAO inhibitors inactive this enzyme, the pressor amines in food or medications are not adequately metabolized, and the exogenous amines remain active to produce hypertension, either directly or by releasing catecholamines that are present in supranormal amounts in nerve endings and the adrenal medulla. Blood pressure can become extremely high, and in rare instances, intracranial bleeding and death may ensue. The risk of hypertensive crisis is believed to be less with phenelzine and possibly isocarboxazid, than with tranylcypromine.

Hypertensive crisis is characterized clinically by an abrupt rise in blood pressure, accompanied by severe headache, frequently occipital in location, or chest pain; diaphoresis; fever; palpitations; tachycardia or bradycardia; visual disturbance; or labored breathing. Stiff neck and nausea or vomiting may occur. Hypertensive crisis is treated by the intravenous administration of 5 mg of phentolamine (Regitine), a short-acting α-adrenergic blocking agent.

In order to prevent hypertensive crisis, as well as other potentially serious side effects that may result from concomitant ingestion of certain foods and medications, the patient must be educated about those foods and medications that must be scrupulously avoided (see Foods and Medications to be Avoided by Patients Taking MAO Inhibitors). Medication and dietary restrictions should be summarized on a card that the patient should carry at all times. One might well advise patients who are taking MAO inhibitors not to take any medications, including over-the-counter, nonprescription preparations, without consulting a physician. Patients should also be advised to inform their dentist and other physicians that they are taking an MAO inhibitor. It is advisable to provide a list of restricted foods to the person who performs the household cooking and food-purchasing, if different from the patient.

Foods and Medications to Be Avoided by Patients Taking MAO Inhibitors

Foods

Aged or matured cheese

Alcoholic beverages (particularly beer and Chianti wine)

Pickled herring and lox

Liver

Yeast products

Spoiled food, especially meat and fish

Pods of broad beans

Excessive amounts of coffee, cocoa, chocolate, sour cream, figs, raisins, soy sauce, avocados, yogurt, licorice, banana peels

Medications*

Sympathomimetic agents

Narcotic analgesics, particularly meperidine (Demerol)

Antihypertensive agents: Clonidine (Catapres), guanethidine (Ismelin, Esimil), methyldopa (Aldomet), reserpine, and Rauwolfia preparations

* It may be advisable that a patient not take *any* medications, particularly over-the-counter remedies, without consulting a physician.

Interactions With Other Medications

Hypertensive reaction can occur when patients taking an MAO inhibitor use medications containing sympathomimetic compounds, including amphetamine and its derivatives, ephedrine and its derivatives, epinephrine, methylphenidate (Ritalin), and phenylpropranolamine. These substances may be present in appetite-reduction or weight-reduction preparations; cough, cold, or decongestant preparations; hay fever remedies; sinus medications; and antiasthmatic inhalants. Additionally, if a patient is already taking an MAO inhibitor, the addition of a tricyclic antidepressant or another MAO inhibitor is contraindicated.

Some clinical studies suggest that the use of a tricyclic antidepressant and an MAO inhibitor in combination may be useful in treating medication-resistant depressed patients. It is not routinely recommended, however, and if it is done, both types of antidepressants are started together at low doses that are increased very gradually, with the final dosages of each drug being lower than the usual dosages for each agent when used alone.

The MAO inhibitors potentiate the effects of both local and general anesthetics, and elective surgery should be postponed for at least 2 weeks after a patient has stopped taking an MAO inhibitor. If emergency surgery must be performed, the anesthesiologist must sharply reduce the doses of anesthetic agents and of narcotics, since much smaller amounts of these medications can produce the desired anesthetic or analgesic effects, and standard doses will likely produce toxic reactions. The use of meperidine (Demerol) is contraindicated for patients taking MAO inhibitors because of the possibility of severe hyperpyrexic reactions, circulatory collapse, and death.

MAO inhibitors potentiate the effects of oral hypoglycemic agents, insulin, L-dopa, alcohol, and phenothiazines. Reduced doses of these agents may be used. However, the antihypertensive agents clonidine (Catapres), guanethidine (Ismelin, Esimil), methyldopa (Aldomet), reserpine, and Rauwolfia preparations should be avoided.

Other Side Effects

Among the more frequent side effects reported by patients taking MAO inhibitors are sedation, myoclonus (particularly during sleep), and dizziness associated with orthostatic hypotension. Some patients may also report insomnia, nausea, or dry mouth. Occasionally, hypomania may occur, and bipolar patients should already be receiving lithium prior to the addition of an MAO inhibitor. Anticholinergic effects of the MAO inhibitors are less frequent than with the tricyclic antidepressants and are generally less troublesome. As a group, the MAO inhibitors are less likely to interfere with cardiac conduction than are the tricyclic antidepressants. Orthostatic hypotension is common, and tachycardia, bradycardia, and palpitations may occur.

Less frequent side effects of the MAO inhibitors include perspiration, hypoglycemia, arthralgia, urinary frequency or urgency, difficulty in urination, constipation, weakness, fatigue, blurred vision, skin rash, anorgasmia, ejaculatory impairment, and hepatic toxicity.

The MAO inhibitors should not be prescribed for patients with advanced cardiovascular, hepatic, or renal disease, or for those with pheochromocytoma or a history of cerebrovascular accidents.

Overdoses

The symptoms of an overdose of an MAO inhibitor include confusion, agitation, hallucinations, hyperreflexia, hyperpyrexia, and convulsions. Both hypertension and hypotension have been reported. Coma can eventually ensue. Treatment involves conservative measures to maintain normal temperature, respiration, blood pressure, and electrolyte balance. Acidification of the urine may increase the renal excretion of the MAO inhibitor, and forced diuresis or dialysis may be considered.

Lithium

The major use of lithium carbonate, available generically and under various brand names, is in the prophylaxis (prevention) and treatment of bipolar disorder. It resolves manic symptoms more specifically than the antipsychotic medications and is effective in reducing the frequency and severity of manic episodes and, to a lesser extent, of depressive episodes in patients with bipolar disorder. Lithium may prevent depression in some patients with recurrent major depressive episodes (recurrent unipolar depression), but this use is not approved by the Food and Drug Administration. Antidepressant medications are often as effective as lithium in this group of patients and are associated with fewer adverse effects. Additionally, schizoaffective disorder may, in some patients, be a variant or atypical form of bipolar disorder, and lithium may be useful, either alone or in conjunction with an antipsychotic medication, in the treatment of these patients.

The mechanism of action by which lithium exerts its mood-stabilizing effects is not known. Speculations concerning its mechanism of action have been based on observations of lithium's ability to affect biochemical and physiologic processes mediated by a number of physiologically important ions and compounds, including sodium, potassium, calcium, magnesium, cyclic AMP, and the neurotransmitters norepinephrine and serotonin.

Prior to the initation of lithium therapy, it is advisable to obtain a careful medical history and to perform a physical examination. Prelithium laboratory studies should include a complete blood count (CBC), urinalysis, blood urea nitrogen (BUN), serum creatinine, electrolytes, and baseline thyroid function tests (T_3, T_4, thyrotropin [TSH]). If indicated by either the medical history or physical examination, an ECG should be performed. These baseline studies are obtained because of lithium's ability to alter normal physiologic states, the adequate functioning of which must be determined prior to lithium treatment. For example, adequate kidney function is an important prerequisite because the elimination of lithium from the body occurs almost entirely through renal excretion. Other laboratory tests are indicated because lithium treatment may be associated with leukocytosis, hypothyroidism, nephrogenic diabetes insipidus, and arrhythmias; or it may result in toxicity in the presence of sodium depletion or dehydration.

Lithium carbonate is available in 300-mg tablets or capsules, and a 300-mg slow-release tablet is available as well. The starting dosage of lithium is generally 300 mg three or four times a day. Subsequent increases in dosages are made by adding a full or half tablet. The daily dose of lithium should be adjusted to achieve a serum level of approximately 1 mEq/L in patients who are acutely manic. For maintenance treatment with lithium, the serum lithium level can be adjusted to between 0.8 mEq and 1 mEq/L, although some patients may not require a serum level of more than 0.6 mEq/L, and dosage should be individualized. Patients who are in the manic phase of their illness may require larger daily doses of lithium to achieve the same therapeutic serum level than when they were euthymic or depressed. Conversely, patients who are no longer manic may require a decrease in their daily dose of lithium in order to minimize side effects or toxicity. In order to obtain meaningful serum lithium levels, blood samples should be obtained 12 hours after the last dose of lithium has been taken.

Unlike other psychotropic medications, lithium has a relatively short half-life, usually between 18 and 24 hours in healthy, nongeriatric adults. Since it takes four or five half-lives to reach steady state, 4 or 5 days should elaspe before determining the serum lithium level associated with a given dose of lithium. Lithium should be taken in divided doses because of its short half-life and in order to avoid large fluctuations in serum levels which, if they are high, may result in undesirable side effects. The relatively short half-life of lithium indicates that if a patient misses a full day of lithium treatment, the serum lithium level will have decreased by half by the following day. The half-life of lithium depends on kidney function, particularly on the glomerular filtration rate (GFR), which diminishes with age. Consequently, low daily doses of lithium may be indicated in the elderly, in whom lithium's half-life may be as long as 30 or more hours. Additionally, elderly patients may be especially sensitive to a given blood level or have several medical illnesses; these factors, too, may indicate the use of low doses and extra caution in the prescription of lithium for elderly patients.

In acutely manic patients, lithium may not become effective for 1 to 2 weeks. Consequently, management of this phase of bipolar disorder often requires the concomitant use of an antipsychotic agent. The dose of the antipsychotic agent, which is administered while lithium therapy is being initiated and while adequate serum lithium levels are being achieved, is gradually decreased as the mania disappears. It is desirable that treatment continue, if possible, with lithium alone. In the acute phase of mania, serum lithium levels may be obtained once or twice a week.

Patients and their families should be educated about lithium, its common side effects, and the importance of taking it regularly even when the patient is feeling well, because of its ability to prevent further episodes. Patients should know that sweating, or fevers associated with flulike illnesses, and the dehydration that may accompany hot weather or exercise may result in toxicity, initially manifest by nausea, diarrhea, and tremor.

After the manic symptoms have remitted, the patient's lithium level should be checked within 1 or 2 weeks. A lower lithium level at that time may suggest a problem in compliance or may reflect dietary changes, particularly in sodium content, following discharge from the hospital. Following stabilization of mood and the achievement of stable serum levels, lithium levels may be checked once a month for a year and every 3 to 6 months thereafter. Certainly, a lithium level should be obtained immediately in patients whose mood is changing, either toward mania or depression. Kidney function should be checked with at least a BUN or serum creatinine, and preferably by measuring creatinine clearance, every 6 months. Thyroid function should be checked once a year.

General Side Effects

Common side effects of lithium are polyuria, polydipsia, hand tremor, gastrointestinal discomfort, and weight gain. In most patients, these side effects are benign and may require no special attention. If significant at nontoxic lithium levels, hand tremor is sometimes improved with low doses of propranolol (Inderal). The mechanism by which weight gain occurs is unclear, and patients may be advised to watch their diets and count calories.

The use of lithium during the first trimester of pregnancy is contraindicated. While the overall incidence of fetal abnormalities associated with lithium is 11% vs 3% in the general population, this may be a function of increased reporting of abnormalities in infants of lithium-treated mothers. Nevertheless, the abnormalities are clustered around malformations of the heart and great vessels, for example, Ebstein's malformation of the tricuspid valve. Beyond the first trimester, the usual daily dose of lithium may have to be increased because of the normal increase in GFR occurring during pregnancy. Toward the end of pregnancy, however, the elevated GFR decreases, and toxicity may occur if the lithium dose is not reduced again. One may decide to lower the dose or stop lithium entirely several days prior to the time of anticipated delivery in order to avoid myotonia or a hypothyroid state in the infant, although these effects tend to disappear without treatment. Since lithium can be transmitted in breast milk, breast-feeding by lithium-treated mothers should be discouraged.

Renal Side Effects

Polyuria and polydipsia are frequent side effects of lithium treatment. In general, these side effects are benign and reversible and do not warrant discontinuing lithium treatment. Occasionally, nephrogenic diabetes insipidus may develop with the excretion of 3 or more liters of urine per day; it is reversible also. An item of concern is the occurrence, in up to 20% of patients, of permanent lithium-induced morphological changes in the kidney, affecting glomeruli, tubules, and interstitial tissue. Fortunately, to date there have been no reports of lithium-associated deaths due to azotemia.

Thyroid Side Effects

Lithium inhibits several steps in the synthesis and metabolism of thyroid hormones. A small percentage of patients may develop either signs of hypothyroidism or a goiter. Approximately one third of patients develop increased serum levels of TSH. Such changes can usually be treated readily and are reversible if lithium is discontinued.

Cardiovascular Side Effects

Minor electrocardiographic changes may occur in patients treated with lithium. Although adverse cardiovascular side effects are uncommon with lithium treatment, conduction abnormalities, including first-degree atrioventricular block, have occurred. Occasionally, particularly in elderly patients, sick-sinus syndrome, manifest by syncope and pulse rates of 50 beats per minute, have been reported. Under conditions of lithium toxicity, atrial fibrillation, ventricular tachycardia, and atrioventricular block may occur.

Central Nervous System Side Effects

Some patients taking lithium report sluggishness that may not be related to their desire to lower the dose of lithium in order to experience some degree of hypomania. Additionally, some patients may report difficulties with concentration or memory, effects that are generally not persistent.

Many patients develop a fine hand tremor that may diminish over time. If the tremor is significant, propranolol may be beneficial. This fine tremor should be distinguished from the coarse tremor associated with lithium toxicity.

Other Side Effects

When lithium is first initiated, some patients may report nausea, anorexia, abdominal discomfort, or diarrhea; these symptoms generally do not persist, but they should be differentiated from signs of toxicity by determining the serum lithium level. Some degree of leukocytosis is commonly seen.

Occasionally, patients may develop mild diabetes mellitus, and parathyroid adenomas have been relatively rarely reported. Skin rashes sometimes occur, including chronic folliculitis, and psoriasis may be exacerbated with lithium treatment.

Interactions With Other Medications

The thiazide diuretics, in particular, can result in increased and even toxic serum lithium levels. Moderate increases in lithium levels can occur with concomitant use of lithium and a potassium-retaining diuretic. Osmotic and carbonic anhydrase-inhibiting diuretics may result in diminished lithium levels secondary to increased lithium excretion. Diuretics may be used in conjunction with lithium as long as one is cautious and adjusts the daily dose of lithium to compensate for changes in serum level resulting from use of these agents.

The nonsteroidal anti-inflammatory agents are prostaglandin synthetase inhibitors, and they affect the renal tubular mechanism which returns lithium from tubular filtrate to blood. These agents, including ibuprofen (Motrin), indomethacin (Indocin), phenylbutazone (Butazolidin), and naproxen (Naprosyn), can increase serum lithium levels.

Toxicity and Overdoses

Toxic reactions occurring at serum lithium levels of 1.5 mEq/L should be distinguished from the side effects of lithium, which occur at subtherapeutic lithium levels when the medication is first begun. The early symptoms of toxicity are similar to the side effects and include gastric distress, anorexia, vomiting, diarrhea, and a fine hand tremor. At toxic serum lithium levels, the gastrointestinal symptoms generally appear early. At the same time, or shortly thereafter, neuromuscular symptoms appear and these include sedation, sluggishness, muscular weakness, coarse tremor, ataxia, and dysarthria. If toxicity develops further, hyperactive deep tendon reflexes, choreoathetoid movements, increased muscle tone, impairment of consciousness, and seizures can ensue. Coma may finally occur, with cardiac arrhythmias and conduction abnormalities, and can be fatal.

Acute toxicity occurring in the absence of overdose can be managed most often by discontinuing lithium. If a large overdose has been taken, however, management should include the use of an emetic or nasogastric suction, the monitoring and maintenance of vital functions, attention to hydration and electrolyte balance, and the use of an osmotic diuretic. Aminophylline and alkalinization of the urine can increase lithium clearance. In extreme instances, dialysis can be employed.

Carbamazepine: A Possible Alternative for Lithium Nonresponders

Carbamazepine (Tegretol), a tricyclic compound similar in chemical structure to imipramine, is a commonly used anticonvulsant medication. Although it is not currently approved by the Food and Drug Administration for psychiatric indications, many clinicians have begun to use carbamazepine for both acute and maintenance treatment of bipolar patients who have not responded satisfactorily to lithium or who are unable to take lithium because of intolerable side effects or medical contraindications. Clinical studies have found a moderate to great amelioration of acute mania in approximately 50% of patients and a moderate to good antidepressant response in 50% of patients in the depressed phase of bipolar disorder. The antimanic effects of carbamazepine generally occur within the first week of treatment, while an antidepressant effect may not be evident until after 2 weeks of treatment. Several of the patients studied had not responded to lithium. Additionally, some smaller studies have suggested that the combined use of lithium and carbamazepine may be effective in bipolar patients who have not responded to either agent alone.

The usual maintenance dose of carbamazepine for patients with bipolar disorder is 400 mg to 800 mg/day. Although there is no clear relationship between carbamazepine dose and plasma concentration, plasma carbamazepine levels can be maintained between 6 μg and 12 μg/ml.

Carbamazepine does not have the renal or thyroid side effects associated with lithium. The most frequent side effects are drowsiness, dizziness, lassitude, headache, nausea, and rashes. Most of these reactions are transient and may respond to a reduction in dose. Hyponatremia may occur, and reticulocytosis has been reported.

The most dangerous side effects of carbamazepine are agranulocytosis, aplastic anemia, and thrombocytopenia, which may all be fatal. It is important to follow the manufacturer's recommendations for regular laboratory tests, including CBC with differential, reticulocyte and platelet counts, electrolytes, serum iron, and periodic evaluations of liver and renal function. Patients with abnormal baseline values on these laboratory tests should not receive carbamazepine. The medication is contraindicated in patients with previous bone marrow depression or hypersensitivity to carbamazepine or to the tricyclic antidepressants. MAO inhibitors should not be used in conjunction with carbamazepine.

Antianxiety Medications

The major use of the antianxiety medications, preeminently the benzodiazepines, is in the treatment of generalized anxiety disorder. Panic disorders are more amenable to treatment with the tricyclic antidepressant imipramine (Tofranil) or the MAO inhibitor phenelzine (Nardil), although one benzodiazepine, alprazolam (Xanax), has also been reported to be effective in these conditions. Phobic and obsessive–compulsive disorders are generally treated with psychotherapy or various behavioral techniques, although the antianxiety agents may be used during the course of treatment.

The benzodiazepines are the most widely prescribed antianxiety agents and have replaced the barbiturates and meprobamate in the treatment of anxiety. Among the guidelines advocated by the American Medical Association for the use of the benzodiazepines are that these agents should be used for relieving severe symptoms, not minor complaints; that the underlying disorder (*e.g.*, hyperthyroidism or mitral valve prolapse) be diagnosed and treated before settling for only symptomatic relief; that the benzodiazepines be avoided in patients who have a history of abuse or misuse of drugs or alcohol; and that the prescribed quantity of these agents be limited to a modest dose that is appropriate for use until the next visit.

A specific benzodiazepine receptor has been discovered in the CNS, and the affinities of benzodiazepines in binding to this receptor reflect their relative clinical potencies in relieving anxiety. The receptor is closely linked to other receptors for the neurotransmitter, γ-aminobutyric acid. Although the existence of a benzodiazepine receptor suggests that these medications might be mimicking or blocking an endogenous substance, such a substance has not yet been found.

The selection of a benzodiazepine agent for use is made by comparing the type of anxiety experienced by the patient with the pharmacokinetic properties, particularly the rate of absorption and duration of action, of the available medications (Table 23-5). For example, if anxiety is sustained at high levels, a benzodiazepine with a long half-life may be preferred. If anxiety is episodic and can be anticipated, benzodiazepines that are reasonably rapidly absorbed and that have shorter durations of action can be helpful when taken approximately 30 minutes before the patient encounters the anxiety-provoking situation.

Both diazepam (Valium) and chlordiazepoxide (Librium) form three active metabolites, at least one of which, desmethyldiazepam, is longer-lasting than the parent compounds, with an elimination half-life of 36 to 200 hours. This metabolite, desmethyldiazepam, is common not only to chlordiazepoxide and diazepam, but is shared by prazepam (Centrax), halazepam (Paxipam), and clorazepate

Table 23-5
Benzodiazepine Antianxiety Agents

Generic Name	Trade Name	Relative Potency†	Rate of Absorption‡	Half-life (Hours)
Alprazolam	Xanax	1	3	10–15
Chlordiazepoxide*	Librium	20	3	6–30
Clorazepate*	Tranxene	15	2	36–200
Diazepam*	Valium	10	1	20–100
Halazepam*	Paxipam	40	3	50–100
Lorazepam	Ativan	2	3	10–20
Oxazepam	Serax	30	4	4–15
Prazepam*	Centrax	20	5	36–200

* Metabolized to desmethyldiazepam (half-life = 36–200 hours)
† The approximate number of milligrams of each agent equivalent to 10 milligrams of diazepam
‡ Rated on a 1–5 scale (1, most rapid; 5, slowest)

(Tranxene). Alprazolam (Xanax) has one active metabolite, α-hydroxyalprazolam, and is classified as having an intermediate duration of action. Oxazepam (Serax) and lorazepam (Ativan) have no active metabolites, are conjugated with glucuronic acid prior to excretion, and are shorter-acting benzodiazepines.

The rate of elimination of a benzodiazepine is important in terms of drug accumulation when multiple doses are given. If a medication has a short elimination half-life, most of the previously administered dose is eliminated prior to the administration of the next dose, so drug accumulation is minimal. This apparent advantage of the short-acting compounds may be disadvantageous for noncompliant patients, since they may experience a rapid reappearance of symptoms if doses are inadvertently missed or if medication is stopped abruptly. For some patients, the long-acting benzodiazepines can be administered once a day for antianxiety therapy. Very short-acting benzodiazepines must be given two to three times a day.

Drug absorption may also be a factor in selecting a benzodiazepine. Because of its more rapid absorption, clorazepate (Tranxene) generates desmethyldiazepam much more rapidly than does prazepam (Centrax). Clinically, there may be large single-dose effects of clorazepate because of the high, early blood level peak. Some patients, who perceive this as prompt onset of clinical efficacy, may view this effect as beneficial; other patients may experience it negatively. A spectrum of absorption rates is available: diazepam and clorazepate are rapidly absorbed; chlordiazepoxide, alprazolam, and lorazepam have intermediate-range absorption rates; prazepam and oxazepam are slowly absorbed.

Caution should be used in prescribing benzodiazepines to elderly patients, and initial doses should be approximately half of those recommended for the general adult population. The half-life of the longer-acting benzodiazepines is prolonged and their total metabolic clearance is reduced because of diminished hepatic biotransformation in patients 60 years of age and older. Agents with short half-lives (*e.g.*, oxazepam), and that do not require extensive liver metabolism prior to excretion may be more suitable for elderly patients.

Dosage of benzodiazepines is established by attempting to maximize clinical response in conjunction with a tolerable, minimum level of side effects.

The duration of treatment with a benzodiazepine agent may be only 1 or 2 weeks for an acutely anxious patient. If the anxiety is chronic and severe, the duration of treatment may be prolonged and, sometimes, indefinite.

The benzodiazepines have become the standard treatment for the management of alcohol withdrawal. Typically, 50 mg of chlordiazepoxide (Librium) is administered orally four times a day until withdrawal symptoms have been controlled. Subsequently, the daily dose is gradually reduced over a 5- to 10-day period. Unless a patient cannot take oral medications because, for example, of protracted vomiting, intramuscular injections of benzodiazepines should be avoided because they have no pharmacokinetic advantage over oral administration and may be erratically absorbed.

Alprazolam (Xanax) has been reported in some studies to have antidepressant activity comparable to that of the tricyclic agents. However, the use of Xanax for the treatment of depression is not an approved indication, and further investigation is necessary.

Patients must be warned about the occurrence of severe CNS depressant effects with a combination of alcohol and benzodiazepines. Several other drug interactions are noteworthy. Heavy smoking tends to increase benzodiazepine metabolism and may necessitate higher doses. Diazepam administration results in elevation of phenytoin (Dilantin) and digoxin levels. Disulfiram (Antabuse) used concomitantly with diazepam or chlordiazepoxide increases the levels of these agents. Antacids may slow the absorption of the benzodiazepines. Cimetidine (Tagamet) increases plasma levels of the longer-acting benzodiazepines, although recent findings suggest that the increase, at least for diazepam, is of minimal clinical importance.

Side Effects

The principal side effects of the benzodiazepines are drowsiness, light-headedness, dizziness, ataxia, fatigue, and muscular weakness, all of which are related to CNS depressant activity. Drowsiness is the most common side-effect and is the prime reason for cautioning patients against using heavy machinery or operating an automobile.

Several studies have suggested that there is an increased risk of congenital malformations associated with the use of benzodiazepines during the first trimester of pregnancy; hence, their use during this period of time should be avoided. Benzodiazepines can pass through the placenta and may affect newly delivered infants. Since benzodiazepines can also enter breast milk and oversedate an infant, breast-feeding should not be encouraged.

Occasionally, patients taking benzodiazepines may develop *paradoxical* reactions, including hostility, aggressiveness, or agitation.

Because of their very high therapeutic index, the benzodiazepines alone rarely result in fatalities when taken in overdose. However, fatalities can occur when benzodiazepines and alcohol are consumed together in large amounts.

Although tolerance develops to the sedative effects of the benzodiazepines, it is uncertain whether tolerance to their antianxiety effects occurs.

Withdrawal Reactions

The clinical manifestations of the benzodiazepine abstinence syndrome, implying some degree of physical dependence, resemble those that occur with sedatives (including barbiturates) and with alcohol, but show some differences in duration and degree. The fall in the blood levels of benzodiazepines with long half-lives is gradual, and levels low enough to precipitate the abstinence syndrome occur later after withdrawal of the medication, usually between the third and sixth day. Additionally, the symptoms and signs last for a shorter time and are less florid. The minor form of withdrawal reaction may be manifested by anxiety, insomnia, dizziness, and anorexia, which are common symptoms of the anxiety state for which the benzodiazepine may have originally been prescribed. It may, therefore, be impossible to decide on clinical grounds whether this state represents abstinence or a recurrence of the previous disorder. If medication has been given for less than 1 month at traditional dosage, abstinence is extremely unlikely. However, if larger doses have been given for longer periods of time, the benzodiazepine should be readministered at the previous dose level for a few days and then gradually withdrawn over a period of 1 to 2 weeks. Return of the symptoms suggests that the underlying anxiety disorder continues to exist.

Occasionally, benzodiazepine withdrawal can result in more severe reactions, including psychosis and seizures.

It is advisable to taper the benzodiazepines gradually, by 5% to 10% of the daily dose, before they are discontinued.

Hypnotic Medications

The term *insomnia* indicates a relative inability to sleep that consists of difficulty falling asleep, difficulty staying asleep, early final awakening, or a combination of these complaints. It is a symptom that can occur during the course of numerous psychiatric disorders. In general, sleep disturbances that occur as part of the clinical pictures of the affective, anxiety, or schizophrenic disorders can be alleviated with medications specifically indicated for treatment of these disorders, rather than hypnotic agents. Furthermore, transient insomnia related to specific situational circumstances, medical conditions, or pharmacologic agents, and situational insomnia related to major life stresses may remit spontaneously without the need for medication. Nonpharmacologic measures to promote better sleep hygiene are often helpful to patients with insomnia. The use of hypnotic medication should be used only as an adjunct to other primary therapeutic modalities, including educational, behavioral, and psychotherapeutic approaches to the treatment of sleep disturbances.

When hypnotic medications are indicated as an adjunctive treatment for insomnia, the benzodiazepine agents are the medications of choice. Barbiturates should be excluded from the pharmacotherapy of insomnia because they have a high potential for drug dependence, drug-withdrawal insomnia, and for respiratory depression and lethality when taken in overdose. Of concern in some patients is the interaction of barbiturates with anticoagulants. Chloral hydrate (Noctec) may be a useful hypnotic for a few nights; however, it has been reported to produce dependence readily, and severe toxicity (renal and liver) has occurred at ten times the hypnotic dose. Additionally, chloral hydrate can stimulate liver microsomal enzymes to metabolize other drugs more rapidly, and trichloroacetic acid, a metabolite of chloral hydrate, may displace other medications that are bound to plasma proteins.

The benzodiazepine hypnotics are preferred to chloral hydrate and the barbiturates because they have a wide safety margin and have a far lower risk of physical dependence associated with their use.

Among the other available agents, glutethimide (Doriden) is not particularly effective in comparative studies, may produce powerful anticholinergic side effects, and has a very high rate of fatalities in overdose (high lipid solubility and anticholinergic activity). Methyprylon (Noludar) produces severe respiratory depression and coma when taken in overdose. Methaqualone (Quaalude) use results in physical dependence with a rapid tolerance to its hypnotic effect. Ethchlorvynol (Placidyl) can produce physical dependence and has a relatively low safety margin. None of these agents can be recommended for the treatment of insomnia.

Three benzodiazepines are currently being marketed specifically for the treatment of insomnia: flurazepam (Dalmane), temazepam (Restoril), and triazolam (Halcion). The differences among the three agents derive largely from differences in their pharmacokinetic properties, including the rate at which they are absorbed and the rate at which they are metabolized and eliminated (Table 23-6).

Table 23-6
Kinetic Characteristics of Benzodiazepine Hypnotics

Generic Name (Trade Name)	Active Compounds in Blood	Rate of Absorption or Appearance	Rate of Elimination (Half-Life Range)
Flurazepam (Dalmane)	Hydroxyethyl-flurazepam	Rapid	Rapid
	Flurazepam aldehyde	Rapid	Rapid
	Desalkyl-flurazepam	Slow	Slow (40–150 hrs)
Temazepam (Restoril)	Temazepam	Slow	Intermediate (10–20 hrs)
Triazolam (Halcion)	Triazolam	Intermediate	Ultra-rapid (1.5–5 hrs)

Flurazepam

Flurazepam (Dalmane) has a complex pharmacokinetic profile. Flurazepam itself appears in the systemic circulation in trace or nonmeasurable amounts, and is essentially a precursor for other substances. Two metabolites of flurazepam, hydroxyethyl-flurazepam and flurazepam aldehyde, appear in the blood immediately following a single oral dose, are pharmacologically active, and probably contribute to the induction of sleep. These two metabolites each have half-lives of 2 to 3 hours, are very rapidly eliminated, and fall to undetectable levels between 8 and 12 hours after drug administration.

Desalkylflurazepam, a third metabolite accounting for only 4% to 7% of the average dose measured in plasma, has a long half-life of 40 to 150 hours. It appears in blood more slowly, is eliminated more slowly, and accumulates during chronic treatment.

To sum up the pharmacokinetics of flurazepam, the drug acts as a mixture of short-acting and long-acting substances. This profile is potentially favorable because drug elimination after the drug has been stopped is gradual, thereby attenuating or preventing withdrawal or rebound effects, including rebound insomnia, an intense worsening of sleep above predrug baseline levels that may follow the withdrawal of shorter-acting benzodiazepines. On the other hand, accumulation of the desalkyl metabolite may cause some degree of drowsiness or impairment of performance during the day. However, these clinical effects do not parallel the actual increase in metabolite concentrations in plasma, because of adaptation or tolerance that offset, at least partially, the potential clinical sequelae of drug accumulation.

Flurazepam shortens sleep latency (the time it takes to fall asleep), decreases nocturnal awakenings, increases total sleep time, and decreases awake time. Some studies report daytime sedation and some impairment of psychomotor performance during regular use of flurazepam 30 mg per night. This is offset at least partially by tolerance, and can be alleviated or eliminated by using 15-mg doses. At the recommended dose of 15 mg, flurazepam is safe for use in elderly patients. It produces no enzyme induction.

Temazepam

Temazepam (Restoril) has no active metabolites and is largely excreted as a glucuronide in the urine. It has an intermedate half-life of 10 to 20 hours and produces an intermediate degree of accumulation during multiple dosage. After oral administration of the hard gelatin capsule preparation of temazepam available in the United States, the absorption of temazepam from the gastrointestinal (GI) tract and its rate of appearance in plasma is slow. The mean time of peak concentration is 2½ hours after the time of administration, which is consistent with clinical studies showing that temazepam has minimal efficacy in sleep-latency insomnia. In other words, temazepam has little effect on the time it takes to fall asleep, although it does decrease the number of awakenings and increase the total sleep time. The package insert for temazepam states that there is "no significant reduction in sleep latency." Clearly, temazepam is not ideal for patients with insomnia characterized primarily by prolonged sleep latency, especially when the drug is taken at bedtime.

Perhaps the 15-mg or 30-mg dose could be taken 1 to 2 hours before bedtime. Some, but not all studies, have reported rebound insomnia with temazepam. Its intermediate degree of accumulation may make it less likely to impair motor and intellectual functioning the next day.

A clinical advantage of temazepam over flurazepam or triazolam in elderly individuals has not been established in controlled studies. Temazepam, unlike flurazepam, does not interact with cimetidine through competition for the cytochrome P450 oxidase hepatic enzyme system; consequently, cimetidine does not increase plasma levels of temazepam.

Triazolam

Triazolam (Halcion) is marketed in scored tablets of 0.25 mg and 0.5 mg; 0.125 mg is the dose suggested for use in the elderly. It has two active metabolites that occur at very low concentrations: α-hydroxytriazolam and 4-hydroxytriazolam. The absorption rate of triazolam is considered to be intermediate, with mean peak plasma concentration occurring 1.3 hours after administration. Its elimination half-life is extremely rapid; therefore, the extent of accumulation during multiple doses will be negligible, and there seem to be no significant carry-over effects such as daytime drowsiness or hangover the following day (*i.e.*, impaired coordination, clumsiness). However, decrements on cognitive and visual–motor tasks are demonstrable during the 8 hours after triazolam administration, which could be important if the patient awakens during the night. It has no effect on plasma warfarin (Coumadin) levels or prothrombin time; preliminary data suggest that old age or cimetidine cause only a small change in triazolam half-life. Triazolam is effective in shortening sleep latency, decreasing nocturnal awakenings, increasing sleep time, and decreasing awake time.

At the present time, reports of rebound insomnia with triazolam remain mixed, although some well-controlled studies have reported marked rebound insomnia after stopping triazolam, with a 160% increase in total awake time above baseline.

Also of concern at this time are reports of anterograde amnesia occurring in patients treated with triazolam, *rebound alertness,* which may represent *hyperalertness* or *rebound anxiety* the following day, *early morning insomnia,* with patients not sleeping all night and awakening earlier than desired, and decreased effectiveness or tolerance to triazolam's hypnotic effect within 2 weeks of nightly administration.

Side Effects

In general, the side effects of the benzodiazepine hypnotic agents are the same as those associated with other benzodiazepines, and patients should be cautioned about them, including the possibility of sleepiness the following day. Patients should be advised to avoid driving or operating machinery if daytime drowsiness occurs.

Patients who are at particular risk for adverse effects with hypnotic drugs include those with respiratory difficulty or impaired renal function, patients who are pregnant or elderly, and those who are alcoholic. All of the available hypnotics may exhibit toxic effects when combined with alcohol or other CNS-depressant drugs.

Bibliography

Davidson JRT: When and how to use MAO inhibitors. Drug Therapy 13: 197, 1983

Davis JM, Janicak P, Chang S, Klerman K: Recent advances in the pharmacologic treatment of the schizophrenic disorders. In Grinspoon L (ed): Psychiatry 1982 Annual Review. Washington, DC, American Psychiatric Press, 1982

Greenblatt DJ, Divoll M, Abernethy DR, Shader RI: Benzodiazepine hypnotics: Kinetic and therapeutic options. Sleep 5:S18, 1982

Greenblatt DJ, Shader RI, Abernethy DR: Current status of benzodiazepines. N Engl J Med 309:354, 410, 1983

Jefferson JW, Greist JH, Ackerman DL: Lithium Encyclopedia for Clinical Practice. Washington, DC, American Psychiatric Press, 1983

Jeste DV, Wyatt RJ: Understanding and Treating Tardive Dyskinesia. New York, Guilford Press, 1982

Kales A, Soldatos CR, Bixler EO, Kales JD: Rebound insomnia and rebound anxiety: A review. Pharmacology 26:121, 1983

Perel JM: Tricyclic antidepressant plasma levels, pharmacokinetics, and clinical outcome. In Grinspoon L (ed): Psychiatry Update, Vol II. Washington, DC, American Psychiatric Press, 1983

Post RM, Uhde TW, Ballenger JC, Squillace KM: Prophylactic efficacy of carbamazepine in manic–depressive illness. Am J Psychiatry 140:1602, 1983

Risch SC, Groom GP, Janowsky DS: Interfaces of psychopharmacology and cardiology. J Clin Psychiatry 42:23, 47, 1981

Richard D. Weiner

24 Electroconvulsive Therapy

Electroconvulsive therapy (ECT) is the psychiatric use of electrically induced seizures to produce a therapeutic remission in certain patients, particularly those suffering major depressive episodes. The purpose of this chapter is to help the reader to understand what ECT is, how it is used, what its potential benefits and risks are, and what its role should be in contemporary psychiatric practice.

In the early part of the 20th century, there was very little that could be done therapeutically for severely ill psychiatric patients. The great strides that had taken place in the development of psychodynamically oriented psychotherapy were of little practical value for such patients. Their therapy at that time consisted predominantly of supportive psychotherapy, hospitalization, and restraints. A number of valiant attempts were made to discover new means of dealing with this major public health problem, very few of which have remained to this day. These include the use of fever therapy, for which a Nobel Prize was won, and insulin coma therapy. In the mid 1930s, building on erroneous data that implied that schizophrenia and epilepsy were incompatible, Lazlo Meduna, a Hungarian psychiatrist, injected camphor into schizophrenics to elicit major motor seizures. To his peers' amazement, and perhaps even to his own, a number of remarkable clinical remissions occurred following a series of such "treatments." A synthetic analogue of camphor, pentylenetetrazol (Metrazol), was quickly developed, and the use of pharmacoconvulsive therapy spread rapidly into psychiatric practice throughout the world over the next 1 to 2 years.

Pharmacoconvulsive therapy, unfortunately, was not a simple technique. Dose-response characteristics were very erratic, with responses ranging from no seizure at all to status epilepticus. In addition, when they did occur, seizures were typically ushered in by a painful series of myoclonic jerks that were poorly tolerated by the patients. In the late 1930s, Ugo Cerletti and Lucino Bini, Italian neuropsychiatrists, learned of Meduna's technique while they were involved in experimental investigations of epilepsy. As part of their research, they had been using electrical stimulation of the scalps of animals as an experimental model for producing major motor seizures. Impressed by the simplicity of such a technique, they decided to use electrical stimulation instead of the pentylenetetrazol to produce seizures in their clinical population. As the reader might guess, Cerletti and Bini found their technique to be as effective as the pharmacoconvulsive technique, easier to use, and more easily tolerated by patients. By 1940 electroconvulsive therapy (ECT), as it is now called, had become a widely used component of psychiatric treatment on a worldwide scale.

The use of ECT reached its peak during the 1940s and early 1950s, when it was the predominant form of available somatic treatment. As with any new and powerful treatment modality, it was tried on patients suffering from a wide variety of conditions. It was discovered that its greatest effectiveness was in cases of severe depressive conditions, although clear efficacy was also demonstrated for schizophrenia and mania, which will be discussed later. Over the years a number of refinements in ECT technique were made, beginning with the use of anesthesia, oxygenation, and muscular relaxation, all of which greatly increased the safety and patient acceptability of this form of treatment. Additional modifications in ECT technique in terms of the nature of the electrical stimulus and the precise location of the stimulus electrodes have also been made, though with continued controversy about their relative merits. With the evolution of antidepressant and neuroleptic drugs in the 1950s, ECT began to shift from a first-line treatment to a more secondary role, though in recent years this decline in use, at least in the United States, appears to have begun to level out.

In 1976 close to 90,000 courses of treatment were reported in the United States, where an average of 4% of psychiatric inpatients presently receive ECT, the vast majority of which is for the treatment of major depressive episode. Some countries report very little use of ECT, whereas others, such as Great Britain and Sweden, report that this treatment modality is used on an even more frequent basis than in the United States. Although early in its history ECT was used particularly heavily in large state hospitals, the focus of United States ECT use has now shifted to the private sector.

Electroconvulsive Technique

Patients referred for ECT treatment are generally, though not exclusively, inpatients. Pretreatment evaluation includes a full medical examination and history, standard laboratory tests, x-rays of the spine, electrocardiogram (ECG), and, in some centers, a baseline electroencephalogram (EEG). Any medical abnormalities that might predispose a patient to increased risk receive appropriate medical consultations. Because of its nature, the use of ECT requires informed consent. Patients and their families are told, in terms that can be understood by the layperson, about the nature of the treatments, their likely benefits, and any risks that may be involved. Whenever possible, ongoing psychotropic medications, or for that matter, any medications that are not absolutely necessary, are discontinued prior to the treatments.

When the pretreatment evaluation has been completed, arrangements are made to begin the actual course of ECT. Treatments are typically given three times a week in a specially equipped treatment room, which is staffed by psychiatric, anesthetic, and nursing personnel and includes resources for providing anesthesia, oxygenation, and, if necessary, resuscitation. The treatments are typically given in the early morning following an overnight fast. Prior to each treatment, the patient is given a parenteral anticholinergic preparation such as atropine or glycopyrrolate, both to minimize orotracheal secretions and to prevent postictal bradycardias from occurring. The patient is brought into the treatment room and placed on his back on a comfortable bed or stretcher. An intravenous line is placed, and light anesthesia is provided by a fast-acting barbiturate such as methohexital (typical dose, 60 mg). Following the onset of anesthesia, muscular relaxation is initiated by the use of succinylcholine (typical dose, 60 mg). Positive pressure oxygenation by face mask is provided, beginning at least by the onset of paralysis, and continuing until the resumption of normal spontaneous breathing, except for the time of passage of the electrical stimulus.

A variety of different types of stimulus electrode types and placements exist. In the United States most psychiatrists use stainless steel disk electrodes of up to 2 inches in diameter. These are coupled to the skin with an electrolyte gel or paste and applied either by hand or by using a headband. It is crucial to prepare the skin properly in order to assure good electrical contact, and the large size of the electrodes prevents the possibility of skin burns under such conditions. With the standard type of electrode placement, called *bilateral ECT* (*BL*), each of the two stimulus electrodes is located roughly midway and slightly above the line connecting the external canthi with the tragus of the ear. This location provides for direct stimulation across frontotemporal areas.

Beginning in the mid 1940s, but not becoming widespread until the 1960s and 1970s, the use of stimulation over the nondominant cerebral hemisphere (usually the right) was found to be associated with considerably less adverse central nervous system (CNS) sequelae. It should be pointed out, however, that controversy about the relative efficacy of unilateral ECT (UL) continues to this day. Most psychiatrists believe that unilateral nondominant ECT is generally as effective as bilateral ECT, though there may be some patients for whom this is not the case. A number of current research investigations are attempting to resolve this issue. The preferred location for UL ECT involves the placement of a frontotemporal electrode as described earlier, and the location of a second electrode just lateral to the vertex of the head in the right centroparietal region. It is usually helpful to clip underlying hair from this area to ensure adequate electrical contact.

As alluded to earlier, a variety of types of electrical stimulation have been used to evoke seizures with ECT. It should be recognized that there is considerable variability in the seizure threshold from patient to patient, probably as a result of differences in scalp and skull properties as well as differences in underlying cerebral excitability. The standard ECT stimulus is the line frequency 60-Hz sine wave, with a typical stimulus intensity setting of 140 volts (root mean square [RMS]) for 0.6 second. The low-energy brief pulse stimulus has also become widespread in the United States in recent years, and requires approximately one third as much stimulus energy to produce a seizure. Interestingly, very little of the electrical stimulus actually passes through the brain, due to the shunting of the current through the scalp and the high resistance of the skull.

As noted earlier, the production of generalized seizure activity is the *sine qua non* of an adequate ECT treatment. Hence, the psychiatrist must have some way to note its presence, and because very brief seizures are probably not optimally effective, he should also note the duration of seizure activity. With the dose of muscle relaxant agents generally used, complete relaxation is not present, allowing an estimate to be made of the presence and duration of the motor components of seizure activity. Preventing the flow of succinylcholine to one of the forearms by using a blood pressure cuff pumped up to above systolic pressure is one means that has sometimes been used to make a more accurate assessment of seizure-related motor activity. The electromyogram (EMG) has also been used for that purpose. A number of studies, however, have shown that the actual electroencephalographic correlates of ictal activity often last as long as tens of seconds after the disappearance of observable motor activity. For this reason, it has been suggested that at least one and preferably more channels of the electroencephalogram (EEG) be monitored. Typical EEG seizure durations vary considerably, but for most patients they are in the range of 40 to 80 seconds. Still, it should be noted that EEG monitoring adds to the complexity of the treatments, and is not a trivial technique, because seizure endpoint can sometimes be quite difficult to assess, particularly with unilateral ECT. Quite recently, the presence of the well-known immediate postictal bradycardia has been used as an aid in determining seizure endpoint.

In the United States, ECT treatments are typically given three times a week. There is some evidence that unilateral ECT can be tolerated on a more frequent basis. For patients who develop a prominent organic brain syndrome over the course of the treatments, the frequency of application of ECT can be decreased.

The number of ECT treatments should be based only on clinical response. Usually the treatments can be stopped after a plateau in therapeutic response is attained. This plateau generally occurs after 5 to 10 treatments in depressed patients and those suffering from mania or catatonic schizophrenia, and after 15 to 25 treatments for those suffering from most other types of schizophrenia. Some clinicians have believed that unilateral ECT may require more treatments than bilateral ECT, but this idea is still controversial and may reflect inadequate attention to technical factors. If a depressed patient does not respond at all after 8 to 10 treatments, it is generally safe to assume that there will be no further clinical response, and then to terminate the treatment course. In view of the much larger number of treatments that are sometimes required in schizophrenic patients, the endpoint for treatment nonresponders in such cases is considerably higher.

With regard to the level of clinical response achieved, it must be remembered that a course of ECT, while often dramatically effective in producing a therapeutic remission, does not in itself have any prophylactic effect. It is incumbent on the treating psychiatrist, therefore, to use some form of maintenance therapy (usually psychopharmacologic), whenever possible, so as to help prevent relapse. The use of maintenance ECT itself, typically starting at one treatment a month, is only infrequently used at the present time, and its effectiveness has not been adequately investigated.

How Electroconvulsive Therapy Works

Generalized seizure activity produces both electrophysiologic and neurochemical activation of many CNS structures. As with psychopharmacologic antidepressant therapy, an increased turnover in norepinephrine and a related down-regulation in β-adrenergic receptors are known byproducts of ECT. Monoaminergic pathways from the ictally activated diencephalon to both limbic and hypothalamic areas could very well serve as sources of the mediation of the therapeutic changes in mood and vegetative symptomatology that transpire over a successful ECT course. Still, ECT-related changes in other CNS chemical constituents (*e.g.*, enkephalins and other neuropeptides, amino acid neurotransmitters such as gamma-aminobutyric acid [GABA], and neuroendocrines) are being investigated with regard to their potential etiologic significance.

Indications

It has already been mentioned that the major indications for ECT are major depressive disorders, manic episodes, and schizophrenia, particularly the acute form. The more a depressed patient fulfills the Diagnostic and Statistical Manual of Mental Disorders, 3rd ed (DSM-III) criteria for major depressive episode with melancholia (*i.e.*, pervasive depressed mood with vegetative features), the more likely is a dramatic therapeutic response. ECT is effective in 80% to 90% of such cases. The more atypical or neurotic the characteristics of the patient's history and presentation, the less likely is a marked beneficial effect. ECT is as effective in drug nonresponders as it is in those who receive ECT without benefit of initial psychopharmacologic intervention. The presence of psychotic ideation as part of the depressive syndrome in no way decreases the likelihood of beneficial effects, as is not the case with antidepressant drugs, because they are not very effective in the majority of such cases. The presence of advanced age, even when associated with a mild to moderate degree of dementia, does not lessen ECT's efficacy. The presence of adverse CNS effects may be slightly elevated in such a population, but probably not to the extent of the increased risk that is encountered with drug use. Despite its very potent efficacy in major depressive episodes, however, ECT has become, as already described, a second-line treatment modality, with its major use in those patients who either have not responded to a trial of psychopharmacologic agents, or who cannot tolerate the effects of the wait associated with them.

ECT is known to be quite effective in terminating episodes of mania, although since the advent of lithium use, the use of ECT is rarely necessary. Still, it can be a lifesaving measure in extreme cases. It should be mentioned that ECT may precipitate a switch from depression to hypomania, and in such cases the ECT is usually stopped and the hypomania treated pharmacologically.

The present role of ECT in schizophrenia is not well defined. For the purpose of prognosis with ECT treatment, it is perhaps most appropriate to consider schizophrenia as consisting of two empirically defined groups. The first of these contains individuals who, while suffering from severe psychotic episodes, tend to reintegrate quickly and to do relatively well between episodes. Patients falling into this group generally do quite well with ECT, with perhaps a 40% to 80% success rate. Patients in the second schizophrenic category, however, whose conditions are much more pervasive, with prominent residual symptomatology present between psychotic episodes, respond poorly to ECT, with perhaps only a 5% to 10% success rate. Despite this pessimistic view, however, it must also be pointed out that there have been some dramatic successes with ECT in a few cases.

Contraindications

Many psychiatrists feel that contraindications to ECT are relative rather than absolute. One can break down such contraindications to ECT into two general areas, functional and biological. In terms of functional contraindications, patients with clinical conditions other than those in which ECT is clearly indicated should not receive this form of therapy. This is particularly true in the case of patients with dysthymic disorder complicated by obsessive or hysterical features. These patients will frequently experience deterioration during ECT and may complain bitterly thereafter about the adverse behavioral effects, such as confusion and amnesia, which readily become incorporated into their maladaptive neurotic schemas.

Patients with a variety of medical conditions are at increased risk with ECT. Those with significant cardiovascular disease, be it cardiac ischemia, hypertension, or another disease, are more prone to adverse sequelae because of the very prominent transient fluctuations in cardiovascular dynamics that occur during and shortly after the electrically induced seizures. Such patients should receive careful pre-ECT evaluation by appropriate medical specialists, with particular attention paid to any modifications in the ECT procedure that might be necessary.

Other patients for which ECT is associated with significantly increased risk are those who suffer from space-occupying cerebral lesions. The transient increase in cerebral blood flow and the relative breakdown in the blood–brain barrier that occurs at the time of the ECT treatments may evoke a fulminant cerebral decompensation in such cases. Despite these caveats, however, it is interesting to note that most medical conditions are not associated with increased risk with ECT.

Risks

The mortality rate of ECT has been variously estimated as between one per thousand and one per ten thousand patients. Death usually occurs because of cardiovascular insufficiency, with pulmonary decompensation and acute CNS insults also occasionally being factors. The level of overall risk is not significantly more than that associated with general anesthesia itself.

As alluded to earlier, the systemic risks associated with ECT are most prominent in the cardiovascular area. The dramatic increased cardiac demand associated with the seizures may produce ischemic effects in susceptible patients. In addition, ictal and postictal fluctuations in autonomic tone can elicit arrhythmias of various sorts, particularly premature ventricular contractions during the immediate postictal period. Only rarely, however, are these of clinical significance, and the need for active treatment of these events is extremely rare. A related cardiovascular effect is the transient rise in systolic pressure observed with ECT. Although very prominent, this rise is almost always well-tolerated by the patient. Attempts to decrease baseline systolic pressure are indicated, however, in patients with severe ongoing hypertensive disease.

The advent of muscular relaxation with ECT has led to a virtual disappearance of musculoskeletal injuries related to the motor components of the ictus. Occasional muscle pains are still reported, but probably relate to the fasciculations produced by the succinylcholine. Contractions of the jaw muscles sometimes occur as a result of direct electrical depolarization, and flexible bite blocks are therefore used to avoid trauma to oral tissues. With proper application of stimulus electrodes, the risk of skin burns is extremely low.

The most frequently cited and the most controversial types of adverse effects associated with ECT are in the area of CNS function, and these effects are similar to those occurring in patients with spontaneous grand mal epilepsy. Some level of acute organic brain syndrome frequently occurs over a course of ECT treatments, manifested by confusion and other signs. Occasionally, a full-blown organic delirium may be present. These symptoms, when present, usually disappear over a period of days (or rarely, weeks) following termination of the course of treatments. The most common behavioral manifestation of CNS dysfunction with ECT, however, is amnesia.

A typical patient receiving ECT will develop some difficulty in retaining newly learned material during and immediately following the course of ECT treatments. In addition, some erratic selective loss of memories from before the onset of ECT treatments may also be present. This loss is most notable for events that occurred closest in time to the index hospitalization. The degree of amnesia varies enormously from patient to patient, and depends greatly on other factors, which will be described. In most patients, amnestic symptomatology disappears over a period of several days or weeks following termination of the ECT course, and is not of concern to them. Still, there have been a number of complaints by patients and their families of more persistent losses, despite the fact that objective testing does not tend to bear these out.

There is no question but that unilateral nondominant ECT produces much less of a memory deficit than does bilateral ECT. To a lesser degree, the same can also be said about the use of low-energy stimuli such as the brief pulse. In both cases, this smaller memory deficit is probably due to a less intensely generalized ictus. A recent investigation in our laboratory has indicated that pulse unilateral nondominant ECT is hardly at all associated with amnesia. The same investigation, on the other hand, noted the presence of apparent autobiographical memory deficits as late as 6 months post-ECT in patients receiving bilateral treatments.

If one looks at the EEG of patients who received ECT, comparing post-treatment recordings with those done at baseline, some degree of pathologic EEG slowing is often present. As with amnesia, such findings generally disappear within a period of days to weeks following termination of the course of treatments, although rare persistent increases may be present at times. As is also the case with ECT-induced amnesia, the degree of EEG slowing depends on the type of electrode placement and stimulus wave form used with the treatments.

There has been some concern over the years that electrically stimulating the brain to produce seizures may induce spontaneous epilepsy. The reported data regarding incidence of spontaneous seizures following ECT, however, do not bear out such fears. In fact, ECT may actually have an anticonvulsant action, consistent with the fact that the electrical seizure threshold rises over a typical course of treatments. Rarely however, one can be confronted with the problem of prolonged seizures or even status epilepticus at the time of the treatments, and adequate preparations for acute management of such crises should always be made.

Risk–Benefit Considerations

In appropriately selected cases, ECT is extremely effective. It is as effective as the available treatment alternatives, if not more so. Despite this fact, ECT may be associated with prominent transient, and at times even persistent CNS deficits, manifested chiefly by organic delirium and amnesia, at least in those patients receiving bilateral ECT. For those receiving low-energy unilateral nondominant ECT, however, the degree and the duration of CNS dysfunction, may be extremely mild. The systemic risks associated with ECT are surprisingly benign, in any case.

In deciding whether or not to recommend ECT in any given case, one must also carefully consider the anticipated risks and benefits associated with treatment alternatives. These treatment alternatives, in the situations for which ECT is generally considered, are psychopharmacologic agents of various types. In most cases, the decision will generally be to try the drugs first and to use ECT if an adequate therapeutic response is not obtained or if it does not occur in sufficient time, or if severe adverse effects or clinical deterioration occur. In certain populations, particularly the elderly, the relative risk–benefit considerations of ECT vs drugs may be shifted in favor of ECT, particularly if low-energy unilateral nondominant ECT is available.

Conclusions

ECT is a much-maligned but dramatically effective treatment modality that is particularly useful in patients with severe major depressive episodes, though it can also be quite effective in selected cases of mania and schizophrenia. When ECT is properly used, its risks are probably significantly fewer than generally believed. At the same time, however, ECT constitutes an invasive form of treatment that is associated with some degree of risk, especially in terms of CNS dysfunction, and therefore considerable thought should be given before the decision for ECT referral is made.

Some researchers have claimed that the risks associated with ECT are, even given the objective findings expressed in the available literature, of sufficient concern that psychiatrists should abandon its use, pointing out that only a small minority of patients are fully refractory to treatment alternatives. Others, however, who have seen the dramatic reversal of miserable, debilitating, and at times even life-threatening depressive episodes with the use of ECT are not so inclined to do away with this treatment modality. In 1976 a referendum of sorts was held among members of the American Psychiatric Association on the issue of ECT, with the vast majority of psychiatrists expressing the view that ECT still retains an important place in contemporary psychiatric practice.

Bibliography

Abrams R, Essman WB (eds): Electroconvulsive Therapy: Biological Foundations and Clinical Applications. New York, SP Medical Scientific Books, 1982

American Psychiatric Association Task Force on ECT: Task Force Report 14: Electroconvulsive Therapy. Washington, DC, American Psychiatric Association, 1978

Fink M: Convulsive Therapy: Theory and Practice. New York, Raven Press, 1979

Gleen MD, Weiner RD: Electroconvulsive Therapy: A Programmed Text. Washington, American Psychiatric Press (in press)

Kalinowsky LB, Hippius, H, Klein HE: Biological Treatments in Psychiatry. New York, Grune & Stratton, 1982

Lerer B, Weiner RD, Belmaker RH, ECT: Basic Mechanisms. London, John Libbey, 1984

Palmer RL (ed): Electroconvulsive Therapy: An Appraisal. London, Oxford University Press, 1981

Scovern AW, Kilmann PR: Status of ECT: A review of the outcome literature. Psychol Bull 87:260–303, 1980

Small JG, Small IF: Electroconvulsive therapy update. Psychopharmacol Bull 17:29–42, 1981

Weiner RD: Does electroconvulsive therapy cause brain damage? Behav Brain Sci 7:1–53, 1984

Index